Table of Contents

INTRODUCTION 1

HOW TO MANAGE DIABETES IF YOU HAVE JUST BEEN DIAGNOSED 4
    Recommendations for Type 1 Diabetes 4
    Recommendations for Type 2 Diabetes 5
    How to Break Free of Your Sugar Habit 5

A HEALTHY MEAL CAN HELP REDUCE THE EFFECTS OF DIABETES 9

THE BASICS OF MEAL PREP 13

BREAKFAST 17

1)	Berry-Oat Breakfast Bars	17
2)	Whole-Grain Breakfast Cookies	17
3)	Blueberry Breakfast Cake	17
4)	Whole-Grain Pancakes	17
5)	Buckwheat Grouts Breakfast Bowl	18
6)	Peach Muesli Bake	18
7)	Steel-Cut Oatmeal Bowl with Fruit and Nuts	18
8)	Whole-Grain Dutch Baby Pancake	18
9)	Mushroom, Zucchini, and Onion Frittata	19
10)	Spinach and Cheese Quiche	19
11)	Spicy Jalapeno Popper Deviled Eggs	19
12)	Lovely Porridge	19
13)	Salty Macadamia Chocolate Smoothie	19
14)	Basil and Tomato Baked Eggs	20
15)	Cinnamon and Coconut Porridge	20
16)	An Omelet of Swiss chard	20

17)	Cheesy Low-Carb Omelet	20
18)	Yogurt And Kale Smoothie	20
19)	Bacon and Chicken Garlic Wrap	20
20)	Grilled Chicken Platter	21
21)	Parsley Chicken Breast	21
22)	Mustard Chicken	21
23)	Balsamic Chicken 1	21
24)	Greek Chicken Breast	21
25)	Chipotle Lettuce Chicken	22
26)	Stylish Chicken-Bacon Wrap	22
27)	Healthy Cottage Cheese Pancakes	22
28)	Avocado Lemon Toast	22
29)	Healthy Baked Eggs	22
30)	Quick Low-Carb Oatmeal	23
31)	Tofu and Vegetable Scramble	23
32)	Breakfast Smoothie Bowl with Fresh Berries	23
33)	Chia and Coconut Pudding	23
34)	Tomato and Zucchini Sauté	24
35)	Steamed Kale with Mediterranean Dressing	24
36)	Vegetable Noodles Stir-Fry	24
37)	Millet Porridge	24
38)	Sweet Potato Waffles	25
39)	Quinoa Bread	25
40)	Veggie Frittata	25
41)	Chicken & Sweet Potato Hash	25
42)	Strawberry & Spinach Smoothie	26
43)	Quinoa Porridge Recipe 1	26

DIABETIC MEAL PREP COOKBOOK FOR BEGINNERS(2021 Edition)

800+ Delicious Recipes. A 4-Week Meal Plan To Manage Newly Diagnosed Type 2 And Prediabetes. With An Easy Guide To Understand And Living Better With Diabetes

Lory Ramos

© **Copyright 2021 - All rights reserved.**

The content contained within this book may not be reproduced, duplicated or transmitted without direct written permission from the author or the publisher.

Under no circumstances will any blame or legal responsibility be held against the publisher, or author, for any damages, reparation, or monetary loss due to the information contained within this book. Either directly or indirectly.

Legal Notice:

This book is copyright protected. This book is only for personal use. You cannot amend, distribute, sell, use, quote or paraphrase any part, or the content within this book, without the consent of the author or publisher.

Disclaimer Notice:

Please note the information contained within this document is for educational and entertainment purposes only. All effort has been executed to present accurate, up to date, and reliable, complete information. No warranties of any kind are declared or implied. Readers acknowledge that the author is not engaging in the rendering of legal, financial, medical or professional advice. The content within this book has been derived from various sources. Please consult a licensed professional before attempting any techniques outlined in this book.

By reading this document, the reader agrees that under no circumstances is the author responsible for any losses, direct or indirect, which are incurred as a result of the use of information contained within this document, including, but not limited to, — errors, omissions, or inaccuracies.

44)	Bell Pepper Pancakes	26
45)	Tofu Scramble	26
46)	Apple Omelet	27
47)	Spiced Overnight Oats	27
48)	Almond & Berry Smoothie	27
49)	Keto Low Carb Crepe	27
50)	Cinnamon Oat Pancakes	27
51)	Healthy Carrot Muffins	28
52)	Keto Creamy Bacon Dish	28
53)	Egg "dough" In A Pan	28
54)	Eggs Florentine	28
55)	Cucumber & Yogurt	28
56)	Eggs Baked In Peppers	29
57)	Easy Egg Scramble	29
58)	Strawberry Puff Pancake	29
59)	Egg Porridge	29
60)	Breakfast Parfait	29
61)	Oatmeal Blueberry Pancakes	29
62)	Bulgur Porridge	30
63)	Turkey-broccoli Brunch Casserole	30
64)	Low-carb Omelet	30
65)	Apple & Cinnamon Pancake	30
66)	Guacamole Turkey Burgers	30
67)	Ham And Goat Cheese Omelet	30
68)	Banana Matcha Breakfast Smoothie	31
69)	Basil And Tomato Baked Eggs	31
70)	Cream Cheese Pancakes	31

71)	Mashed Cauliflower	31
72)	Quinoa Porridge Recipe 2	31
73)	Vanilla Mixed Berry Smoothie	31
74)	Granola With Fruits	32
75)	Egg Muffins	32
76)	Eggs On The Go	32
77)	Breakfast Mix	32
78)	Vegetable Omelet	32
79)	Vegetable Frittata	32
80)	Egg-veggie Scramble	33
81)	Veggie Fritters	33
82)	Millet Porridge	33
83)	Tofu & Zucchini Muffins	33
84)	Savory Keto Pancake	33
85)	Buckwheat Porridge	33
86)	Breakfast Sandwich	34
87)	Eggplant Omelet	34
88)	Breakfast Muffins	34

LUNCH 35

89)	Sweet Potato, Kale, and White Bean Stew	35
90)	Slow Cooker Two-Bean Sloppy Joes	35
91)	Lighter Eggplant Parmesan	36
92)	Coconut-Lentil Curry	36
93)	Stuffed Portobello with Cheese	37
94)	Lighter Shrimp Scampi	37
95)	Maple-Mustard Salmon	37
96)	Chicken Salad with Grapes and Pecans	37

97)	Lemony Salmon Burgers	38
98)	Caprese Turkey Burgers	38
99)	Pasta Salad	38
100)	Chicken, Strawberry, And Avocado Salad	38
101)	Lemon-Thyme Eggs	38
102)	Spinach Salad with Bacon	38
103)	Pea and Collards Soup	39
104)	Spanish Stew	39
105)	Creamy Taco Soup	39
106)	Chicken with Caprese Salsa	39
107)	Balsamic-Roasted Broccoli	39
108)	Hearty Beef and Vegetable Soup	39
109)	Cauliflower Muffin	40
110)	Ham and Egg Cups	40
111)	Cauliflower Rice with Chicken	40
112)	Turkey with Fried Eggs	40

DINNER 41

113)	Salmon with Asparagus	41
114)	Shrimp in Garlic Butter	41
115)	Cobb Salad	41
116)	Seared Tuna Steak	41
117)	Beef Chili	41
118)	Greek Broccoli Salad	41
119)	Cheesy Cauliflower Gratin	42
120)	Strawberry Spinach Salad	42
121)	Cauliflower Mac & Cheese	42
122)	Easy Egg Salad	42

123)	Baked Chicken Legs	42
124)	Creamed Spinach	42
125)	Stuffed Mushrooms	43
126)	Vegetable Soup	43
127)	Misto Quente	43
128)	Garlic Bread	43
129)	Bruschetta	43
130)	Cauliflower Potato Mash	43
131)	Cream Buns with Strawberries	44
132)	Blueberry Buns	44
133)	French toast in Sticks	44
134)	Muffins Sandwich	44
135)	Bacon BBQ	44
136)	Stuffed French toast	45
137)	Scallion Sandwich	45
138)	Lean Lamb and Turkey Meatballs with Yogurt	45
139)	Air Fried Section and Tomato	45
140)	Cheesy Salmon Fillets	46

SALAD 47

141)	Tuna Salad Recipe 1	47
142)	Roasted Portobello Salad	47
143)	Shredded Chicken Salad	47
144)	Broccoli Salad 1	47
145)	Cherry Tomato Salad	47
146)	Ground Turkey Salad	48
147)	Asian Cucumber Salad	48
148)	Cauliflower Tofu Salad	48

149)	Scallop Caesar Salad	48
150)	Chicken Avocado Salad	48
151)	California Wraps	49
152)	Chicken Breast Salad	49
153)	Sunflower Seeds and Arugula Garden Salad	49
154)	Supreme Caesar Salad	49
155)	Tabbouleh- Arabian Salad	49

APPETIZERS AND SALADS 50

156)	Broccoli Salad 2	50
157)	Tenderloin Grilled Salad	50
158)	Barley Veggie Salad	50
159)	Spinach Shrimp Salad	50
160)	Sweet Potato and Roasted Beet Salad	51
161)	Potato Calico Salad	51
162)	Mango and Jicama Salad	51
163)	Asian Crispy Chicken Salad	51
164)	Kale, Grape and Bulgur Salad	51
165)	Strawberry Salsa	52
166)	Garden Wraps	52
167)	Party Shrimp	52
168)	Zucchini Mini Pizzas	52
169)	Garlic-Sesame Pumpkin Seeds	52
170)	Tuna Salad Recipe 2	52

POULTRY 53

173)	Chicken with Chickpeas	54
174)	Chicken & Broccoli Bake	54

175)	Meatballs Curry	54
176)	Chicken, Oats & Chickpeas Meatloaf	55
177)	Herbed Turkey Breast	55
178)	Turkey with Lentils	55
179)	Stuffed Chicken Breasts Greek-style	55
180)	Chicken & Tofu	56
181)	Chicken & Peanut Stir-Fry	56
182)	Honey Mustard Chicken	56
183)	Lemon Garlic Turkey	56
184)	Chicken & Spinach	56
185)	Balsamic Chicken 2	57
186)	Greek Chicken Lettuce Wraps	57
187)	Lemon Chicken with Kale	57

MEAT ... 58

188)	Pork Chops with Grape Sauce	58
189)	Roasted Pork & Apples	58
190)	Pork with Cranberry Relish	58
191)	Sesame Pork with Mustard Sauce	58
192)	Steak with Mushroom Sauce	59
193)	Steak with Tomato & Herbs	59
194)	Barbecue Beef Brisket	59
195)	Beef & Asparagus	59
196)	Italian Beef	60
197)	Lamb with Broccoli & Carrots	60
198)	Rosemary Lamb	60
199)	Mediterranean Lamb Meatballs	60
200)	Shredded Beef	60

201)	Classic Mini Meatloaf	61
202)	Skirt Steak With Asian Peanut Sauce	61
203)	Roasted Pork Loin With Grainy Mustard Sauce	61
204)	Meatballs In Tomato Gravy	61
205)	Garlic-braised Short Rib	62
206)	Pulled Pork	62
207)	Rosemary-garlic Lamb Racks	62
208)	Irish Pork Roast	62
209)	Lamb & Chickpeas	63
210)	Braised Lamb with Vegetables	63
211)	Beef Salad	63
212)	Beef Curry	63
213)	Beef with Barley & Veggies	64
214)	Beef with Broccoli	64
215)	Pan Grilled Steak	64
216)	Lamb Stew Recipe 1	64
217)	Lamb Curry	65
218)	Yummy Meatballs in Tomato Gravy	65
219)	Spiced Leg of Lamb	66
220)	Baked Lamb & Spinach	66
221)	Pork Salad	66
222)	Pork with Bell Peppers	67
223)	Roasted Pork Shoulder	67
224)	Pork Chops in Peach Glaze	67
225)	Ground Pork with Spinach	68

FISH AND SEAFOOD 69

226)	Baked Salmon with Garlic Parmesan Topping	69

227)	Blackened Shrimp	69
228)	Cajun Catfish	69
229)	Cajun Flounder & Tomatoes	69
230)	Cajun Shrimp & Roasted Vegetables	69
231)	Cilantro Lime Grilled Shrimp	70
232)	Crab Frittata	70
233)	Crunchy Lemon Shrimp	70
234)	Grilled Tuna Steaks	70
235)	Red Clam Sauce & Pasta	70
236)	Salmon Milano	71
237)	Shrimp & Artichoke Skillet	71
238)	Tuna Carbonara	71
239)	Mediterranean Fish Fillets	71
240)	Lemony Salmon	71
241)	Shrimp with Green Beans	72
242)	Crab Curry	72
243)	Mixed Chowder	72
244)	Mussels in Tomato Sauce	72
245)	Citrus Salmon	72
246)	Herbed Salmon	73
247)	Salmon in Green Sauce	73
248)	Braised Shrimp	73
249)	Shrimp Coconut Curry	73
250)	Trout Bake	73
251)	Sardine Curry	74
252)	Swordfish Steak	74
253)	Lemon Sole	74

254)	Tuna Sweet corn Casserole	74
255)	Lemon Pepper Salmon	74
256)	Almond Crusted Baked Chili Mahi Mahi	74
257)	Salmon & Asparagus	75
258)	Halibut with Spicy Apricot Sauce	75
259)	Popcorn Shrimp	75
260)	Shrimp Lemon Kebab	75
261)	Grilled Herbed Salmon with Raspberry Sauce & Cucumber Dill Dip	76
262)	Tarragon Scallops	76
263)	Garlic Shrimp & Spinach	76
264)	Herring & Veggies Soup	76
265)	Salmon Soup	77
266)	Salmon Curry	77
267)	Salmon with Bell Peppers	77
268)	Shrimp Salad	78
269)	Shrimp & Veggies Curry	78
270)	Shrimp with Zucchini	78
271)	Shrimp with Broccoli	79
272)	Grilled Salmon with Ginger Sauce	79
273)	Swordfish with Tomato Salsa	79
274)	Salmon & Shrimp Stew	79
275)	Salmon Baked	80

SIDE DISH 81

276)	Lemon Garlic Green Beans	81
277)	Brown Rice & Lentil Salad	81
278)	Mashed Butternut Squash	81
279)	Cilantro Lime Quinoa	81

280)	Oven-Roasted Veggies	81
281)	Vegetable Rice Pilaf	82
282)	Curry Roasted Cauliflower Florets	82
283)	Mushroom Barley Risotto	82
284)	Braised Summer Squash	82
285)	Parsley Tabbouleh	82
286)	Garlic Sautée d Spinach	82
287)	French Lentils	83
288)	Grain-Free Berry Cobbler	83
289)	Spicy Spinach	83
290)	Herbed Asparagus	83
291)	Lemony Brussels Sprout	84
292)	Gingered Cauliflower	84
293)	Roasted Broccoli	84
294)	Garlicky Cabbage	84
295)	Stir Fried Zucchini	85
296)	Green Beans with Tomatoes	85

SOUPS AND STEWS 86

297)	Kidney Bean Stew	86
298)	Cabbage Soup	86
299)	Pumpkin Spice Soup	86
300)	Cream of Tomato Soup	86
301)	Shiitake Soup	86
302)	Spicy Pepper Soup	86
303)	Zoodle Won-Ton Soup	86
304)	Broccoli Stilton Soup	86
305)	Lamb Stew Recipe 2	87

306)	Irish Stew	87
307)	Sweet And Sour Soup	87
308)	Meatball Stew	87
309)	Kebab Stew	87
310)	French Onion Soup	87
311)	Meatless Ball Soup	87
312)	Fake-On Stew	87
313)	Chickpea Soup	88
314)	Chicken Zoodle Soup	88

SMOOTHIES & JUICES 89

315)	Strawberry Smoothie	89
316)	Berry Mint Smoothie	89
317)	Greenie Smoothie	89
318)	Coconut Spinach Smoothie	89
319)	Oats Coffee Smoothie	89
320)	Veggie Smoothie	89
321)	Avocado Smoothie	89
322)	Orange Carrot Smoothie	90
323)	Blackberry Smoothie	90
324)	Key Lime Pie Smoothie	90
325)	Cinnamon Roll Smoothie	90
326)	Strawberry Cheesecake Smoothie	90
327)	Peanut Butter Banana Smoothie	90
328)	Avocado Turmeric Smoothie	90
329)	Blueberry Smoothie	91
330)	Matcha Green Smoothie	91

DESSERTS ... 92

331) Slow Cooker Peaches ... 92
332) Pumpkin Custard 1 ... 92
333) Blueberry Lemon Custard Cake ... 92
334) Sugar Free Carrot Cake ... 92
335) Sugar Free Chocolate Molten Lava Cake ... 93
336) Chocolate Quinoa Brownies ... 93
337) Blueberry Crisp ... 93
338) Maple Custard ... 93
339) Raspberry Cream Cheese Coffee Cake ... 94
340) Pumpkin Pie Bars ... 94
341) Dark Chocolate Cake ... 94
342) Lemon Custard ... 94
343) Coffee & Chocolate Ice Cream ... 95
344) Choco Banana Bites ... 95
345) Blueberries with Yogurt ... 95
346) Roasted Mangoes ... 95
347) Figs with Yogurt ... 95
348) Grilled Peaches ... 95
349) Fruit Salad ... 95
350) Strawberry & Watermelon Pops ... 96
351) Frozen Vanilla Yogurt ... 96
352) Spinach Sorbet ... 96
353) Avocado Mousse ... 96
354) Strawberry Mousse ... 96
355) Blueberries Pudding ... 96
356) Raspberry Chia Pudding ... 97

357)	Brown Rice Pudding	97
358)	Lemon Cookies	97
359)	Yogurt Cheesecake	97
360)	Flourless Chocolate Cake	98
361)	Raspberry Cake With White Chocolate Sauce	98
362)	Ketogenic Lava Cake	98
363)	Ketogenic Cheese Cake	99
364)	Cake with Whipped Cream Icing	99
365)	Walnut-Fruit Cake	99
366)	Ginger Cake	100
367)	Ketogenic Orange Cake	100
368)	Lemon Cake	100
369)	Cinnamon Cake	101
370)	Chocolate & Raspberry Ice Cream	101
371)	Mocha Pops	101
372)	Fruit Kebab	101
373)	Salad Preparation	101

MORE RECIPES 102

374)	Chili Chicken Wings	102
375)	Garlic Chicken Wings	102
376)	Spinach Cheese Pie	102
377)	Tasty Harissa Chicken	102
378)	Roasted Balsamic Mushrooms	102
379)	Roasted Cumin Carrots	103
380)	Tasty & Tender Brussels Sprouts	103
381)	Sautéed Veggies	103
382)	Mustard Green Beans	103

383)	Zucchini Fries	103
384)	Broccoli Nuggets	103
385)	Zucchini Cauliflower Fritters	104
386)	Roasted Chickpeas	104
387)	Peanut Butter Mousse	104
388)	Coffee Mousse	104

VEGETARIAN 105

389)	Baked Beans	105
390)	Grains Combo	105
391)	Black Beans	105
392)	Lentils Chili	106
393)	Quinoa in Tomato	106
394)	Barley Pilaf	106
395)	Baked Veggies Combo	106
396)	Mixed Veggie Salad	107
397)	Tofu with Brussels Sprout	107
398)	Beans, Walnuts & Veggie Burgers	107

DIABETIC AIR FRYER RECIPES 108

399)	Hard Boiled Eggs	108
400)	Breakfast Egg Rolls	108
401)	Scrambled Eggs	108
402)	Lemon Dill Scallops	108
403)	Herb Mushrooms	108
404)	Omelette with Cheese And Onion	108
405)	Radish Hash Browns	109
406)	Spinach Frittata	109

407)	Omelette Frittata with Cheese and Mushrooms	109
408)	Asparagus Frittata	109
409)	Breakfast Jalapeno Muffins	109
410)	Mushroom and Spinach Frittata	109
411)	Avocado Egg Rolls	110
412)	Air Fryer Eggs (Perfect)	110
413)	Bacon and Eggs	110
414)	Breakfast Soufflé	110
415)	Whole 30 Air fryer Muffins	110
416)	Bacon Egg Muffins	110
417)	Sausage Cheese Mix	111
418)	Kale Omelet	111
419)	Super Easy Crispy Bacon	111
420)	French Toast	111
421)	French Toast Sticks	111
422)	French Toast Sticks (Ver.2)	111
423)	Mushroom Leek Frittata	111
424)	French Toast Sticks With Berries	112
425)	Breakfast Egg Muffins	112
426)	Cheese Pie	112
427)	Spinach Egg Breakfast	112
428)	Parmesan Breakfast Casserole	112
429)	Vegetable Quiche	113
430)	Tomato Mushroom Frittata	113
431)	Breakfast Egg Tomato	113
432)	Healthy Mix Vegetables	113
433)	Broccoli Frittata	113

434)	Tasty Salsa Chicken	113
435)	Perfect Breakfast Frittata	114
436)	Buttery Scallops	114
437)	Sausage Egg Cups	114
438)	Cheese Stuff Peppers	114
439)	Roasted Pepper Salad	114
440)	Breakfast Casserole Delicious	114
441)	Huevos Rancheros	115
442)	Flourless Broccoli Cheese Quiche	115
443)	Asparagus Cheese Strata	115
444)	Almond Crunch Granola	115
445)	Breakfast Burrito	116
446)	Pumpkin Oatmeal with Raisins	116
447)	Mushroom and Black Bean Burrito	116
448)	Yogurt Raspberry Cake	116
449)	Turkey Egg Casserole	116
450)	Mixed Berry Dutch Pancake	117
451)	Jalapeño Potato Hash	117
452)	Bacon and Egg Sandwiches	117
453)	Spinach and Tomato Egg Cup	117
454)	Egg Muffins with Bell Pepper	117
455)	Tomato and Spinach Egg Cup	118
456)	Egg and Cheese Pockets	118
457)	Leftovers Bubble and Squeak	118
458)	Baked Mini Spinach Quiches	118
459)	Cheesy Garlic Bread	118
460)	Fried Ravioli	119

#	Title	Page
461)	Fast Food Hot Dogs	119
462)	Taco Dogs	119
463)	Pizza Dogs	119
464)	Pizza with Salami and Mushrooms	119
465)	Amazing XXL burger	120
466)	Quick Blend Mexican Chicken Burgers	120
467)	Chicken Spiedie Recipe	120
468)	Simple Grilled American Cheese Sandwich	120
469)	Fried Pizza Sticks	120
470)	Five Cheese Pull Apart Bread	121
471)	Grilled Cheese	121
472)	Cheese Burger	121
473)	Chicken Burgers	121
474)	Chicken Avocado Burgers	121
475)	Veggie Burgers	122
476)	Cauliflower Veggie Burger Recipe	122
477)	Falafel Burger	122
478)	Vegan Lentil Burgers	122
479)	Spanakopita Bites	123
480)	Fried Calzones	123
481)	Reuben Calzones	123
482)	Popcorn	124
483)	Mexican-Style Corn on the Cob	124
484)	Salt and Vinegar Chickpeas	124
485)	Curry Chickpeas	124
486)	Buffalo-Ranch Chickpeas	125
487)	Baja Fish Taco Recipe	125

488)	Lighten up Empanadas	125
489)	Whole-Wheat Pizzas	125
490)	Hot Dogs	126
491)	Crunchy Corn Dog Bites	126
492)	Crispy Veggie Quesadillas	126
493)	Homemade Sausage Rolls	126
494)	Feta Cheese Dough Balls	127
495)	Flourless Crunchy Cheese Straws	127
496)	Baked Camembert Cheese with Soldiers	127
497)	Low-Fat Mozzarella Cheese Sticks and marinara sauce	127
498)	Homemade Mozzarella Sticks (ver. 2)	128
499)	Fried Mozzarella Sticks	128
500)	Feta Triangles	128
501)	Cheese and Onion Nuggets	128
502)	Airfryer Cheese and Bacon Fries	128
503)	Roasted Pepper Rolls	129
504)	Mini Peppers with Goat Cheese	129
505)	Mini Frankfurters in Pastry	129
506)	Mini Quiche Wedges	129
507)	Air fryer Pizza Hut Bread Sticks	130
508)	Healthy Flapjacks Recipe	130
509)	Air Fryer Chewy Granola Bars	130
510)	Roasted Corn	130
511)	Banana Chips	130
512)	Corn Tortilla Chips	131
513)	Bacon Cashews	131
514)	Pumpkin Seeds	131

#	Title	Page
515)	Spiced Nuts	131
516)	Salted Nuts	131
517)	Low Carb Roasted Nuts	131
518)	Frugal Cheesy Homemade Garlic Bread	132
519)	Budget Friendly Air fryer Mini Cheese Scones	132
520)	Bruschetta Recipe	132
521)	Two Ingredient Croutons	132
522)	Vegan Croutons	132
523)	Garlic Bread Recipe	133
524)	British Fish and Chip Shop Healthy Battered Sausage and Chips	133
525)	Pigs In a Blanket	133
526)	Chicken Breasts in a Bag	133
527)	Stuffed Chicken Breasts (Mexican-Style)	134
528)	Chicken Wings in Nandos Marinade	134
529)	Herb Seasoned Turkey Breast	134
530)	Delicious Rotisserie Chicken	134
531)	Chicken Wings in Orange Sauce	134
532)	Spicy Asian Chicken Thighs	135
533)	Spicy and Crispy Chicken Wing Drumettes	135
534)	Turkey Scotch Eggs	135
535)	Air-Fried Chicken Drumettes	135
536)	Wings in a Peach-Bourbon Sauce	136
537)	Spicy Drumsticks with Barbecue Marinade	136
538)	Chicken Quesadillas	136
539)	Coconut and Turmeric Chicken	136
540)	Sandwich	137
541)	Chick-fil- A Chicken Sandwich	137

542)	Chicken Popcorn	137
543)	Delicious & Easy Meatballs	138
544)	Garlic Parmesan Breaded Fried Chicken Wings	138
545)	Quick & Easy Chicken Breast	138
546)	Spicy Air-Fried Chicken Thighs	138
547)	Simply Fried Chicken Thighs	139
548)	Buttermilk Chicken Thighs	139
549)	Bacon-Wrapped Chicken Breasts	139
550)	Air-Fried Chicken Popcorn	139
551)	Spicy Buffalo Chicken Wings	139
552)	Classic Chicken Wings	140
553)	Sweet Garlicky Chicken Wings	140
554)	BBQ Chicken Wings	140
555)	Flavorful Fried Chicken	140
556)	Easy Chicken Nuggets	140
557)	Buffalo Style Skinny Chicken Wings	140
558)	Italian Seasoned Chicken Tenders	141
559)	Lemon Pepper Chicken Wings	141
560)	Easy and Delicious Whole Chicken	141
561)	Barbeque Chicken Wings	141
562)	Southern Chicken Drumsticks	141
563)	Nando's Chicken Drumsticks	142
564)	Spicy Air Fryer Chicken Breasts	142
565)	Balsamic Glazed Chicken Breasts	142
566)	Buffalo Chicken Breasts	143
567)	Syn Free Slimming World Chicken Tikka	143
568)	Air Fried Chicken Schnitzel	143

569)	Thai Mango Chicken	143
570)	Philadelphia Herby Chicken Breasts	144
571)	Lemon Pepper Chicken Breasts	144
572)	Panko Breaded, Chicken Parmesan, Marinara Sauce	144
573)	Chicken Parmesan and Fries	144
574)	Crumbed Chicken Tenderloins	145
575)	Chicken Tenders	145
576)	Spatchcock Chicken	145
577)	General Tso's Chicken	146
578)	Southern-Style Chicken	146
579)	Rotisserie Chicken	146
580)	Thai Peanut Chicken Egg Rolls	147
581)	Friendly Airfryer Whole Chicken	147
582)	KFC Chicken in the Air Fryer	147
583)	KFC Easy Chicken Strips in the Air Fryer	147
584)	KFC Popcorn Chicken in the Air Fryer	147
585)	Everything Bagel Chicken Strips	148
586)	Buffalo Chicken Strips	148
587)	Flourless Cordon Bleu	148
588)	Jamaican Chicken Meatballs	149
589)	Chicken Fried Rice	149
590)	Crispy Fried Spring Rolls	149
591)	Turkey Spicy Rolled Meat	149
592)	Turkey Breast Glazed with Maple Mustard	150
593)	Turkey Goujons and Sweet Chilli Dip	150
594)	Brazilian Mini Turkey Pies	150
595)	Turkey Spring Rolls	150

596)	Sizzling Turkey Fajitas Platter	151
597)	Turkey Stuffed Bread Recipe	151
598)	Leftover Turkey Muffins	151
599)	Turkey Curry Samosas	151
600)	Leftover Turkey and Cheese Calzone	152
601)	Thanksgiving Turkey Sandwich Recipe	152
602)	Airfryer Turkish Cheese and Leek Koftas	152
603)	Steak in the Air Fryer 1	152
604)	Steak in the Air Fryer 2	152
605)	Rib Eye Steak	153
606)	Herb and Cheese-Stuffed Burgers	153
607)	Bunless Burgers	153
608)	Air Fryer Meatloaf	153
609)	Peppercorns	154
610)	Fried Meatballs in Tomato Sauce	154
611)	Roasted Stuffed Peppers	154
612)	Air Fryer Party Meatballs	154
613)	Mustard Honey Beef Balls	155
614)	Easy Spring Rolls	155
615)	Beef Wellington	155
616)	Pork Tenderloin with Bell Pepper	155
617)	Air-Fried Pork Dumplings with Dipping Sauce	156
618)	Pork Chops	156
619)	Crispy Breaded Pork Chops	156
620)	Breaded Pork Chops (ver. 2)	156
621)	Balsamic Smoked Pork Chops	157
622)	Garlic Butter Pork Chops	157

#	Recipe	Page
623)	Turkey and Cheese Calzone	157
624)	Country Fried Steak	157
625)	Tender Juicy Smoked BBQ Ribs	158
626)	Chinese Take Out Sweet 'N Sour Pork	158
627)	Bourbon Bacon Cinnamon Rolls	158
628)	Rosemary Sausage Meatballs	158
629)	Air-Fried Meatloaf	159
630)	Chinese Pineapple Pork	159
631)	Chinese Kebabs and Rice	159
632)	Air Fryer Bacon	159
633)	Drunken Ham with Mustard	159
634)	Roasted Rack of Lamb with a Macadamia Crust	160
635)	Meatballs with Feta	160
636)	Air Fryer Lamb Burgers	160
637)	Fish and Chips	160
638)	Fish Fingers	161
639)	Fish and Fries	161
640)	Fish and Chips	161
641)	Slimming World Beer Battered Fish and Chips Recipe	161
642)	Chili Lime Tilapia Healthy	162
643)	Fried Catfish 3 Ingredient	162
644)	Air-Fried Crumbed Fish	162
645)	Five Ingredient Super Simple Fisherman's Fishcakes	162
646)	Grilled Fish Fillet with Pesto Sauce	162
647)	Sesame Seeds Fish Fillet	163
648)	Thai Fish Cakes with Mango Salsa	163
649)	Air Fryer Salmon	163

650)	Salmon and Fennel Salad	163
651)	Tandoori Salmon with Refreshing Raita	164
652)	Salmon Patties	164
653)	Air-Grilled Honey-Glazed Salmon	164
654)	Grilled Cajun Salmon	164
655)	Chili Tuna Puff	164
656)	Tuna Patties	165
657)	Shrimp Spring Rolls and Sweet Chili Sauce	165
658)	Coconut Shrimp and Apricot	165
659)	Coconut Shrimp and Lime Juice	165
660)	Lemon Pepper Shrimp	166
661)	Bang Bang Air Fryer Shrimp	166
662)	Crispy Nachos Prawns	166
663)	Scampi Shrimp and Chips	166
664)	Gambas 'Pil Pil' with Sweet Potato	166
665)	Fried Hot Prawns with Cocktail Sauce	167
666)	Crispy Airfryer Coconut Prawns	167
667)	King Prawns in Ham with Red Pepper Dip	167
668)	Crispy Crabstick Crackers	167
669)	Wasabi Crab Cakes	168
670)	Flourless Truly Crispy Calamari Rings	168
671)	Scallops Wrapped In Bacon	168
672)	Air Fryer Egg in a Hole	168
673)	Traditional Welsh Rarebit	168
674)	French Toast Soldiers	169
675)	Cheese Toastie	169
676)	Breakfast Potatoes	169

677)	Breakfast Toad-in-the-Hole Tarts	169
678)	Green Tomato BLT	169
679)	Home Bakery Cornish Pasty Recipe	170
680)	Flaky Buttermilk Biscuits	170
681)	Easy Pull Apart Bread	170
682)	Pumpkin Bread	170
683)	Rock Buns	171
684)	Buttery Dinner Rolls	171
685)	Hot Cross Buns	171
686)	Rich Fruit Scones	171
687)	Strawberry Scones	172
688)	Three Ingredient Shortbread Fingers	172
689)	Yorkshire Pudding Recipe	172
690)	Crispy Risotto Balls	172
691)	Sticky Mushroom Rice	172
692)	Cool Green Beans	173
693)	Spicy Green Beans	173
694)	Falafel	173
695)	Macaroni and Cheese Toasties in the Air fryer	173
696)	Macaroni and Cheese Mini Quiche Recipe	174
697)	Patatas Bravas	174
698)	Rosemary Potato Wedges	174
699)	Baked Potatoes	174
700)	Garlic and Parsley Baby Potatoes	174
701)	Airfryer Crispy Roasted Onion Potatoes	175
702)	Rosemary Roast Potatoes	175
703)	Potato Hay	175

704)	Easy Potato Gratin	175
705)	Make Loaded Potatoes	175
706)	Small Jacket Potatoes with Rosemary	175
707)	Stuffed Potatoes	176
708)	Potato-Skin Wedges	176
709)	Restaurant Style Garlic Potatoes	176
710)	Roasted Paprika Potatoes with Greek Yoghurt	176
711)	Potato Latkes Bites	177
712)	Hassleback Potatoes	177
713)	Homemade Fries	177
714)	The Best Ever Air Fryer Fries	177
715)	Parmesan Truffle Oil Fries	177
716)	Five Guys Cajun Fries	178
717)	Skin on French Fries	178
718)	Garlic Sweet Potato Fries	178
719)	Flourless Mashed Potato Cakes	178
720)	Hash Brown Recipe	178
721)	Tex-Mex Hash Browns	179
722)	Poutine	179
723)	Sweet Potato Fries	179
724)	Spicy Sweet Potato Wedges	179
725)	Crispy Crunchy Sweet Potato Fries	179
726)	Sweet Potato Chips	180
727)	Sweet Potato Hash	180
728)	Sweet Potato Tots	180
729)	Big Fat Veggie Fritters	180
730)	Carrot and Pumpkin Recipes	180

731)	Honey Roasted Carrots	180
732)	Shoestring Carrots	181
733)	Slimming World Carrot Fritters	181
734)	Oil Free Pumpkin French Fries	181
735)	Oil Free Sticky Pumpkin Wedges	181
736)	Spiced Pumpkin	181
737)	Pumpkin Tortilla Chips	182
738)	Butternut Squash Roasties	182
739)	Avocado Fries	182
740)	Avocado Slices Recipe	182
741)	Avocado On Toast	182
742)	Avocado Egg Boat	182
743)	Air Fried Guacamole	183
744)	Zucchini Chips	183
745)	Flourless Mini Zucchini Fritter Bites	183
746)	Guilt-Free Ranch Zucchini Chips	183
747)	Baked Zucchini Fries	184
748)	Zucchini Rounds	184
749)	Zucchini Fritters	184
750)	Zucchini Gratin	184
751)	Broccoli with Cheese Sauce	184
752)	Roasted Broccoli and Cauliflower	185
753)	Roasted Cauliflower	185
754)	Buffalo Cauliflower	185
755)	Buffalo Cauliflower Bites (ver. 2)	185
756)	Orange Sesame Cauliflower	185
757)	Honey Glazed Cauliflower Bites	186

758)	Spicy Cauliflower Stir-Fry	186
759)	Cauliflower Cheese Tater Tots	186
760)	Cauliflower Rice Stuffed Peppers Budget Recipe	186
761)	Sprouts Breaded Mushrooms	187
762)	Mushroom Croquettes or Meat Croquettes	187
763)	Stuffed Mushrooms with Sour Cream	187
764)	Shiitake Mushroom Chips	187
765)	Stuffed Garlic Mushrooms	187
766)	Stuffed Portobello Mushrooms	188
767)	Button Mushroom Melt	188
768)	Brussels Sprouts	188
769)	Garlic-Rosemary Brussels Sprouts	188
770)	Brussels Sprouts with Bacon	188
771)	Onion Rings	189
772)	Onion Rings With Comeback Sauce	189
773)	Roasted Parsnips	189
774)	Curry Parsnip Fries	190
775)	Celery Root Fries	190
776)	Everything Bagel Kale Chips	190
777)	Vegan Stuffed Bell Peppers	190
778)	Roasted Peppers (Bell Peppers)	190
779)	Green Salad with Roasted Pepper	190
780)	Grilled Tomatoes	191
781)	Stuffed Tomatoes and Broccoli	191
782)	Air Fryer Pickles	191
783)	Spicy Dill Pickle Fries	191
784)	Ratatouille	191

785)	Ratatouille Italian-Style	192
786)	Air-Fried Asparagus	192
787)	Asparagus Fries	192
788)	Roasted Okra	192
789)	Tasty Peanut Butter Bars	192
790)	Crustless Pie	193
791)	Cinnamon Ginger Cookies	193
792)	Chia Chocolate Cookies	193
793)	Pumpkin Cookies	193
794)	Vanilla Coconut Cheese Cookies	193
795)	Cheese Butter Cookies	193
796)	Pumpkin Custard 2	193
797)	Cranberry Almond Cake	193
798)	Choco Fudge Cake	194
799)	Chocolate Coconut Cake	194
800)	Chocolate Custard	194
801)	Almond Cinnamon Mug Cake	194
802)	Yummy Brownies	194

30 DAY MEAL PLAN 195

CONCLUSION 198

INDEX 201

Introduction

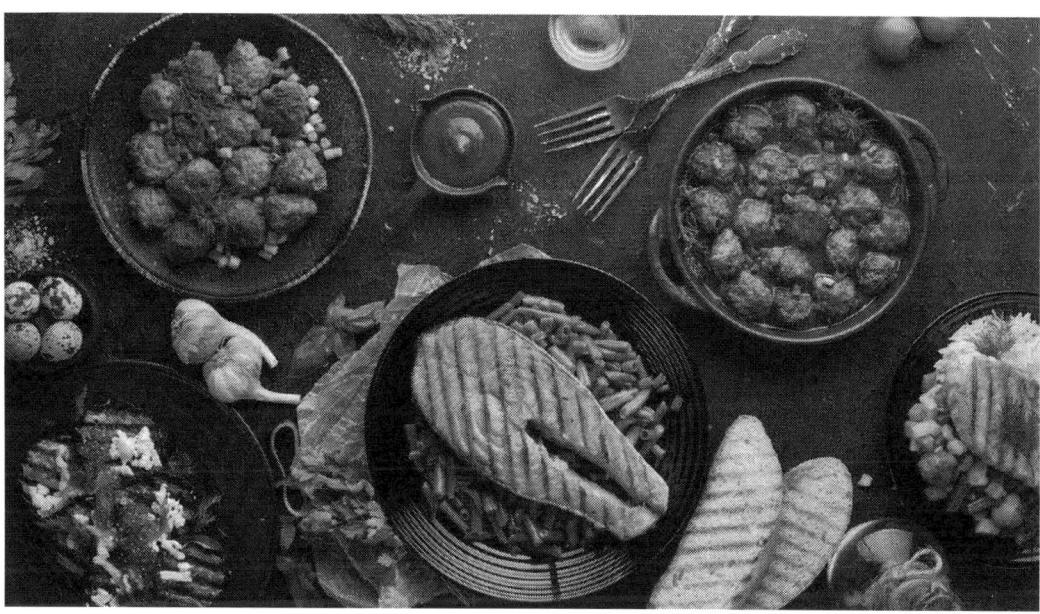

The Benefits of the Diabetes Meal Prep

Meal planning is extremely helpful in many practical ways, but one of its greatest benefits is on a person's health, particularly if it combines healthy balanced food and proper portion control.

Benefit # 1 - It helps improve your general health

Whether or not you have a medical condition, meal planning can help you improve your overall health when the meals provide all the macro and micronutrients your body needs. It also helps you avoid saturated fats and processed sugars, which is what most people would reach for if they're hungry and just want something satisfying.

Benefit # 2 - It ensures that you can eat on time

Preparing your meals in advance helps manage hunger pains. Missing a meal or delaying it can cause your blood sugar level to drop too low, a condition otherwise known as hypoglycemia.

Hypoglycemia can cause shaking, disorientation, and irritability. You may even have a seizure if your blood sugar level gets any lower. Having your meal already prepared ensures that you can always eat on time and, therefore, decrease the risk of low blood glucose.

Benefit # 3 - It lowers your risk of heart disease

Diabetes increases the risk of heart disease. With the help of a dietician, planning your meals can help you reduce this risk. Because meal prep reduces the time you need to spend in the kitchen, you'll have more opportunities to exercise and do other activities that promote a healthier lifestyle.

Benefit # 4 - It lowers your risk of cancer

Diabetes also increases the risk of all forms of cancer. While experts are still unable to identify the exact link between these two conditions, they expect that it has something to do with insulin resistance and obesity. Cancer patients are advised to pursue a healthy lifestyle, which includes eating a balanced diet and getting adequate exercise. Because these activities are also encouraged among diabetics, the risk of cancer is lowered.

Benefit # 5 - It helps you maintain healthy body weight

Again, portion control plays a part in this area. Even if you eat healthy food, overindulging can lead to an unhealthy weight gain, which can make it harder to control your blood sugar level.

If left unchecked, this could lead to high blood sugar levels or hyperglycemia, which can cause various complications that include heart and liver damage as well as the loss of kidney function.

It's important to note that while meal planning can help keep the effects of diabetes under control, you and your dietician still need to conduct a periodic review of its effectiveness and make changes whenever necessary.

How to identify if you have Diabetes

The early signs of diabetes include:

- Hunger and fatigue

When your body consumes food, it converts it into glucose so that the cells can use it for energy. The body needs insulin so that the cells can take in the glucose. Without enough insulin or if the cells are unable to use insulin, the body does not get any energy, making you feel tired as well as hungry all the time.

- Excessive thirst and urination

Usually, a person pees from four to seven times a day. But with people who suffer from diabetes pee a lot more. This also makes you thirsty more frequently.

- Dry mouth and itchy skin

When the body uses fluids to create urine, it has less moisture to keep the mouth and skin from drying.

- Blurry vision

Changes in the body's fluid levels can inflame the lens of the eyes, making it more difficult for the eyes to focus.

Symptoms of type-2 diabetes include:

- Yeast infections
- Slow-healing wounds
- Pain in the muscles
- Numbness of legs and feet

Symptoms of type-1 diabetes are the following:

- Unexplained weight loss
- Nausea and vomiting

As for gestational diabetes, there are no symptoms. The condition is only determined during prenatal screening.

How to Manage Diabetes If You Have Just Been Diagnosed

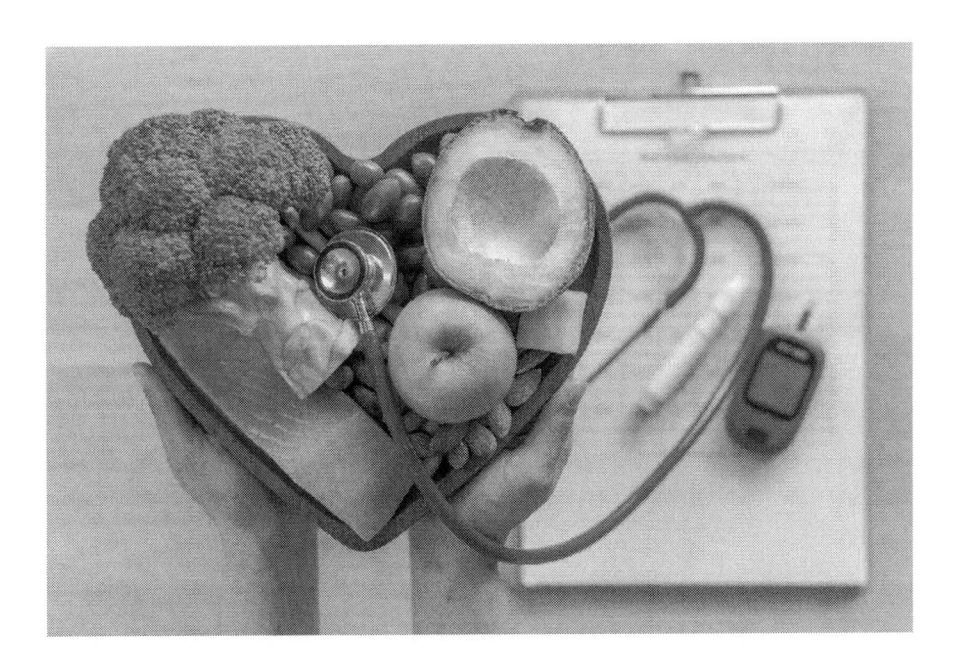

Recommendations for Type 1 Diabetes

If you have type 1 diabetes, there are certain methods of treatment that you can use that will help you to manage yourself better. You will have very specific goals that are put out for you to help with the management of your disease. You will be expected to, for example, make sure that you are managing your blood sugar and pressure. According to the experts at Kaiser Permanente, an American nationwide healthcare provider and the largest nonprofit health plan throughout the US, blood sugar should follow these guidelines to be considered well controlled:

Timing	Target
Before meals	80-130 mg/dL
2 hours after meals	160 mg/dL
Bedtime	80-130 mg/dL
3 a.m.	80-130 mg/dL

When diagnosed with type 1 diabetes, you will find that a lot changes. You need to be able to change how you are living your life. In particular, you must change up your diet, make sure that exercise is a priority, and make sure that you are consuming the highest amounts of healthy foods possible. You will be recommended to make sure that you are providing yourself with as much good, healthy foods as possible, and you will want to keep your weight healthy. Keep in mind that type 1 diabetes is permanent—there is no way to cure it. However, you will need to treat yourself with insulin on a regular basis. You must make sure that you are giving yourself insulin, either through injections or pumps, to make sure that your body is able to function regardless of what you eat. Without providing your body that insulin, you will not be able to regulate that blood sugar. Your doctor will focus mostly on teaching you what it will take for you to know what it is that your body needs at any given time based on the foods that you are eating. If you know that blood sugar rises after eating, you know that you need to also inject yourself with insulin.

However, the amount of insulin that you inject varies greatly from person to person, as well as based on the carbs that you consumed.

Recommendations for Type 2 Diabetes

As with type 1 diabetes, type 2 comes with very similar recommendations. You will need to make sure that you are managing your health in general, but you will also be recommended to be more mindful of the foods that you are eating. You may also be recommended to work to lose weight. This is because type 2 diabetes is entirely controllable through just diet and exercise. You will be able to treat yourself without the need for insulin because the problem is not that you don't have insulin at all—the problem is that your body isn't responding to it.

Your diet will be more strictly monitored on type 2 diabetes, and it will be harder to keep it in line if you are not treating yourself carefully. However, because you can effectively reverse this disease over time with the right diet, it is one that is highly favored over other options.

How to Break Free of Your Sugar Habit

So, maybe you're at risk of diabetes, or maybe you already have it but don't know what you can do to lessen your sugar consumption habits. The good news is it isn't that bad to break these habits. It can take a while, and you need willpower, but if you have that, you should be able to fight off the habits as well. All you have to do is be willing to make some significant changes to your diet.

Ultimately, people are hardwired to desire sugar—when we didn't have easy access to sugar, we needed to want as many carbs as possible to keep ourselves healthy and alive; the carbs would help us to create fats. They would also help to keep us full. However, nowadays, because we don't have to forage or hunt and gather for food, we have our own problems. Nowadays, the problem is that food is too easy to find. Because it is so readily available, you run into the problem of potentially storing up too much fat as a direct result. However, you can learn to prevent this from being a problem.

We are hardwired to want to go for those sugary choices. Most animals are—studies have shown that animals will go out of their way to choose sugar over cocaine in lab tests. However, sugar is not good for us in excess, as we have established thus far. This means that you will need to be mindful of what you are doing to prevent yourself from getting ill. You will need to figure out how you can make sure that you do not unintentionally poison yourself with too much sugar. Now, let's look at what goes into breaking that habit—or even that addiction in some cases.

A Brief Guide to Eliminating Sugar

First, before we begin, consider the fact that sugar comes in all sorts of forms. It comes in the form of sucrose and fructose. Lactose and maltose are two others. Sucrose can be found, as well. As you can see, hover, they all end in "-ose." That is the sign that you are looking at a sugar if you don't see the actual word written in front of you. Because sugars come in so many different forms, it can be difficult to truly eliminate them. It can be impossible for you to figure out what you will need to do to prevent yourself from getting ill from these effects—you will need to make sure that you are working hard to ensure that your diet is well-managed. Ultimately, if you are able to recognize these different forms of sugar, you will be able to prevent yourself from eating things that aren't going to help you.

As an additional note before we begin, consider the fact that you don't need to cut out all forms of sugar—you just want to cut it out when it is added to your diet. This means that it is okay to eat whole food that breaks down into carbs—but you don't want to eat something that is laden with high fructose corn syrup. Eating foods that are loaded up with sugars can be a huge problem, and most people don't even realize that they are doing it—they just do so because they think that since the word sugar isn't on the ingredient list, they are safe to eat it without a concern.

If you are ready to cut out sugar from your diet, there are a few steps that you should follow to help yourself do so. These aren't necessarily difficult to do, but many people find that it is hard to stick to it. They get caught up in the cravings, or they give into the withdrawals that they feel when they do cut them out. Your body gets used to those higher levels of sugar in your diet and comes to rely on them; when you cut them out, you are likely to run into some symptoms as your body has to develop and adjust to its new normal.

Cutting sugar by tossing out added sugar sources the first step to making sure that you can eliminate sugar is to take the time to genuinely cut it out in the first place. If you have added sugar options in your home, such as white and brown sugars, or also eliminating the honey. If you are going to make yourself coffee or tea, you want to make sure that you aren't adding these. At first, make sure that you do so gradually. You want to start out by cutting the amounts of sugar in half and slowly weaning down over the period of a couple of weeks. This is what is best for you.

Cut out liquid sugars

All too often, people drink sugars that they don't even realize. Soda is one of the biggest sources of sugar that we get. Additionally, you can see that adding honey or sugar to coffees and teas is another common source, as is drinking juice. None of these are very healthy options; you need to make sure that you are cutting out those sugars over time. Coffee and tea are fine, so long as you are mindful of the sugars that you put into them.

Choose fresh fruits

If you want something sweet, go for fruit, but still, be mindful. Fresh fruit is usually the best for you, but you can also go for unsweetened frozen fruit or even canned fruit if it is in water or natural juices. Make sure that you avoid the fruit that is canned in heavy syrups; this is a common source of sugars that people don't realize that they are using. You can also use fruit as a natural sweetener. If you are going to use a sweetener of some sort for yogurt, cereals, or oatmeal, this is a great option for you. Fruit is a great option to flavor your teas or water as well if you are someone that's used to sweetened and flavored drinks.

Always compare food labels

When you look at your food labels, make sure that you choose those that have the lowest amounts of added sugars. Many foods are naturally going to have carbohydrates in them—and that's okay in moderation. You must make sure that you are cutting out those high added sugar foods to keep yourself healthy. This means that if you have a food with 22 grams of sugar and 18 are added, and you can also choose a food that has 25 grams of sugar with just 4 or 5 added the second food is going to be the healthier choice because it doesn't involve adding any natural sugars.

Extracts for flavor

Instead of relying on sweeteners like sugar, you can use extracts like vanilla or lemon to add some richness and flavor without the calories.

Non-nutritive sweeteners

If you just can't cut the sugar entirely, you can make it a point to limit the sugar that you do consume, switching it out with non-nutritive sweeteners. However, treat this as a crutch rather than a permanent option. It is better for you to just keep things natural and avoid adding any sweeteners entirely.

Substitute or replace it

If you are cooking something, there are several options that you can use as a way of avoiding the sugar entirely. You could use spices to enhance the foods instead of using sweeteners. You can also use ingredients such as applesauce to replace sugar and fats in many baking dishes as a nice way to cut out the added sugars.

A Healthy Meal Can Help Reduce the Effects of Diabetes

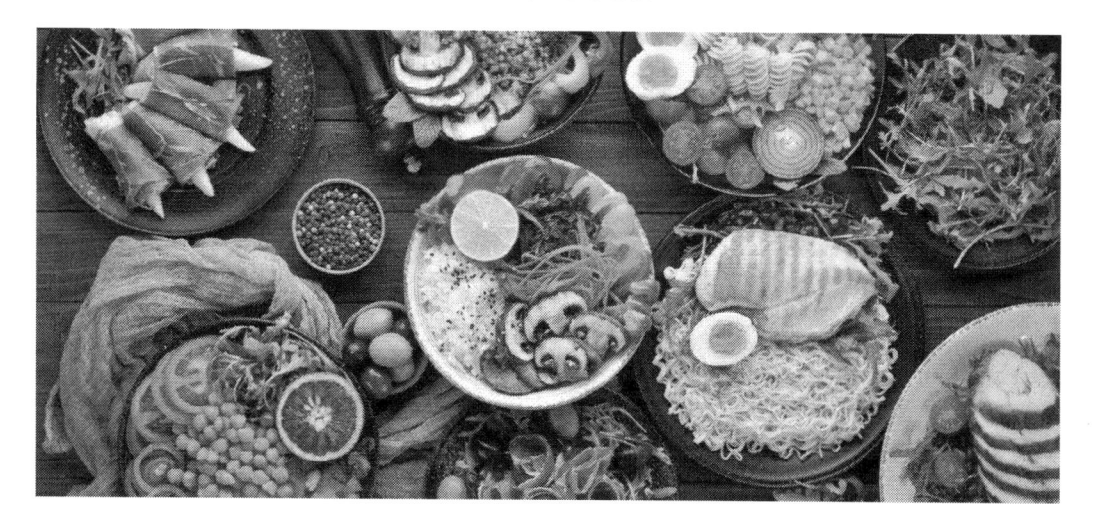

Relationship between Meals and Your Blood Sugar

Your daily meals have a direct effect on your body's blood glucose levels. Some foods raise blood glucose more than others while some other foods do not (have minimal effects on blood sugar levels. Therefore, managing what you eat, knowing their calorie content, knowing what they contain and how they affect your glucose levels and your body is very important. Basically, three major classes of food appear in most of our meals or diets. They include carbohydrates, fats and proteins. Vegetables, fruits and fiber appear much less in meals and diets. An understanding of these food classes and their effects on the body is very important.

Proteins

Proteins are important parts of our diet. In an experiment where Protein of the same quantity and carbohydrate of the same quantity is taking by two individuals at the same time, the individual who took the carbohydrate would most likely get hungry first. This shows how important they are. They help to create satiety. Proteins mildly contribute to the glucose (sugar levels) in the body, and are usually increased in most diabetes meal plans. Proteins are equally the building blocks of the body, and generally help the body to recover from stress and ailments.

Generally, to create a balanced diet (in relation to diabetes). These three classes should be included, albeit in differing quantities.

Vegetables and fruit

Vegetables and fruits are very helpful in the creation of balanced diabetes meal plans. They help in flushing and cleansing the body. They equally contain many vitamins and minerals that help in regulating blood sugar levels in the body. They can equally be used as snacks, because most of them contain fibers. Hence, they can easily cause satiety. Fruits equally contain natural sugars that are less harmful to the body.

Artificial Sweeteners and Weight

As a diabetic, it is generally recommended that you avoid artificial sweeteners or drinks that have artificial sweeteners. They might seem insignificant, but over time they can cause serious harm to the body.

Recent research has shown that despite the fact sweeteners are very low in kilojoules; they can actually make you gain weight. A standardized review studied all published randomized controlled trials and investigative studies on body weight. The review discovered that the use of artificial sweeteners led to a significant increase in body weight.

Generally, sweeteners are divided into two. They are nutritive and non-nutritive. Ongoing research from scientists indicates that non- nutritive sweeteners might be inconsequential, especially when the user does not take additional processed food. It is however advised that sweeteners should be avoided, as much as possible.

Some sweetener protagonists argue that the quantity used is usually set aside. They believe that some of these findings are biased. That most of them based their calculations on doses that are never used. They believe that the quantity of sweeteners used is negligible.

Whether these findings are true or not, it is generally advised that individuals (especially diabetics), should avoid diabetes as much as possible.

Check What You Drink

Drinks are equally an important part of our diet. For good health and optimum fitness, the body requires between thirty-five and forty-five milliliters of fluid for each kilo of weight every day.

There might be alterations based on gender, level of physical activity, body composition and the weather. For example, the common Australian lady weighs about 70 kg on average, while an Australian man weighs an average of 80 kg. Therefore, a typical lady needs 2.5 to 3.2 liters, and a man about 3.0 to 3.9 liters of fluid every day. All fluids don't have to come from drinks; however, as around 750 milliliter comes from our food and an extra 250 milliliter comes from the metabolism of food. So, on average, girls ought to aim to drink 1.5 to 2.2 liters and men ought to aim to drink 2.0 to 2.9 liters every day.

With such a large amount of drinks available now, it is understandable if you get confused (on what to drink. Your choice depends on your personal circumstances and health status.

Water

Plain water is the best drink to quench your thirst: it's refreshing and provides zero kilojoules, and a number of minerals. Pure water doesn't have any taste, though the minerals that are generally found in water naturally (for example, fluoride), will have an effect on its flavor. If water flavor is a problem for you, attempt using a water apparatus or adding a slice or 2 of lemon or lime.

Depending on the supply, drinking water typically contains little amounts of metallic element, potassium, metal and metal, and is appropriate for individuals with polygenic disease (diabetes)

Diet soft drinks

People with diabetes will benefit from a diet or low sugar and soft drinks, however they ought to not consume them on a routine. This is often as a result of sugar-based beverages which are acidic and frequent consumption could increase the danger of developing high sugar levels. There's proof that subbing regular soft drinks with a proper diet or low-joule varieties can facilitate health recovery in some individuals.

Fruit juices and fruit drinks

Fruit juices and fruit drinks may be enjoyed often, however ideally not on a routine. They supply kilojoules, vitamin C, dietary fiber and sugar. Fruit juices and drinks are acidic and also are a supply of possible sugar for the cariogenic bacterium; therefore, frequent consumption of those drinks could increase the danger of developing diseases...

Fruit juices and drinks raise glucose levels in individuals with diabetes. On average, they supply twenty-two g of sugar per 250 milliliters serve. Fruit juices made of low-GI fruit and most fruit drinks have a reduced glycemic index (GI), whereas a 250-milliliter serve of most varieties features a medium glycemic load (GL).

Fruit juices are related to an increased risk of type 2 diabetes in empirical studies. This association is also thanks to their kilojoules content, which can contribute to weight gain, and glycemic load, which can contribute to duct gland stress. Higher-quality analysis is additionally needed to prove this association.

Regular sugar-sweetened soft drink

Sugar-sweetened soft drinks are related to associate to magnified increase in the occurrence of diabetes empirical studies. Like fruit juices and drinks, this association is also thanks to the sugar content of those drinks, which can contribute to weight gain, and their glycemic load, whichcan contribute to duct gland stress.

Alcohol

While alcohol isn't a necessary nutrient, it's however enjoyed by the bulk of adults living in the world today. Alcohol provides twenty-nine kJ of energy for each gram consumed — second solely to fats in energy density. Once consumed, alcohol is then absorbed into the blood from the abdomen and bowel. It doesn't need any digestion, and may consequently induce the acquainted feelings of high spirits among minutes if it's consumed on an empty abdomen.

Alcohol is metabolized within the liver, however there's a limit to what quantity it will handle — about (or 1 1/2 normal drinks) per hour. Therefore, excess amounts will cause a buildup of sugar within the blood if you drink over one or two normal drinks per hour.

Other Food Tips:

Take your meals at regular time intervals

Taking meals at regular intervals helps the body to regulate blood sugar. Our bodies are adaptive and intelligent. Over time they learn to expertly manage and process these foods, because they already know what to expect. Hence food processing (in the body) becomes faster and efficient.

Monitor your food portions

The quantity of food you eat is an important part of diabetes management. Portion sizes are usually dependent on the level of a patient's diabetes (blood sugar level). Equally portions are directly related to an individual's weight. Heavier persons tend to eat more. Any decrease in food portions should be done gradually.

Canada's Food Guide suggests one way to plan your portions. Half of your plate should be filled with vegetables and fruits. It should be more vegetables than fruit because, vegetables have less sugar. The other half of your plate should be between proteins and carbohydrates. Portion control is very important in diabetes control. For overweight diabetes patients, this might be the fastest way to lose weight and regulate blood sugar.

The Basics of Meal Prep

It is time for us first to look into the basics of being able to prep and plan your meals to help keep your diet on track. Being able to prep and plan your meals can help you greatly with making sure that you stay healthy and to ensure that your food is nourishing your body the right way. We are going to address topics such as how to choose healthy foods at the store and how you should be working to stock your kitchen. You will also see what goes into planning a diet, how you can determine what the right foods for your meal plan will be, and you will be introduced to meal prepping—the idea that you can create your meals and even start with parts of your meals in advance so that you can cut down the cooking time when it's time to eat.

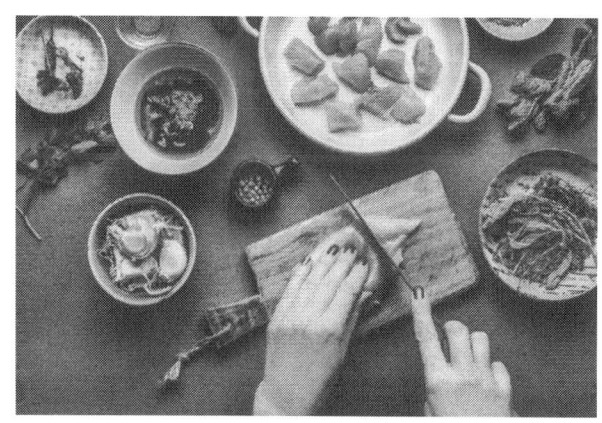

The Foods to Choose at the Store

It's easy for you to think that you are making a good choice for your food, only to realize that the choice that you did make is actually not very practical or healthy at all. In particular, when we see all of these different foods that claim on their packaging that they are healthy or complete, we can run into a very simple problem—we buy things without actually knowing what is in them.

However, you can avoid that problem just by learning what you should be looking for when you are shopping. Consider these points when you are making your shopping plans:

•   Always read the nutrition label: No matter what the front box says, make sure that you always take the time to figure out what is actually inside the foods that you pick up. Double-check how healthy the food that you are looking at actually is. Make sure that you check the label—and compare it to other options as well. Take the time to compare the ingredients and choose those that have the lowest amounts of sodium, unhealthy fats, and sugars.

•   Avoid tricky Ingredients a lot of ingredients that are in your food are hidden under other names. You might not see sugar on the top three ingredients—but is high fructose

corn syrup up there? Or any other of the –ose ingredients? That ending is specific to sugars, and if you know that it is high in one of the other –ose endings, you know that it is actually high in sugar, even if it doesn't say sugar.

- If fresh produce isn't available, always choose frozen: When you have to choose between no produce and frozen produce, you should choose the frozen. If you can't get frozen, choose canned, but make sure that you choose options that are lower in sodium and added sugars or syrups.

- Opt for whole-grain Ingredients when you go shopping; make sure that you choose those whole-grain options. Pasta, bread, crackers, and all sorts of other foods all come in whole-grain forms that will help you enjoy them without getting those high blood sugar spikes.

- If you can't pronounce the ingredients, avoid it: Take a look at the ingredient names. You need to make sure that you are eating mostly healthy whole foods, and that means making sure that you should actually recognize the names of what you are eating.

Stocking Your Kitchen

Of course, any good meal plan is only as good as the kitchen that it is cooked in, and that means that you need to make sure that you are giving yourself plenty of good foods that will keep you full for longer. We're going to take a look at several of the essential food items that you can keep in your kitchen at all times. Consider these the basics that you should keep constantly stocked on top of anything else that you may decide that you want to eat based on your meal plan.

Whole grains to keep on hand

- Whole wheat flours and oats
- Brown rice
- Whole wheat bread, cereals, and pasta
- Quinoa

Beans and legumes to keep on hand

- Variety of canned beans (red, pinto, garbanzo, etc.)
- Dried lentils and peas

Healthy fats to keep on hand

- No sugar added nut butter
- Olive oil

- Coconut oil
- Canola oil
- Avocado oil

Canned fruits and veggies to keep on hand

- Tomatoes (diced and sauced)
- Green beans
- Artichokes

Fresh produce to keep on hand

- In-season produce
- Citrus fruits of choice
- Avocados
- Onions
- Sweet potatoes
- Spinach
- Kale
- Broccoli
- Zucchini
- Squash
- Tomatoes

Protein sources to keep on hand

- Canned salmon or tuna in water, not oil
- Chicken breast
- Fresh meats of choice
- Eggs

Snacks to keep on hand

- Whole-grain crackers (low-carb)
- Multi-grain chips
- Seeds and nuts (unsalted)
- Popcorn

Seasonings to keep on hand

- Garlic
- Herbs and spices to limit salt content

How to Meal Plan

Now consider that you will need to plan out your meals to make sure that you stick to the right tasks at hand. Making your shopping list and avoiding the frustration of figuring out what you are going to eat is all simplified with one simple task: Meal planning.

When you meal plan, you make yourself a menu for the week. You make it so that you are able to find the meals that will work for you to make sure that you are eating foods that will be healthy, but also so that you don't unnecessarily buy foods that you don't actually need. To meal plan, all you need to do, then, is writing down what you will eat that week.

Breakfasts, lunches, dinners, and snacks should all be planned out. When you do that and make sure that you know what it is that you want to eat, you can then assemble your shopping list. When you have that shopping list, you buy only what you need, meaning that you save money and avoid waste!

Your meal plan should incorporate meals with similar ingredients so that you can either reuse the same bunch of ingredients, or it may contain leftovers intentionally to slow down how much you have to cook. We will look at how to create a 30-day meal plan.

When you have your meal plan, you have a few simple benefits—you are able to meal prep, for example. You can make sure that you prepare ingredients in advance if it works better for your schedule. When you do this, you can make meals that might have a lot of prep actually work better during days that are actually quite busy. Say you want to eat enchiladas for dinner, for example, but you are going to be busy. The best way to make that work is to prep what you can before that. When you know what you will be eating, you know that you can prep the foods that you want in advance and know that you aren't just taking a shot in the dark.

BREAKFAST

1) Berry-Oat Breakfast Bars

Ingredients:

- 2 cups fresh raspberries or blueberries
- 2 tablespoons sugar
- 2 tablespoons freshly squeezed lemon juice
- 1 tablespoon cornstarch
- 1/2 cups rolled oats
- 1/2 cup whole-wheat flour
- 1/2 cup walnuts
- ¼ cup chia seeds
- ¼ cup extra-virgin olive oil
- ¼ cup honey
- 1 large egg

Direction: Preparation Time: 10 minutes
Cooking Time: 25 minutes Servings: 12

- Preheat the oven to 350F.
- In a small saucepan over medium heat, stir together the berries, sugar, lemon juice, and cornstarch. Bring to a simmer. Reduce the heat and simmer for 2 to 3 minutes, until the mixture thickens.
- In a food processor or high-speed blender, combine the oats, flour, walnuts, and chia seeds. Process until powdered. Add the olive oil, honey, and egg. Pulse a few more times, until well combined. Press half of the mixture into a 9-inch square baking dish.
- Spread the berry filling over the oat mixture. Add the remaining oat mixture on top of the berries. Bake for 25 minutes, until browned.
- Let cool completely, cut into 12 pieces, and serve. Store in a covered container for up to 5 days.

Nutrition: Calories: 201; Total fat: 10g; Saturated fat: 1g; Protein: 5g; Carbs: 26g; Sugar: 9g; Fiber: 5g; Cholesterol: 16mg; Sodium: 8mg

2) Whole-Grain Breakfast Cookies

Ingredients:

- cups rolled oats
- 1/2 cup whole-wheat flour
- ¼ cup ground flaxseed
- 1 teaspoon baking powder
- 1 cup unsweetened applesauce
- 2 large eggs
- 2 tablespoons vegetable oil
- 2 teaspoons vanilla extract
- 1 teaspoon ground cinnamon
- 1/2 cup dried cherries
- ¼ cup unsweetened shredded coconut
- 2 ounces dark chocolate, chopped

Direction: Preparation time: 20 minutes
Cooking time: 10 minutes Servings: 18 cookies

- 1. Preheat the oven to 350F.
- 2. In a large bowl, combine the oats, flour, flaxseed, and baking powder. Stir well to mix.
- 3. In a medium bowl, whisk the applesauce, eggs, vegetable oil, vanilla, and cinnamon. Pour the wet mixture into the dry mixture, and stir until just combined.
- 4. Fold in the cherries, coconut, and chocolate. Drop tablespoon-size balls of dough onto a baking sheet. Bake for 10 to 12 minutes, until browned and cooked through.
- 5. Let cool for about 3 minutes, remove from the baking sheet, and cool completely before serving. Store in an airtight container for up to 1 week.

Nutrition: Calories: 136; Total fat: 7g; Saturated fat: 3g; Protein: 4g; Carbs: 14g; Sugar: 4g; Fiber: 3g; Cholesterol: 21mg; Sodium: 11mg

3) Blueberry Breakfast Cake

Ingredients:

FOR THE TOPPING
- ¼ cup finely chopped walnuts
- 1/2 teaspoon ground cinnamon
- 2 tablespoons butter, chopped into small pieces
- 2 tablespoons sugar
- or frozen blueberries

FOR THE CAKE
- Nonstick cooking spray
- 1 cup whole-wheat pastry flour
- 1 cup oat flour
- ¼ cup sugar
- 2 teaspoons baking powder
- 1 large egg, beaten
- 1/2 cup skim milk
- 2 tablespoons butter, melted
- 1 teaspoon grated lemon peel
- 2 cups fresh

Direction: Preparation time: 15 minutes
Cooking time: 45 minutes Servings: 12

TO MAKE THE TOPPING
- In a small bowl, stir together the walnuts, cinnamon, butter, and sugar. Set aside.

TO MAKE THE CAKE
- Preheat the oven to 350F. Spray a 9-inch square pan with cooking spray. Set aside.
- In a large bowl, stir together the pastry flour, oat flour, sugar, and baking powder.
- Add the egg, milk, butter, and lemon peel, and stir until there are no dry spots.
- Stir in the blueberries, and gently mix until incorporated. Press the batter into the prepared pan, using a spoon to flatten it into the dish.
- Sprinkle the topping over the cake.
- Bake for 40 to 45 minutes, until a toothpick inserted into the cake comes out clean, and serve.

Nutrition: Calories: 177; Total fat: 7g; Saturated fat: 3g; Protein: 4g; Carbs: 26g; Sugar: 9g; Fiber: 3g; Cholesterol: 26mg; Sodium: 39mg

4) Whole-Grain Pancakes

Ingredients:

- 2 cups whole-wheat pastry flour
- 4 teaspoons baking powder
- 2 teaspoons ground cinnamon
- 1/2 teaspoon salt
- 2 cups skim milk, plus more as needed
- 2 large eggs
- 1 tablespoon honey
- Nonstick cooking spray
- Maple syrup, for serving
- Fresh fruit, for serving

Direction: Preparation time: 10 minutes
Cooking time: 15 minutes Servings: 4 to 6

- In a large bowl, stir together the flour, baking powder, cinnamon, and salt.
- Add the milk, eggs, and honey, and stir well to combine. If needed, add more milk, 1 tablespoon at a time, until there are no dry spots and you has a pourable batter.
- Heat a large skillet over medium-high heat, and spray it with cooking spray.
- Using a ¼-cup measuring cup, scoop 2 or 3 pancakes into the skillet at a time. Cook for a couple of minutes, until bubbles form on the surface of the pancakes, flip, and cook for 1 to 2 minutes more, until golden brown and cooked through. Repeat with the remaining batter.
- Serve topped with maple syrup or fresh fruit.

Nutrition: Calories: 392; Total fat: 4g; Saturated fat: 1g; Protein: 15g; Carbs: 71g; Sugar: 11g; Fiber: 9g; Cholesterol: 95mg; Sodium: 396mg

5) Buckwheat Grouts Breakfast Bowl

Ingredients:

- 3 cups skim milk
- 1 cup buckwheat grouts
- ¼ cup chia seeds
- 2 teaspoons vanilla extract
- 1/2 teaspoon ground cinnamon
- Pinch salt
- 1 cup water
- 1/2 cup unsalted pistachios
- 2 cups sliced fresh strawberries
- ¼ cup cacao nibs (optional)

Direction: Preparation time: 5 minutes, plus overnight to soak
Cooking time: 10 to 12 minutes **Servings:** 4

- ✓ In a large bowl, stir together the milk, groats, chia seeds, vanilla, cinnamon, and salt. Cover and refrigerate overnight.
- ✓ The next morning, transfer the soaked mixture to a medium pot and add the water. Bring to a boil over medium-high heat, reduce the heat to maintain a simmer, and cook for 10 to 12 minutes, until the buckwheat is tender and thickened.
- ✓ Transfer to bowls and serve, topped with the pistachios, strawberries, and cacao nibs (if using).

Nutrition: Calories: 340; Total fat: 8g; Saturated fat: 1g; Protein: 15g; Carbs: 52g; Sugar: 14g; Fiber: 10g; Cholesterol: 4mg; Sodium: 140mg

6) Peach Muesli Bake

Ingredients:

- Nonstick cooking spray
- 2 cups skim milk
- 1 1/2 cups rolled oats
- 1/2 cup chopped walnuts
- 1 large egg
- 2 tablespoons maple syrup
- 1 teaspoon ground cinnamon
- 1 teaspoon baking powder
- 1/2 teaspoon salt
- 2 to 3 peaches, sliced

Direction: Preparation time: 10 minutes
Cooking time: 40 minutes **Servings:** 8

- ✓ Preheat the oven to 375F. Spray a 9-inch square baking dish with cooking spray. Set aside.
- ✓ In a large bowl, stir together the milk, oats, walnuts, egg, maple syrup, cinnamon, baking powder, and salt. Spread half the mixture in the prepared baking dish.
- ✓ Place half the peaches in a single layer across the oat mixture.
- ✓ Spread the remaining oat mixture over the top. Add the remaining peaches in a thin layer over the oats. Bake for 35 to 40 minutes, uncovered, until thickened and browned.
- ✓ Cut into 8 squares and serve warm.

Nutrition: Calories: 138; Total fat: 3g; Saturated fat: 1g; Protein: 6g; Carbs: 22g; Sugar: 10g; Fiber: 3g; Cholesterol: 24mg; Sodium: 191mg

7) Steel-Cut Oatmeal Bowl with Fruit and Nuts

Ingredients:

- 1 cup steel-cut oats
- 2 cups almond milk
- ¾ cup water
- 1 teaspoon ground cinnamon
- ¼ teaspoon salt
- 2 cups chopped fresh fruit, such as blueberries, strawberries, raspberries, or peaches
- 1/2 cup chopped walnuts
- ¼ cup chia seeds

Direction: Preparation time: 5 minutes
Cooking time: 20 minutes **Servings:** 4

- ✓ In a medium saucepan over medium-high heat, combine the oats, almond milk, water, cinnamon, and salt. Bring to a boil, reduce the heat to low, and simmer for 15 to 20 minutes, until the oats are softened and thickened.
- ✓ Top each bowl with 1/2 cup of fresh fruit, 2 tablespoons of walnuts, and 1 tablespoon of chia seeds before serving.

Nutrition: Calories: 288; Total fat: 11g; Saturated fat: 1g; Protein: 10g; Carbs: 38g; Sugar: 7g; Fiber: 10g; Cholesterol: 0mg; Sodium: 329mg

8) Whole-Grain Dutch Baby Pancake

Ingredients:

- 2 tablespoons coconut oil
- 1/2 cup whole-wheat flour
- ¼ cup skim milk
- 3 large eggs
- 1 teaspoon vanilla extract
- 1/2 teaspoon baking powder
- ¼ teaspoon salt
- ¼ teaspoon ground cinnamon
- Powdered sugar, for dusting

Direction: Preparation time: 5 minutes
Cooking time: 25 minutes **Servings:** 4

- ✓ Preheat the oven to 400F.
- ✓ Put the coconut oil in a medium oven-safe skillet, and place the skillet in the oven to melt the oil while it preheats.
- ✓ In a blender, combine the flour, milk, eggs, vanilla, baking powder, salt, and cinnamon. Process until smooth.
- ✓ Carefully remove the skillet from the oven and tilt to spread the oil around evenly.
- ✓ Pour the batter into the skillet and return it to the oven for 23 to 25 minutes, until the pancake puffs and lightly browns.
- ✓ Remove, dust lightly with powdered sugar, cut into 4 wedges, and serve.

Nutrition: Calories: 195; Total fat: 11g; Saturated fat: 7g; Protein: 8g; Carbs: 16g; Sugar: 1g; Fiber: 2g; Cholesterol: 140mg; Sodium: 209mg

9) Mushroom, Zucchini, and Onion Frittata

Ingredients:

- 1 tablespoon extra-virgin olive oil
- 1/2 onion, chopped
- 1 medium zucchini, chopped
- 1 1/2 cups sliced mushrooms
- 6 large eggs, beaten
- 2 tablespoons skim milk
- Salt
- Freshly ground black pepper
- 1 ounce feta cheese, crumbled

Direction: Preparation time: 10 minutes
Cooking time: 20 minutes Servings: 4

- ✓ Preheat the oven to 400F.
- ✓ In a medium oven-safe skillet over medium-high heat, heat the olive oil.
- ✓ Add the onion and sauté for 3 to 5 minutes, until translucent.
- ✓ Add the zucchini and mushrooms, and cook for 3 to 5 more minutes, until the vegetables are tender.
- ✓ Meanwhile, in a small bowl, whisk the eggs, milk, salt, and pepper. Pour the mixture into the skillet, stirring to combine, and transfer the skillet to the oven. Cook for 7 to 9 minutes, until set.
- ✓ Sprinkle with the feta cheese, and cook for 1 to 2 minutes more, until heated through.
- ✓ Remove, cut into 4 wedges, and serve.

Nutrition: Calories: 178; Total fat: 13g; Saturated fat: 4g; Protein: 12g; Carbs: 5g; Sugar: 3g; Fiber: 1g; Cholesterol: 285mg; Sodium: 234mg

10) Spinach and Cheese Quiche

Ingredients:

- Nonstick cooking spray
- 8 ounces Yukon Gold potatoes, shredded
- 1 tablespoon plus 2 teaspoons extra-virgin olive oil, divided
- 1 teaspoon salt, divided
- Freshly ground black pepper
- 1 onion, finely chopped
- 1 (10-ounce) bag fresh spinach
- 4 large eggs
- 1/2 cup skim milk
- 1 ounce Gruyere cheese, shredded

Direction: Preparation time: 10 minutes, plus 10 minutes to rest
Cooking time: 50 minutes Servings: 4 to 6

- ✓ Preheat the oven to 350F. Spray a 9-inch pie dish with cooking spray. Set aside.
- ✓ In a small bowl, toss the potatoes with 2 teaspoons of olive oil, 1/2 teaspoon of salt, and season with pepper. Press the potatoes into the bottom and sides of the pie dish to form a thin, even layer. Bake for 20 minutes, until golden brown. Remove from the oven and set aside to cool.
- ✓ In a large skillet over medium-high heat, heat the remaining 1 tablespoon of olive oil.
- ✓ Add the onion and sauté for 3 to 5 minutes, until softened.
- ✓ By handfuls, add the spinach, stirring between each addition, until it just starts to wilt before adding more. Cook for about 1 minute, until it cooks down.
- ✓ In a medium bowl, whisk the eggs and milk. Add the Gruyère, and season with the remaining 1/2 teaspoon of salt and some pepper. Fold the eggs into the spinach. Pour the mixture into the pie dish and bake for 25 minutes, until the eggs are set.
- ✓ Let rest for 10 minutes before serving.

Nutrition: Calories: 445; Total fat: 14g; Saturated fat: 4g; Protein: 19g; Carbs: 68g; Sugar: 6g; Fiber: 7g; Cholesterol: 193mg; Sodium: 773mg

11) Spicy Jalapeno Popper Deviled Eggs

Ingredients:

- 4 large whole eggs, hardboiled
- 2 tablespoons Keto-Friendly mayonnaise
- ¼ cup cheddar cheese, grated
- 2 slices bacon, cooked and crumbled
- 1 jalapeno, sliced

Direction: Preparation Time: 5 minutes
Cooking Time: 5 minutes Servings: 4

- ✓ Cut eggs in half, remove the yolk and put them in bowl
- ✓ Lay egg whites on a platter
- ✓ Mix in remaining ingredients and mash them with the egg yolks
- ✓ Transfer yolk mix back to the egg whites
- ✓ Serve and enjoy!

Nutrition: Calories: 176; Fat: 14g; Carbohydrates: 0.7g; Protein: 10g

12) Lovely Porridge

Ingredients:

- 2 tablespoons coconut flour
- 2 tablespoons vanilla protein powder
- 3 tablespoons Golden Flaxseed meal
- 1 and 1/2 cups almond milk, unsweetened
- Powdered erythritol

Direction: Preparation Time: 15 minutes
Cooking Time: Nil Servings: 2

- ✓ Take a bowl and mix in flaxseed meal, protein powder, coconut flour and mix well
- ✓ Add mix to the saucepan (placed over medium heat)
- ✓ Add almond milk and stir, let the mixture thicken
- ✓ Add your desired amount of sweetener and serve

Nutrition: Calories: 259; Fat: 13g; Carbohydrates: 5g; Protein: 16g

13) Salty Macadamia Chocolate Smoothie

Ingredients:

- 2 tablespoons macadamia nuts, salted
- 1/3 cup chocolate whey protein powder, low carb
- 1 cup almond milk, unsweetened

Direction: Preparation Time: 5 minutes
Cooking Time: Nil Servings: 1

- ✓ Add the listed ingredients to your blender and blend until you have a smooth mixture
- ✓ Chill and enjoy it!

Nutrition: Calories: 165; Fat: 2g; Carbohydrates: 1g; Protein: 12g

14) Basil and Tomato Baked Eggs

Ingredients:

- 1 garlic clove, minced
- 1 cup canned tomatoes
- ¼ cup fresh basil leaves, roughly chopped
- 1/2 teaspoon chili powder
- 1 tablespoon olive oil
- 4 whole eggs
- Salt and pepper to taste

Direction: Preparation Time: 10 minutes
Cooking Time: 15 minutes Servings: 4

- ✓ Preheat your oven to 375 degrees F
- ✓ Take a small baking dish and grease with olive oil
- ✓ Add garlic, basil, tomatoes chili, olive oil into a dish and stir
- ✓ Crackdown eggs into a dish, keeping space between the two
- ✓ Sprinkle the whole dish with salt and pepper
- ✓ Place in oven and cook for 12 minutes until eggs are set and tomatoes are bubbling
- ✓ Serve with basil on top
- ✓ Enjoy!

Nutrition: Calories: 235; Fat: 16g; Carbohydrates: 7g; Protein: 14g

15) Cinnamon and Coconut Porridge

Ingredients:

- 2 cups of water
- 1 cup 36% heavy cream
- 1/2 cup unsweetened dried coconut, shredded
- 2 tablespoons flaxseed meal
- 1 tablespoon butter
- 1 and 1/2 teaspoon stevia
- 1 teaspoon cinnamon
- Salt to taste
- Toppings as blueberries

Direction: Preparation Time: 5 minutes
Cooking Time: 5 minutes Servings: 4

- ✓ Add the listed ingredients to a small pot, mix well
- ✓ Transfer pot to stove and place it over medium-low heat
- ✓ Bring to mix to a slow boil
- ✓ Stir well and remove the heat
- ✓ Divide the mix into equal servings and let them sit for 10 minutes
- ✓ Top with your desired toppings and enjoy!

Nutrition: Calories: 171; Fat: 16g; Carbohydrates: 6g; Protein: 2g

16) An Omelet of Swiss chard

Ingredients:

- 4 eggs, lightly beaten
- 4 cups Swiss chard, sliced
- 2 tablespoons butter
- 1/2 teaspoon garlic salt
- Fresh pepper

Direction: Preparation Time: 5 minutes
Cooking Time: 5 minutes Servings: 4

- ✓ Take a non-stick frying pan and place it over medium-low heat
- ✓ Once the butter melts, add Swiss chard and stir cook for 2 minutes
- ✓ Pour egg into the pan and gently stir them into Swiss chard
- ✓ Season with garlic salt and pepper
- ✓ Cook for 2 minutes
- ✓ Serve and enjoy!

Nutrition: Calories: 260; Fat: 21g; Carbohydrates: 4g; Protein: 14g

17) Cheesy Low-Carb Omelet

Ingredients:

- 2 whole eggs
- 1 tablespoon water
- 1 tablespoon butter
- 3 thin slices salami
- 5 fresh basil leaves
- 5 thin slices, fresh ripe tomatoes
- 2 ounces fresh mozzarella cheese
- Salt and pepper as needed

Direction: Preparation Time: 5 minutes
Cooking Time: 5 minutes Servings: 5

- ✓ Take a small bowl and whisk in eggs and water
- ✓ Take a non-stick Sauté pan and place it over medium heat, add butter and let it melt
- ✓ Pour egg mixture and cook for 30 seconds
- ✓ Spread salami slices on half of egg mix and top with cheese, tomatoes, basil slices
- ✓ Season with salt and pepper according to your taste
- ✓ Cook for 2 minutes and fold the egg with the empty half
- ✓ Cover and cook on LOW for 1 minute
- ✓ Serve and enjoy!

Nutrition: Calories: 451; Fat: 36g; Carbohydrates: 3g; Protein: 33g

18) Yogurt And Kale Smoothie

Ingredients:

- 1 cup whole milk yogurt
- 1 cup baby kale greens
- 1 pack stevia
- 1 tablespoon MCT oil
- 1 tablespoon sunflower seeds
- 1 cup of water

Direction: Servings: 1 Preparation Time: 10 minutes

- ✓ Add listed ingredients to the blender
- ✓ Blend until you have a smooth and creamy texture
- ✓ Serve chilled and enjoy!

Nutrition: Calories: 329; Fat: 26g; Carbohydrates: 15g; Protein: 11g

19) Bacon and Chicken Garlic Wrap

Ingredients:

- 1 chicken fillet, cut into small cubes
- 8-9 thin slices bacon, cut to fit cubes
- 6 garlic cloves, minced

Direction: Preparation Time: 15 minutes
Cooking Time: 10 minutes Servings: 4

- ✓ Preheat your oven to 400 degrees F
- ✓ Line a baking tray with aluminum foil
- ✓ Add minced garlic to a bowl and rub each chicken piece with it
- ✓ Wrap bacon piece around each garlic chicken bite
- ✓ Secure with toothpick
- ✓ Transfer bites to the baking sheet, keeping a little bit of space between them
- ✓ Bake for about 15-20 minutes until crispy
- ✓ Serve and enjoy!

Nutrition: Calories: 260; Fat: 19g; Carbohydrates: 5g; Protein: 22g

20) Grilled Chicken Platter

Ingredients:

- 3 large chicken breast, sliced half lengthwise
- 10-ounce spinach, frozen and drained
- 3-ounce mozzarella cheese, part-skim
- 1/2 a cup of roasted red peppers, cut in long strips
- 1 teaspoon of olive oil
- 2 garlic cloves, minced
- Salt and pepper as needed

Direction: Preparation Time: 5 minutes
Cooking Time: 10 minutes Servings: 6

- ✓ Preheat your oven to 400 degrees Fahrenheit
- ✓ Slice 3 chicken breast lengthwise
- ✓ Take a non-stick pan and grease with cooking spray
- ✓ Bake for 2-3 minutes each side
- ✓ Take another skillet and cook spinach and garlic in oil for 3 minutes
- ✓ Place chicken on an oven pan and top with spinach, roasted peppers, and mozzarella
- ✓ Bake until the cheese melted
- ✓ Enjoy!

Nutrition: Calories: 195; Fat: 7g; Carbohydrates: 3g; Protein: 30g

21) Parsley Chicken Breast

Ingredients:

- 1 tablespoon dry parsley
- 1 tablespoon dry basil
- 4 chicken breast halves, boneless and skinless
- 1/2 teaspoon salt
- 1/2 teaspoon red pepper flakes, crushed
- 2 tomatoes, sliced

Direction: Preparation Time: 10 minutes
Cooking Time: 40 minutes Servings: 4

- ✓ Preheat your oven to 350 degrees F
- ✓ Take a 9x13 inch baking dish and grease it up with cooking spray
- ✓ Sprinkle 1 tablespoon of parsley, 1 teaspoon of basil and spread the mixture over your baking dish
- ✓ Arrange the chicken breast halves over the dish and sprinkle garlic slices on top
- ✓ Take a small bowl and add 1 teaspoon parsley, 1 teaspoon of basil, salt, basil, red pepper and mix well. Pour the mixture over the chicken breast
- ✓ Top with tomato slices and cover, bake for 25 minutes
- ✓ Remove the cover and bake for 15 minutes more
- ✓ Serve and enjoy!

Nutrition: Calories: 150; Fat: 4g; Carbohydrates: 4g; Protein: 25g

22) Mustard Chicken

Ingredients:

- 4 chicken breasts
- 1/2 cup chicken broth
- 3-4 tablespoons mustard
- 3 tablespoons olive oil
- 1 teaspoon paprika
- 1 teaspoon chili powder
- 1 teaspoon garlic powder

Direction: Preparation Time: 10 minutes
Cooking Time: 40 minutes Servings: 4

- ✓ Take a small bowl and mix mustard, olive oil, paprika, chicken broth, garlic powder, chicken broth, and chili
- ✓ Add chicken breast and marinate for 30 minutes
- ✓ Take a lined baking sheet and arrange the chicken
- ✓ Bake for 35 minutes at 375 degrees Fahrenheit
- ✓ Serve and enjoy!

Nutrition: Calories: 531; Fat: 23g; Carbohydrates: 10g; Protein: 64g

23) Balsamic Chicken 1

Ingredients:

- 6 chicken breast halves, skinless and boneless
- 1 teaspoon garlic salt
- Ground black pepper
- 2 tablespoons olive oil
- 1 onion, thinly sliced
- 14 and 1/2 ounces tomatoes, diced
- 1/2 cup balsamic vinegar
- 1 teaspoon dried basil
- 1 teaspoon dried oregano
- 1 teaspoon dried rosemary
- 1/2 teaspoon dried thyme

Direction: Preparation Time: 10 minutes
Cooking Time: 25 minutes Servings: 6

- ✓ Season both sides of your chicken breasts thoroughly with pepper and garlic salt
- ✓ Take a skillet and place it over medium heat
- ✓ Add some oil and cook your seasoned chicken for 3-4 minutes per side until the breasts are nicely browned
- ✓ Add some onion and cook for another 3-4 minutes until the onions are browned
- ✓ Pour the diced up tomatoes and balsamic vinegar over your chicken and season with some rosemary, basil, thyme, and rosemary
- ✓ Simmer the chicken for about 15 minutes until they are no longer pink
- ✓ Take an instant-read thermometer and check if the internal temperature gives a reading of 165 degrees Fahrenheit
- ✓ If yes, then you are good to go!

Nutrition: Calories: 196; Fat: 7g; Carbohydrates: 7g; Protein: 23g

24) Greek Chicken Breast

Ingredients:

- 4 chicken breast halves, skinless and boneless
- 1 cup extra virgin olive oil
- 1 lemon, juiced
- 2 teaspoons garlic, crushed
- 1 and 1/2 teaspoons black pepper
- 1/3 teaspoon paprika

Direction: Preparation Time: 10 minutes
Cooking Time: 25 minutes Servings: 4

- ✓ Cut 3 slits in the chicken breast
- ✓ Take a small bowl and whisk in olive oil, salt, lemon juice, garlic, paprika, pepper and whisk for 30 seconds
- ✓ Place chicken in a large bowl and pour marinade
- ✓ Rub the marinade all over using your hand
- ✓ Refrigerate overnight
- ✓ Pre-heat grill to medium heat and oil the grate
- ✓ Cook chicken in the grill until center is no longer pink
- ✓ Serve and enjoy!

Nutrition: Calories: 644; Fat: 57g; Carbohydrates: 2g; Protein: 27g

25) Chipotle Lettuce Chicken

Ingredients:

- 1 pound chicken breast, cut into strips
- Splash of olive oil
- 1 red onion, finely sliced
- 14 ounces tomatoes
- 1 teaspoon chipotle, chopped
- 1/2 teaspoon cumin
- Pinch of sugar
- Lettuce as needed
- Fresh coriander leaves
- Jalapeno chilies, sliced
- Fresh tomato slices for garnish
- Lime wedges

Direction: Preparation Time: 10 minutes
Cooking Time: 25 minutes Servings: 6

- ✓ Take a non-stick frying pan and place it over medium heat
- ✓ Add oil and heat it up
- ✓ Add chicken and cook until brown
- ✓ Keep the chicken on the side
- ✓ Add tomatoes, sugar, chipotle, cumin to the same pan and simmer for 25 minutes until you have a nice sauce
- ✓ Add chicken into the sauce and cook for 5 minutes
- ✓ Transfer the mix to another place
- ✓ Use lettuce wraps to take a portion of the mixture and serve with a squeeze of lemon
- ✓ Enjoy!

Nutrition: Calories: 332; Fat: 15g; Carbohydrates: 13g; Protein: 34g

26) Stylish Chicken-Bacon Wrap

Ingredients:

- 8 ounces lean chicken breast
- 6 bacon slices
- 3 ounces shredded cheese
- 4 slices ham

Direction: Preparation Time: 5 minutes
Cooking Time: 50 minutes Servings: 3

- ✓ Cut chicken breast into bite-sized portions
- ✓ Transfer shredded cheese onto ham slices
- ✓ Roll up chicken breast and ham slices in bacon slices
- ✓ Take a skillet and place it over medium heat
- ✓ Add olive oil and brown bacon for a while
- ✓ Remove rolls and transfer to your oven
- ✓ Bake for 45 minutes at 325 degrees F
- ✓ Serve and enjoy!

Nutrition: Calories: 275; Fat: 11g; Carbohydrates: 0.5g; Protein: 40g

27) Healthy Cottage Cheese Pancakes

Ingredients:

- 1/2 cup of Cottage cheese (low-fat)
- 1/3 cup (approx. 2 egg whites) Egg whites
- 1/4 cup of Oats
- 1 teaspoon of Vanilla extract
- Olive oil cooking spray
- 1 tablespoon of Stevia (raw)
- Berries or sugar-free jam (optional)

Direction: Preparation Time: 10 minutes
Cooking Time: 15 Servings: 1

- ✓ Begin by taking a food blender and adding in the egg whites and cottage cheese. Also add in the vanilla extract, a pinch of stevia, and oats. Palpitate until the consistency is well smooth.
- ✓ Get a nonstick pan and oil it nicely with the cooking spray. Position the pan on low heat.
- ✓ After it has been heated, scoop out half of the batter and pour it on the pan. Cook for about 2 1/2 minutes on each side.
- ✓ Position the cooked pancakes on a serving plate and cover with sugar-free jam or berries.

Nutrition: Calories: 205 calories per serving Fat – 1.5 g, Protein – 24.5 g, Carbs – 19 g

28) Avocado Lemon Toast

Ingredients:

- Whole-grain bread – 2 slices
- Fresh cilantro (chopped) – 2 tablespoons
- Lemon zest – 1/4 teaspoon
- Fine sea salt – 1 pinch
- Cayenne pepper – 1 pinch
- Chia seeds – 1/4 teaspoon
- Avocado – 1/2
- Fresh lemon juice – 1 teaspoon

Direction: Preparation Time: 10 minutes
Cooking Time: 13 minutes Servings: 2

- ✓ Begin by getting a medium-sized mixing bowl and adding in the avocado. Make use of a fork to crush it properly.
- ✓ Then, add in the cilantro, lemon zest, lemon juice, sea salt, and cayenne pepper. Mix well until combined.
- ✓ Toast the bread slices in a toaster until golden brown. It should take about 3 minutes.
- ✓ Top the toasted bread slices with the avocado mixture and finalize by drizzling with chia seeds.

Nutrition: Calories: 72 calories per serving; Protein – 3.6 g; Fat – 1.2 g; Carbs – 11.6 g

29) Healthy Baked Eggs

Ingredients:

- Olive oil – 1 tablespoon
- Garlic – 2 cloves
- Eggs – 8 large
- Sea salt – 1/2 teaspoon
- Shredded mozzarella cheese (medium-fat) – 3 cups
- Olive oil spray
- Onion (chopped) – 1 medium
- Spinach leaves – 8 ounces
- Half-and-half – 1 cup
- Black pepper – 1 teaspoon
- Feta cheese – 1/2 cup

Direction: Preparation Time: 10 minutes
Cooking Time: 1 hour Servings: 6

- ✓ Begin by heating the oven to 375F.
- ✓ Get a glass baking dish and grease it with olive oil spray. Arrange aside.
- ✓ Now take a nonstick pan and pour in the olive oil. Position the pan on allows heat and allows it heat.
- ✓ Immediately you are done, toss in the garlic, spinach, and onion. Prepare for about 5 minutes. Arrange aside.
- ✓ You can now Get a large mixing bowl and add in the half, eggs, pepper, and salt. Whisk thoroughly to combine.
- ✓ Put in the feta cheese and chopped mozzarella cheese (reserve 1/2 cup of mozzarella cheese for later).
- ✓ Put the egg mixture and prepared spinach to the prepared glass baking dish. Blend well to combine. Drizzle the reserved cheese over the top.
- ✓ Bake the egg mix for about 45 minutes.
- ✓ Extract the baking dish from the oven and allow it to stand for 10 minutes.
- ✓ Dice and serve!

Nutrition: Calories: 323 calories per serving; Fat 22.3 g; Protein 22.6 g; Carbs 7.9 g

30) Quick Low-Carb Oatmeal

Ingredients:

- Almond flour – 1/2 cup
- Flax meal – 2 tablespoons
- Cinnamon (ground) – 1 teaspoon
- Almond milk (unsweetened) – 1 1/2 cups
- Salt – as per taste
- Chia seeds – 2 tablespoons
- Liquid stevia – 10 – 15 drops
- Vanilla extract – 1 teaspoon

Direction: Preparation Time: 10 minutes
Cooking Time: 15 minutes Servings: 2

- ✓ Begin by taking a large mixing bowl and adding in the coconut flour, almond flour, ground cinnamon, flax seed powder, and chia seeds. Mix properly to combine.
- ✓ Position a stockpot on a low heat and add in the dry ingredients. Also add in the liquid stevia, vanilla extract, and almond milk. Mix well to combine.
- ✓ Prepare the flour and almond milk for about 4 minutes. Add salt if needed.
- ✓ Move the oatmeal to a serving bowl and top with nuts, seeds, and pure and neat berries.

Nutrition: Calories: calories per serving; Protein – 11.7 g; Fat – 24.3 g; Carbs – 16.7 g

31) Tofu and Vegetable Scramble

Ingredients:

- Firm tofu (drained) – 16 ounces
- Sea salt – 1/2 teaspoon
- Garlic powder – 1 teaspoon
- Fresh coriander – for garnishing
- Red onion – 1/2 medium
- Cumin powder – 1 teaspoon
- Lemon juice – for topping
- Green bell pepper – 1 medium
- Garlic powder – 1 teaspoon
- Fresh coriander – for garnishing
- Red onion – 1/2 medium
- Cumin powder – 1 teaspoon
- Lemon juice – for topping

Direction: Preparation Time: 10 minutes
Cooking Time: 15 minutes Servings: 2

- ✓ Begin by preparing the ingredients. For this, you are to extract the seeds of the tomato and green bell pepper. Shred the onion, bell pepper, and tomato into small cubes.
- ✓ Get a small mixing bowl and position the fairly hard tofu inside it. Make use of your hands to break the fairly hard tofu. Arrange aside.
- ✓ Get a nonstick pan and add in the onion, tomato, and bell pepper. Mix and cook for about 3 minutes.
- ✓ Put the somewhat hard crumbled tofu to the pan and combine well.
- ✓ Get a small bowl and put in the water, turmeric, garlic powder, cumin powder, and chili powder. Combine well and stream it over the tofu and vegetable mixture.
- ✓ Allow the tofu and vegetable crumble cook with seasoning for 5 minutes. Continuously stir so that the pan is not holding the ingredients.
- ✓ Drizzle the tofu scramble with chili flakes and salt. Combine well.
- ✓ Transfer the prepared scramble to a serving bowl and give it a proper spray of lemon juice.
- ✓ Finalize by garnishing with pure and neat coriander. Serve while hot!

Nutrition: Calories: 238 calories per serving; Carbohydrates – 16.6 g; Fat – 11 g

32) Breakfast Smoothie Bowl with Fresh Berries

Ingredients:

- Almond milk (unsweetened) – 1/2 cup
- Psyllium husk powder – 1/2 teaspoon
- Strawberries (chopped) – 2 ounces
- Coconut oil – 1 tablespoon
- Crushed ice – 3 cups
- Liquid stevia – 5 to 10 drops
- Pea protein powder – 1/3 cup

Direction: Preparation Time: 10 minutes
Cooking Time: 5 minutes Servings: 2

- ✓ Begin by taking a blender and adding in the mashed ice cubes. Allow them to rest for about 30 seconds.
- ✓ Then put in the almond milk, shredded strawberries, pea protein powder, psyllium husk powder, coconut oil, and liquid stevia. Blend well until it turns into a smooth and creamy puree.
- ✓ Vacant the prepared smoothie into 2 glasses.
- ✓ Cover with coconut flakes and pure and neat strawberries.

Nutrition: Calories: 166 calories per serving; Fat – 9.2 g; Carbs – 4.1 g; Protein – 17.6 g

33) Chia and Coconut Pudding

Ingredients:

- Light coconut milk – 7 ounces
- Liquid stevia – 3 to 4 drops
- Kiwi – 1
- Chia seeds – ¼ cup
- Clementine – 1
- Shredded coconut (unsweetened)

Direction: Preparation Time: 10 minutes
Cooking Time: 5 minutes Servings: 2

- ✓ Begin by getting a mixing bowl and putting in the light coconut milk. Set in the liquid stevia to sweeten the milk. Combine well.
- ✓ Put the chia seeds to the milk and whisk until well-combined. Arrange aside.
- ✓ Scrape the clementine and carefully extract the skin from the wedges. Leave aside.
- ✓ Also, scrape the kiwi and dice it into small pieces.
- ✓ Get a glass vessel and gather the pudding. For this, position the fruits at the bottom of the jar; then put a dollop of chia pudding. Then spray the fruits and then put another layer of chia pudding.
- ✓ Finalize by garnishing with the rest of the fruits and chopped coconut.

Nutrition: Calories: 201 calories per serving; Protein – 5.4 g; Fat – 10 g; Carbs – 22.8 g

34) Tomato and Zucchini Sauté

Ingredients:

- Vegetable oil – 1 tablespoon
- Tomatoes (chopped) – 2
- Green bell pepper (chopped)
- Black pepper (freshly ground) – as per taste
- Onion (sliced)
- 1 Zucchini (peeled) – 2 pounds and cut into 1-inch-thick slices
- Salt – as per taste
- Uncooked white rice – ¼ cup

Direction: Preparation Time: 10 minutes
Cooking Time: 43 minutes Servings: 6

- ✓ Begin by getting a nonstick pan and putting it over low heat. Stream in the oil and allow it to heat through.
- ✓ Put in the onions and sauté for about 3 minutes.
- ✓ Then pour in the zucchini and green peppers. Mix well and spice with black pepper and salt.
- ✓ Reduce the heat and cover the pan with a lid. Allow the veggies cook on low for 5 minutes.
- ✓ While you're done, put in the water and rice. Place the lid back on and cook on low for 20 minutes.

Nutrition: Calories: 94 calories per serving; Fat – 2.8 g; Protein – 3.2 g; Carbs – 16.1 g

35) Steamed Kale with Mediterranean Dressing

Ingredients:

- Kale (chopped) – 12 cups
- Olive oil – 1 tablespoon
- Soy sauce – 1 teaspoon
- Pepper (freshly ground) – as per taste
- Lemon juice – 2 tablespoons
- Garlic (minced) – 1 tablespoon
- Salt – as per taste

Direction: Preparation Time: 10 minutes
Cooking Time: 25 minutes Servings: 6

- ✓ Get a gas steamer or an electric steamer and fill the bottom pan with water. If making use of a gas steamer, position it on high heat. Making use of an electric steamer, place it on the highest setting.
- ✓ Immediately the water comes to a boil, put in the shredded kale and cover with a lid. Boil for about 8 minutes. The kale should be tender by now.
- ✓ During the kale is boiling, take a big mixing bowl and put in the olive oil, lemon juice, soy sauce, garlic, pepper, and salt. Whisk well to mix.
- ✓ Now toss in the steamed kale and carefully enclose into the dressing. Be assured the kale is well-coated.
- ✓ Serve while it's hot!

Nutrition: Calories: 91 calories per serving; Fat – 3.5 g; Protein – 4.6 g; Carbs – 14.5 g

36) Vegetable Noodles Stir-Fry

Ingredients:

- White sweet potato – 1 pound
- Zucchini – 8 ounces
- Garlic cloves (finely chopped) – 2 large
- Vegetable broth – 2 tablespoons
- Salt – as per taste
- Carrots – 8 ounces
- Shallot (finely chopped) – 1
- Red chili (finely chopped) – 1
- Olive oil – 1 tablespoon
- Pepper – as per taste

Direction: Preparation Time: 10 minutes
Cooking Time: 40 minutes Servings: 4

- ✓ Begin by scrapping the carrots and sweet potato. Make Use a spiralizer to make noodles out of the sweet potato and carrots.
- ✓ Rinse the zucchini thoroughly and spiralize it as well.
- ✓ Get a large skillet and position it on a high flame. Stream in the vegetable broth and allow it to come to a boil.
- ✓ Toss in the spiralized sweet potato and carrots. Then put in the chili, garlic, and shallots. Stir everything using tongs and cook for some minutes.
- ✓ Transfer the vegetable noodles into a serving platter and generously spice with pepper and salt.
- ✓ Finalize by sprinkling olive oil over the noodles. Serve while hot!

Nutrition: Calories: 169 calories per serving; Fat 3.7 g; Protein 3.6 g; Carbs – 31.2 g

37) Millet Porridge

Ingredients:

- 1 cup millet, rinsed and drained
- Pinch of salt
- 3 cups water
- 2 tablespoons almonds, chopped finely
- 6-8 drops liquid stevia
- 1 cup unsweetened almond milk
- 2 tablespoons fresh blueberries

Direction: Preparation Time: 10 minutes
Cooking Time: 25 minutes Servings: 4

- ✓ In a nonstick pan, add the millet over medium-low heat and cook for about 3 minutes, stirring continuously.
- ✓ Add the salt and water and stir to combine Increase the heat to medium and bring to a boil.
- ✓ Cook for about 15 minutes.
- ✓ Stir in the almonds, stevia and almond milk and cook for 5 minutes.
- ✓ Top with the blueberries and serve. Meal Prep Tip:
- ✓ Transfer the cooled porridge in an airtight container and preserve in the refrigerator for up to 2 days.
- ✓ Just before serving, reheat in the microwave.
- ✓ Serve with the topping of berries.

Nutrition: Calories 219 Total Fat 4.5 g Saturated Fat 0.6 g Cholesterol 0 mg Total Carbs 38.2 g Sugar 0.6 g Fiber 5 g Sodium 92 mg Potassium 1721 mg Protein 6.4 g

38) Sweet Potato Waffles

Ingredients:

- 1 medium sweet potato, peeled, grated and squeezed
- 1 teaspoon fresh thyme, minced
- 1 teaspoon fresh rosemary, minced
- 1/8 teaspoon red pepper flakes, crushed
- Salt and ground black pepper, as required

Direction: Preparation Time: 10 minutes
Cooking Time: 20 minutes Servings: 2

- ✓ Preheat the waffle iron and then grease it.
- ✓ In a large bowl, add all ingredients and mix till well combined.
- ✓ Place half of the sweet potato mixture into preheated waffle iron and cook for about 8-10 minutes or until golden brown.
- ✓ Repeat with the remaining mixture.
- ✓ Serve warm.

Meal Prep Tip:
- ✓ Store these cooled waffles into an airtight container by placing a piece of wax paper between each waffle.
- ✓ Refrigerate up to 5 days. Reheat in the microwave for about 1-2 minutes.

Nutrition: Calories 72 Total Fat 0.3 g Saturated Fat 0.1 g Cholesterol 0 mg Total Carbs 16.3 g Sugar 4.9 g Fiber 3 g Sodium 28 mg Potassium 369 mg Protein 1.6 g

39) Quinoa Bread

Ingredients:

- 1¾ cups uncooked quinoa, rinsed, soaked overnight and drained
- ¼ cup chia seeds, soaked in ½ cup of water overnight
- ½ teaspoon bicarbonate soda
- Pinch of sea salt
- ½ cup filtered water
- ¼ cup olive oil, melted
- 1 tablespoon fresh lemon juice

Direction: Preparation Time: 10 minutes
Cooking Time: 1½ hours Servings: 12

- ✓ Preheat the oven to 320 degrees F. Line a loaf pan with a parchment paper.
- ✓ In a food processor, add all the ingredients and pulse for about 3 minutes.
- ✓ Transfer the mixture into prepared loaf pan evenly.
- ✓ Bake for about 1½ hours or until a wooden skewer inserted in the center of loaf comes out clean.
- ✓ Remove the pan from oven and place onto a wire rack to cool for about 10-15 minutes.
- ✓ Carefully, remove the bread from the loaf pan and place onto the wire rack to cool completely before slicing.
- ✓ With a sharp knife, cut the bread loaf into desired sized slices and serve.

Meal Prep Tip:
- ✓ In a resealable plastic bag, place the bread and seal the bag after squeezing out the excess air.
- ✓ Set the bread away from direct sunlight and preserve in a cool and dry place for about 1-2 days.

Nutrition: Calories 137 Total Fat 6.5 g Saturated Fat 0.9 g Cholesterol 0 mg Total Carbs 16.9 g Sugar 0 g Fiber 2.6 g Sodium 203 mg Potassium 158 mg Protein 4 g

40) Veggie Frittata

Ingredients:

- 1 tablespoon olive oil
- 1 large sweet potato, peeled and cut into thin slices
- 1 yellow squash, sliced
- 1 zucchini, sliced
- ½ of red bell pepper, seeded and sliced
- ½ of yellow bell pepper, seeded and sliced
- 8 eggs
- Salt and ground black pepper, as required
- 2 tablespoons fresh cilantro, chopped finely

Direction: Preparation Time: 15 minutes
Cooking Time: 25 minutes Servings: 6

- ✓ Preheat the oven to broiler.
- ✓ In a large oven proof skillet, heat the oil over medium-low heat and cook the sweet potato for about 6-7 minutes.
- ✓ Add the yellow squash, zucchini and bell peppers and cook for about 3-4 minutes.
- ✓ Meanwhile, in a bowl, add the eggs, salt and black pepper and beat until well combined.
- ✓ Pour egg mixture over vegetables mixture evenly.
- ✓ Immediately, reduce the heat to low and cook for about 8-10 minutes or until just done.
- ✓ Transfer the skillet in the oven and broil for about 3-4 minutes or until top becomes golden brown.
- ✓ With a sharp knife, cut the frittata in desired size slices and serve with the garnishing of cilantro.

Meal Prep Tip:
- ✓ In a resealable plastic bag, place the cooled frittata slices and seal the bag.
- ✓ Refrigerate for about 2-4 days.
- ✓ Reheat in the microwave on High for about 1 minute before serving.

Nutrition: Calories 143 Total Fat 8.4 g Saturated Fat 2.2 g Cholesterol 218 mg Total Carbs 9.3 g Sugar 4.2 g Fiber 1.1 g Sodium 98 mg Potassium 408 mg Protein 8.9 g

41) Chicken & Sweet Potato Hash

Ingredients:

- 2 tablespoons olive oil, divided
- 1½ pounds boneless, skinless chicken breasts, cubed
- Salt and ground black pepper, as required
- 2 celery stalks, chopped
- 1 medium white onion, chopped
- 4 garlic cloves, minced
- 1 tablespoon fresh oregano, chopped
- 1 tablespoon fresh thyme, chopped
- 2 large sweet potatoes, peeled and cubed
- 1 cup low-sodium chicken broth
- 1 cup scallion, chopped
- 2 tablespoons fresh lime juice

Direction: Preparation Time: 15 minutes
Cooking Time: 35 minutes Servings: 8

- ✓ In a large skillet, heat 1 tablespoon of oil over medium heat and cook the chicken with a little salt and black pepper for about 4-5 minutes.
- ✓ Transfer the chicken into a bowl. In the same skillet, heat the remaining oil over medium heat and sauté celery and onion for about 3-4 minutes.
- ✓ Add the garlic and herbs and sauté for about 1 minute. Add the sweet potato and cook for about 8-10 minutes.
- ✓ Add the broth and cook for about 8-10 minutes.
- ✓ Add the cooked chicken and scallion and cook for about 5 minutes.
- ✓ Stir in lemon juice, salt and serve. Meal Prep Tip: Transfer the cooled hash in an airtight container and preserve in the refrigerator for up to 2 days. Just before serving, reheat in the microwave.

Nutrition: Calories 253 Total Fat 10 g Saturated Fat 2.3 g Cholesterol 76 mg Total Carbs 14 g Sugar 1.2 g Fiber 2.6 g Sodium 92 mg Potassium 597 mg Protein 26 g

42) Strawberry & Spinach Smoothie

Ingredients:

- 1½ cups fresh strawberries, hulled and sliced
- 2 cups fresh baby spinach
- ½ cup fat-free plain Greek yogurt
- 1 cup unsweetened almond milk
- ¼ cup ice cubes

Direction: Preparation Time: 10 minutes Servings: 2

- ✓ In a high-speed blender, add all the ingredients and pulse until smooth. Pour into serving glasses and serve immediately.

Meal Prep Tip:

- ✓ In 2 zip lock bags, divide the strawberries and spinach. Seal the bags and store in the freezer for about 2-3 days.
- ✓ Just before serving, remove from the freezer and transfer into a blender with yogurt, almond milk and ice cubes and pulse until smooth.

Nutrition: Calories 96 Total Fat 2.3 g Saturated Fat 0.2 g Cholesterol 1 mg Total Carbs 12.3 g Sugar 7.7 g Fiber 3.9 g Sodium 144 mg Potassium 428 mg Protein 8.1 g

43) Quinoa Porridge Recipe 1

Ingredients:

- 2 cups water 1 cup dry quinoa, rinsed
- ½ teaspoon organic vanilla extract
- ½ cup unsweetened almond milk
- 10-12 drops liquid stevia
- ¼ teaspoon lemon peel, grated freshly
- ½ teaspoon ground cinnamon
- ½ teaspoon ground nutmeg
- Pinch of ground cloves
- 1 cup fresh mixed berries

Direction: Preparation Time: 10 minutes Cooking Time: 15 minutes Servings: 4

- ✓ In a pan, mix together the water, quinoa and vanilla essence over low heat and cook for about 15 minutes, stirring occasionally.
- ✓ Stir in the almond milk, stevia, lemon peel and spices and immediately, remove from the heat.
- ✓ Top with the berries and serve warm.

Meal Prep Tip:

- ✓ Transfer the cooled porridge in an airtight container and preserve in the refrigerator for up to 2 days.
- ✓ Just before serving, reheat in the microwave. Serve with the topping of berries.

Nutrition: Calories 186 Total Fat 3.3 g Saturated Fat 0.4 g Cholesterol 0 mg Total Carbs 32.3 g Sugar 2.7 g Fiber 4.6 g Sodium 25 mg Potassium 312 mg Protein 6.4 g

44) Bell Pepper Pancakes

Ingredients:

- ½ cup chickpea flour
- ¼ teaspoon baking powder
- Pinch of sea salt Pinch of red pepper flakes, crushed
- ½ cup plus
- 2 tablespoons filtered water
- ¼ cup green bell peppers, seeded and chopped finely
- ¼ cup scallion, chopped finely
- 2 teaspoons olive oil

Direction: Preparation Time: 15 minutes Cooking Time: 8 minutes Servings: 2

- ✓ : In a bowl, mix together flour, baking powder, salt and red pepper flakes.
- ✓ Add the water and mix until well combined.
- ✓ Fold in bell pepper and scallion. In a large frying pan, heat the oil over low heat.
- ✓ Add half of the mixture and cook for about 1-2 minutes per side.
- ✓ Repeat with the remaining mixture.
- ✓ Serve warm.

Meal Prep Tip:

- ✓ Store these cooled pancakes into an airtight container by placing a piece of wax paper between each pancake.
- ✓ Refrigerate up to 4 days.
- ✓ Reheat in the microwave for about 1½-2 minutes.

Nutrition: Calories 232 Total Fat 7.8 g Saturated Fat 1 g Cholesterol 0 mg Total Carbs 32.7 g Sugar 6.4 g Fiber 9.3 g Sodium 132 mg Potassium 566 mg Protein 10 g

45) Tofu Scramble

Ingredients:

- : ½ tablespoon olive oil
- 1 small onion, chopped finely
- 1 small red bell pepper, seeded and chopped finely
- 1 cup cherry tomatoes, chopped finely
- 1½ cups firm tofu, pressed and crumbled
- Pinch of ground turmeric
- Pinch of cayenne pepper
- 1 tablespoon fresh parsley, chopped

Direction: Preparation Time: 15 minutes Cooking Time: 15 minutes Servings: 2

- ✓ : In a skillet, heat the oil over medium heat and sauté the onion and bell pepper for about 4-5 minute.
- ✓ Add the tomatoes and cook for about 1-2 minutes.
- ✓ Add the tofu, turmeric and cayenne pepper and cook for about 6-8 minutes.
- ✓ Garnish with parsley and serve. Meal Prep Tip:
- ✓ Transfer the cooled scramble into an airtight container and refrigerate for up to 3 days.
- ✓ Reheat in microwave before serving.

Nutrition: Calories 213 Total Fat 11.8 g Saturated Fat 2.2 g Cholesterol 0 mg Total Carbs 14.7 g Sugar 8 g Fiber 4.5 g Sodium 31 mg Potassium 872 mg Protein 17.3 g

46) Apple Omelet

Ingredients:

- 4 teaspoons olive oil, divided
- 2 small green apples, cored and sliced thinly
- ¼ teaspoon ground cinnamon
- Pinch of ground cloves
- Pinch of ground nutmeg
- 4 large eggs
- ¼ teaspoon organic vanilla extract
- Pinch of salt

Direction: Preparation Time: 10 minutes Cooking Time: 10 minutes Servings: 3

- ✓ In a large nonstick frying pan, heat 1 teaspoon of oil over medium-low heat. Place the apple slices and sprinkle with spices.
- ✓ Cook for about 4-5 minutes, flipping once halfway through.
- ✓ Meanwhile, in a bowl, add the eggs, vanilla extract and salt and beat until fluffy.
- ✓ Add the remaining oil in the pan and let it heat completely.
- ✓ Place the egg mixture over apple slices evenly and cook for about 3-5 minutes or until desired doneness.
- ✓ Carefully, turn the pan over a serving plate and immediately, fold the omelet.
- ✓ Serve immediately.

Meal Prep Tip:

- ✓ In a resealable plastic bag, place the cooled omelet slices and seal the bag.
- ✓ Refrigerate for about 2-4 days.
- ✓ Reheat in the microwave on High for about 1 minute before serving.

Nutrition: Calories 228 Total Fat 13.2 g Saturated Fat 3 g Cholesterol 248 mg Total Carbs 21.3 g Sugar 16.1 g Fiber 3.8 g Sodium 145 mg Potassium 251 mg Protein 8.8 g

47) Spiced Overnight Oats

Ingredients:

- 2 cups old-fashioned oats
- 1 cup fat-free milk
- 1 tablespoon vanilla extract
- 1 teaspoon liquid stevia extract
- 1 teaspoon ground cinnamon
- ¼ teaspoon ground nutmeg
- ½ cup toasted walnuts, chopped

Direction: Servings: 6 Cooking Time: None

- ✓ Stir together the oats, milk, vanilla extract, liquid stevia extract, cinnamon, and nutmeg in a large bowl. Cover and chill overnight until thick.
- ✓ Stir in the yogurt just before serving and spoon into cups.
- ✓ Top with chopped walnuts and fresh fruit to serve.

Nutrition: Calories 140, Total Fat 7.1g, Saturated Fat 0.5g, Total Carbs 12.7g, Net Carbs 10.4g, Protein 5.6g, Sugar 2.6g, Fiber 2.3g, Sodium 23mg

48) Almond & Berry Smoothie

Ingredients:

- ⅔ cup frozen raspberries
- ½ cup frozen banana, sliced
- ½ cup almond milk (unsweetened)
- 3 tablespoons almonds, sliced flakes (unsweetened)
- ¼ teaspoon ground cinnamon
- ⅛ teaspoon vanilla extract
- ¼ cup blueberries
- 1 tablespoon coconut

Direction: Cooking Time: 0 Minute Servings: 1

- ✓ Put the Ingredients in a blender except coconut flakes. Pulse until smooth.
- ✓ Top with the coconut flakes before serving.

Nutrition: Calories 360 Total Fat 19 g Saturated Fat 3 g Cholesterol 0 mg Sodium 89 mg Carbohydrate 46 g Dietary Fiber 14 g Total Sugars 21 g Protein 9 g Potassium 736 mg

49) Keto Low Carb Crepe

Ingredients:

- 2 eggs 1 egg white
- 1 tbsp unsalted butter
- 1 1/3 tbsp cream cheese
- 2/3 tbsp psyllium husk

Direction: Servings: 2 Cooking Time: 4 Minutes

- ✓ Put all the ingredients in a bowl, except for butter, and then whisk by using a stick blender until smooth and very liquid.
- ✓ Bring out a skillet pan, put it over medium heat, add ½ tbsp butter and when it melts, pour in half of the batter, spread evenly, and cook until the top has firmed.
- ✓ Carefully flip the crepe, then continue cooking for 2 minutes until cooked and then move it to a plate.
- ✓ Add remaining butter and when it melts, cook another crepe in the same manner and then serve.

Nutrition: 118 Cal 9.4 g Fats 6.5 g Protein 1 g Net Carb 0.9 g Fiber

50) Cinnamon Oat Pancakes

Ingredients:

- 1 cup old-fashioned oats
- 1 cup whole-wheat flour
- 2 teaspoons baking powder
- 1 teaspoon salt
- 1 ½ cups fat-free milk
- ¼ cup canola oil
- 2 large eggs, whisked
- 1 teaspoon lemon juice
- ½ to 1 teaspoon liquid stevia extract

Direction: Servings: 6 Cooking Time: 15 Minutes

- ✓ Combine the oats, flour, baking powder, and salt in a medium mixing bowl. In a separate bowl, stir together the milk, canola oil, eggs, lemon juice, and stevia extract.
- ✓ Stir the wet ingredients into the dry until just combined.
- ✓ Heat a large skillet or griddle to medium-high heat and grease with cooking spray.
- ✓ Spoon the batter in ¼ cups into the skillet and cook until bubbles form on the surface.
- ✓ Flip the pancakes and cook to brown on the other side. Slide onto a plate and repeat with the remaining batter.
- ✓ Store the extra pancakes in an airtight container and reheat in the microwave or oven.

Nutrition: Calories 230, Total Fat 11.4g, Saturated Fat 1.3g, Total Carbs 24.3g, Net Carbs 23g, Protein 7.1g, Sugar 3.3g, Fiber 1.3g, Sodium 446mg

51) Healthy Carrot Muffins

Ingredients:

Dry ingredients
- Tapioca starch ¼ cup
- Baking soda – 1 teaspoon
- Cinnamon – 1 tablespoon
- Cloves – ¼ teaspoon

Wet ingredients
- Vanilla extract – 1 teaspoon
- Water – 1 1/2 cups
- Carrots (shredded) – 1 1/2

- Almond flour – 1¾ cups
- Granulated sweetener of choice – 1/2 cup
- Baking powder – 1 teaspoon
- Nutmeg – 1 teaspoon
- Salt – 1 teaspoon
- Coconut oil – 1/3 cup
- Flax meal – 4 tablespoons
- Banana (mashed) – 1 medium

Direction: Servings: 8 Cooking Time: 40 Minutes

- ✓ Begin by heating the oven to 350F. Get a muffin tray and position paper cups in all the moulds.
- ✓ Arrange aside. Get a small glass bowl and put half a cup of water and flax meal.
- ✓ Allow this rest for about 5 minutes. Your flax egg is prepared.
- ✓ Get a large mixing bowl and put in the almond flour, tapioca starch, granulated sugar, baking soda, baking powder, cinnamon, nutmeg, cloves, and salt.
- ✓ Mix well to combine. Conform a well in the middle of the flour mixture and stream in the coconut oil, vanilla extract, and flax egg.
- ✓ Mix well to conform a mushy dough. Then put in the chopped carrots and mashed banana.
- ✓ Mix until well-combined. Make use of a spoon to scoop out an equal amount of mixture into 8 muffin cups.
- ✓ Position the muffin tray in the oven and allow it to bake for about 40 minutes.
- ✓ Extract the tray from the microwave and allow the muffins to stand for about 10 minutes.
- ✓ Extract the muffin cups from the tray and allow them to chill until they reach room degree of hotness and coldness.
- ✓ Serve and enjoy!

Nutrition: Calories: 189 calories per serving; Fat 13.9 g; Protein 3.8 g; Carbs 17.3 g

52) Keto Creamy Bacon Dish

Ingredients:

- ½ tsp dried basil
- ½ tsp minced garlic
- ½ tsp tomato paste
- 2 oz unsalted butter, softened
- 3 slices of bacon, chopped

Direction: Servings: 2 Cooking Time: 5 Minutes

- ✓ Bring out a skillet pan, put it over medium heat, add 1 tbsp butter and when it starts to melts, add chopped bacon and cook for 5 minutes.
- ✓ Then remove the pan from heat, add remaining butter, along with basil and tomato paste, season with salt and black pepper and stir until well mixed.
- ✓ Move bacon butter into an airtight container, cover with the lid, and refrigerate for 1 hour until solid.

Nutrition: 150 Cal 16 g Fats 1 g Protein 0.5 g Net Carb 1 g Fiber

53) Egg "dough" In A Pan

Ingredients:

- ¼ tsp salt
- ½ of medium red bell pepper, chopped
- 1/8 tsp ground black pepper
- 2 eggs
- 2 tbsp chopped chives

Direction: Servings: 2 Cooking Time: 4 Minutes

- ✓ Turn on the oven, then set it to 350 degrees F and let it preheat. In the meantime, crack eggs in a bowl, add remaining ingredients and whisk until combined.
- ✓ Bring out a small heatproof dish, pour in egg mixture, and bake for 5 to 8 minutes until set. When done, cut it into two squares and then serve.

Nutrition: 87 Cal 5.4 g Fats 7.2 g Protein 1.7 g Net Carb 0.7 g Fiber

54) Eggs Florentine

Ingredients:

- 1 cup washed, fresh spinach leaves
- 2 tbsp freshly grated parmesan cheese
- Sea salt and pepper
- 1 tbsp white vinegar
- 2 eggs

Direction: Servings: 2 Cooking Time: 10 Minutes

- ✓ Cook the spinach the microwave or steam until wilted.
- ✓ Sprinkle with parmesan cheese and seasoning.
- ✓ Slice into bite-size pieces
- ✓ Simmer a pan of water and add the vinegar. Stir quickly with a spoon.
- ✓ Break an egg into the center.
- ✓ Turn off the heat and cover until set.
- ✓ Repeat with the second egg. Place the eggs on top of the spinach and serve.

Nutrition: 180 cal.10g fat 7g protein 5g carbs.

55) Cucumber & Yogurt

Ingredients:

- 1 cup low-fat yogurt
- ½ cup cucumber, diced
- ¼ teaspoon lemon zest
- ¼ teaspoon lemon juice
- ¼ teaspoon fresh mint, chopped Salt to taste

Direction: Servings: 1 Cooking Time: 0 Minute

- ✓ Mix all the Ingredients in a jar.
- ✓ Refrigerate and serve.

Nutrition: Calories 164 Total Fat 4 g Saturated Fat 2 g Cholesterol 15 mg Sodium 318 mg Total Carbohydrate 19 g Dietary Fiber 1 g Total Sugars 18 g Protein 13 g Potassium 683 mg

56) Eggs Baked In Peppers

Ingredients:

- 4 medium bell peppers, assorted
- 1 cup shredded low-fat cheddar cheese
- 8 large eggs Salt and pepper
- Fresh chopped parsley, to serve

Direction: Servings: 4 Cooking Time: 25 Minutes

- ✓ Preheat the oven to 400°F and slice the peppers in half.
- ✓ Remove the seeds and pith from each pepper and place them cut-side up in a baking dish large enough to fit them all.
- ✓ Divide the shredded cheese among the pepper halves and crack an egg into each.
- ✓ Season with salt and pepper then bake for 20 to 25 minutes until done to your liking.
- ✓ Garnish with fresh chopped parsley to serve.

Nutrition: Calories 260, Total Fat 16.3g, Saturated Fat 6.6g, Total Carbs 10.9g, Net Carbs 9.3g, Protein 20.8g, Sugar 6.8g, Fiber 1.6g, Sodium 374mg

57) Easy Egg Scramble

Ingredients:

- 2 large eggs
- 1 tablespoon fat-free milk Salt and pepper
- ¼ cup diced green pepper
- 2 tablespoons diced onion
- ¼ cup diced tomatoes

Direction: Servings: 1 Cooking Time: 10 Minutes

- ✓ Whisk together the eggs, milk, salt, and pepper in a small bowl. Heat a medium skillet over medium-high heat and grease with cooking spray.
- ✓ Add the green pepper and onion then cook for 2 to 3 minutes.
- ✓ Spoon the veggies into a bowl then reheat the skillet. Pour in the egg mixture and cook until the eggs start to thicken.
- ✓ Spoon in the cooked veggies and diced tomatoes. Stir the mixture and cook until the egg is set and scrambled. Serve hot.

Nutrition: Calories 170, Total Fat 10.1g, Saturated Fat 3.1g, Total Carbs 6.3g, Net Carbs 4.9g, Protein 13.9g, Sugar 4.1g, Fiber 1.4g, Sodium 152mg

58) Strawberry Puff Pancake

Ingredients:

- 3 eggs, large
- 1/8 teaspoon cinnamon, ground
- 1 cup strawberry, sliced
- 3/4 cup milk, fat-free What you will need from the store cupboard:
- 1 teaspoon vanilla extract
- ¾ cup of all-purpose flour
- 2 tablespoons of butter
- 1 tablespoon cornstarch
- ½ cup of water
- 1/8 teaspoon salt

Direction: Servings: 4 Cooking Time: 20 Minutes

- ✓ Keep the butter in a pie plate and keep in an oven for 4 to 5 minutes. In the meantime, whisk the vanilla, milk, and eggs in a bowl.
- ✓ Take another bowl and bring together the cinnamon, salt, and flour in it. Whisk this into the egg mix until it blends well. Pour this into the plate.
- ✓ Bake for 15 minutes. The sides should be golden brown and crisp. Add the cornstarch in your saucepan.
- ✓ Stir the water in until it turns smooth. Now add the strawberries.
- ✓ Cook while stirring till it thickens. Mash the strawberries coarsely and serve with the pancake.

Nutrition: Calories 277, Carbohydrates 38g, Fiber 2g, Cholesterol 175mg, Total Fat 10g, Protein 9g, Sodium 187mg

59) Egg Porridge

Ingredients:

- 2 organic free-range eggs
- 1/3 cup organic heavy cream without food additives
- 2 packages of your preferred sweetener
- 2 tbsp grass-fed butter ground organic cinnamon to taste

Direction: Servings: 1 Cooking Time: 10 Minutes

- ✓ In a bowl add the eggs, cream and sweetener, and mix together. Melt the butter in a saucepan over a medium heat.
- ✓ Lower the heat once the butter is melted. Combine together with the egg and cream mixture.
- ✓ While Cooking, mix until it thickens and curdles.
- ✓ When you see the first signs of curdling, remove the saucepan immediately from the heat.
- ✓ Pour the porridge into a bowl. Sprinkle cinnamon on top and serve immediately.

Nutrition: 604 cal 45g fat 8g protein 2.8g carbs.

60) Breakfast Parfait

Ingredients:

- 4 oz. unsweetened applesauce
- 6 oz. non-fat and sugar-free vanilla yogurt
- ¼ teaspoon pumpkin pie spice
- ¼ teaspoon honey
- 1 cup low-fat granola

Direction: Servings: 2 Cooking Time: 0 Minute

- ✓ Mix the Ingredients except the granola in a bowl..
- ✓ Layer the mixture with the granola in a cup. Refrigerate before serving

Nutrition: Calories 287 Total Fat 3 g Saturated Fat 1 g Cholesterol 28 mg Sodium 186 mg Total Carbohydrate 57 g Dietary Fiber 4 g Total Sugars2 g Protein 8 g

61) Oatmeal Blueberry Pancakes

Ingredients:

- ½ cup rolled oats
- ½ cup unsweetened almond milk
- ¼ cup unsweetened applesauce
- ¼ cup unsweetened vegan protein powder
- ½ tablespoon flax meal
- 1 teaspoon baking powder
- ½ teaspoon vanilla extract
- ¼ teaspoon baking soda
- ¼ teaspoon ground cinnamon
- 1/8 teaspoon salt
- ½ cup fresh blueberries

Direction: Servings: 4 Cooking Time: 40 Minutes

- ✓ Place all ingredients (except for blueberries) in a food processor and pulse until smooth.
- ✓ Transfer the mixture into a bowl and set aside for 5 minutes. Gently, fold in blueberries.
- ✓ Place a lightly greased medium skillet over medium heat until heated.
- ✓ Place desired amount of the mixture and cook for about 3–5 minutes per side.
- ✓ Repeat with the remaining mixture. Serve warm.

Nutrition: Calories 105 Total Fat 1.8 g Saturated Fat 0.2 g Cholesterol 0 mg Sodium 204 mg Total Carbs 15.4 g Fiber 2.2 g Sugar 5.2 g Protein 8 g

62) Bulgur Porridge

Ingredients:
- 2/3 cup unsweetened soy milk
- 1/3 cup bulgur, rinsed
- Pinch of salt
- 1 ripe banana, peeled and mashed
- 2 kiwis, peeled and sliced

Direction: Servings: 2 Cooking Time: 15 Minutes

- ✓ In a pan, add the soy milk, bulgur, and salt over medium-high heat and bring to a boil.
- ✓ Adjust the heat to low and simmer for about 10 minutes.
- ✓ Remove the pan of bulgur from heat and immediately, stir in the mashed banana.
- ✓ Serve warm with the topping of kiwi slices.

Nutrition: Calories 223 Total Fat 2.3 g Saturated Fat 0.3 g Cholesterol 0 mg Sodium 126 mg Total Carbs 47.5 g Fiber 8.6 g Sugar 17.4 g Protein 7.1 g

63) Turkey-broccoli Brunch Casserole

Ingredients:
- 2-1/2 cups turkey breast, cubed and cooked
- 16 oz. broccoli, chopped and drained
- 1-1/2 cups of milk, fat-free 1 cup cheddar cheese, low-fat, shredded
- 10 oz. cream of chicken soup, low sodium and low fat What you will need from the store cupboard:
- 8 oz. egg substitute
- ¼ teaspoon of poultry seasoning
- ¼ cup of sour cream, low fat
- ½ teaspoon pepper
- 1/8 teaspoon salt 2 cups of seasoned stuffing cubes
- Cooking spray

Direction: Servings: 6 Cooking Time: 20 Minutes

- ✓ Bring together the egg substitute, soup, milk, pepper, sour cream, salt, and poultry seasoning in a big bowl.
- ✓ Now stir in the broccoli, turkey, ¾ cup of cheese and stuffing cubes.
- ✓ Transfer to a baking dish. Apply cooking spray.
- ✓ Bake for 10 minutes. Sprinkle the remaining cheese.
- ✓ Bake for another 5 minutes.
- ✓ Keep it aside for 5 minutes. Serve.

Nutrition: Calories 303, Carbohydrates 26g, Fiber 3g, Sugar 0.8g, Cholesterol 72mg, Total Fat 7g, Protein 33g Cheesy

64) Low-carb Omelet

Ingredients:
- 2 whole eggs
- 1 tablespoon water
- 1 tablespoon butter
- 3 thin slices salami
- 5 fresh basil leaves
- 5 thin slices, fresh ripe tomatoes
- 2 ounces fresh mozzarella cheese
- Salt and pepper as needed

Direction: Servings: 5 Cooking Time: 5 Minutes

- ✓ Take a small bowl and whisk in eggs and water
- ✓ Take a non-stick Sauté pan and place it over medium heat, add butter and let it melt
- ✓ Pour egg mixture and cook for 30 seconds Spread salami slices on half of egg mix and top with cheese, tomatoes, basil slices
- ✓ Season with salt and pepper according to your taste
- ✓ Cook for 2 minutes and fold the egg with the empty half
- ✓ Cover and cook on LOW for 1 minute Serve and enjoy!

Nutrition: Calories: 451; Fat: 36g; Carbohydrates: 3g; Protein:33g

65) Apple & Cinnamon Pancake

Ingredients:
- : ¼ teaspoon ground cinnamon
- 1 ¾ cups Better Baking Mix
- 1 tablespoon oil
- 1 cup water
- 2 egg whites
- ½ cup sugar-free applesauce
- Cooking spray
- 1 cup plain yogurt
- Sugar substitute

Direction: Servings: 4 Cooking Time: 10 Minutes

- ✓ Blend the cinnamon and the baking mix in a bowl.
- ✓ Create a hole in the middle and add the oil, water, egg and applesauce.
- ✓ Mix well. Spray your pan with oil.
- ✓ Place it on medium heat. Pour ¼ cup of the batter.
- ✓ Flip the pancake and cook until golden.
- ✓ Serve with yogurt and sugar substitute.

Nutrition: Calories 231 Total Fat 6 g Saturated Fat 1 g Cholesterol 54 mg Sodium 545 mg Total Carbohydrate 37 g Dietary Fiber 4 g Total Sugars 1 g Protein 8 g Potassium 750 mg

66) Guacamole Turkey Burgers

Ingredients:
- 12 oz. turkey, ground
- 1-1/2 avocados
- 2 teaspoons of juice from a lime
- ½ teaspoon cumin
- 1 red chili, chopped
- What you will need from the store cupboard:
- ½ teaspoon garlic powder
- ½ teaspoon onion powder
- 3 teaspoons of olive oil
- ½ teaspoon salt

Direction: Servings: 3 Cooking Time: 15 Minutes

- ✓ Mix the turkey with the cumin, chili, salt, garlic powder, and onion powder in a medium-sized bowl.
- ✓ Create 3 patties Pour 3 teaspoons olive oil in a skillet and heat over medium heat.
- ✓ Now cook your patties. Make sure that both sides are brown. Make the guacamole in the meantime.
- ✓ Mash together the garlic powder, juice from lime and avocados in a bowl.
- ✓ Add salt for seasoning. Serve the burgers with guacamole on the patties.

Nutrition: Calories 316, Carbohydrates 9g, Fiber 8g, Sugar 0g, Cholesterol 80mg, Total Fat 21g, Protein 24g

67) Ham And Goat Cheese Omelet

Ingredients:
- 1 slice of ham, chopped
- 4 egg whites
- 2 teaspoons of water
- 2 tablespoons onion, chopped
- 1 tablespoon parsley, minced
- What you will need from the store cupboard:
- 2 tablespoons green pepper, chopped
- 1/8 teaspoon pepper
- 2 tablespoons goat cheese, crumbled Cooking spray

Direction: Servings: 1 Cooking Time: 10 Minutes

- ✓ Whisk together the water, pepper and egg whites in a bowl till everything blends well. Stir in the green pepper, ham, and onion.
- ✓ Now heat your skillet over medium heat after applying the cooking spray. Pour in the egg white mix towards the edge.
- ✓ As it sets, push the cooked parts to the center. Allow the uncooked portions to flow underneath.
- ✓ Sprinkle the goat cheese to one side when there is no liquid egg. Now fold your omelet into half.
- ✓ Sprinkle the parsley.

Nutrition: Calories 143, Carbohydrates 5g, Fiber 1g, Sugar 0.3g, Cholesterol 27mg, Total Fat 4g, Protein 21g

68) Banana Matcha Breakfast Smoothie

Ingredients:

- 1 cup fat-free milk
- 1 medium banana, sliced
- ¼ cup frozen chopped pineapple
- ½ cup ice cubes
- 1 tablespoon Matcha powder
- ¼ teaspoon ground cinnamon
- Liquid stevia extract, to taste

Direction: Servings: 1 Cooking Time: None

- ✓ Combine the ingredients in a blender.
- ✓ Pulse the mixture several times to chop the ingredients.
- ✓ Blend for 30 to 60 seconds until smooth and well combined. Sweeten to taste with liquid stevia extract, if desired.
- ✓ Pour into a glass and serve immediately.

Nutrition: Calories 230, Total Fat 0.4g, Saturated Fat 0.1g, Total Carbs 44.9g, Net Carbs 38g, Protein 12.6g, Sugar 30.9g, Fiber 6.9g, Sodium 135mg

69) Basil And Tomato Baked Eggs

Ingredients:

- 1 garlic clove, minced
- 1 cup canned tomatoes
- ¼ cup fresh basil leaves, roughly chopped
- 1/2 teaspoon chili powder
- 1 tablespoon olive oil
- 4 whole eggs
- Salt and pepper to taste

Direction: Servings: 4 Cooking Time: 15 Minutes

- ✓ Preheat your oven to 375 degrees F Take a small baking dish and grease with olive oil
- ✓ Add garlic, basil, tomatoes chili, olive oil into a dish and stir
- ✓ Crackdown eggs into a dish, keeping space between the two
- ✓ Sprinkle the whole dish with salt and pepper
- ✓ Place in oven and cook for 12 minutes until eggs are set and tomatoes are bubbling Serve with basil on top Enjoy!

Nutrition: Calories: 235; Fat: 16g; Carbohydrates: 7g; Protein: 14g

70) Cream Cheese Pancakes

Ingredients:

- 2 oz cream cheese 2 eggs
- ½ tsp cinnamon
- 1 tbsp keto coconut flour
- ½ to 1 packet of Stevia

Direction: Servings: 1 Cooking Time: 5 Minutes

- ✓ Skillet with butter the pan or coconut oil on medium-high. Make them as you would normal pancakes.
- ✓ Cook and flip one side to cook the other side! Top with some butter and/or sugar-free syrup.

Nutrition: 340 cal.30g fat 7g protein 3g carbs

71) Mashed Cauliflower

Ingredients:

- 1 cauliflower head
- 1/8 cup plain yogurt, skim milk or butter 1 red chili, diced
- 1 tomato, sliced ½ chopped onion
- What you will need from the store cupboard: 1 garlic clove, optional Salt and pepper Paprika to taste

Direction: Servings: 6 Cooking Time: 10 Minutes

- ✓ Steam the cauliflower till it becomes tender. You can steam with a garlic clove as well. Now cut your cauliflower into small pieces.
- ✓ Keep in your blender with yogurt, butter or milk.
- ✓ Season with pepper and salt. Whip until it gets smooth. Pour the cauliflower into a small baking dish.
- ✓ Sprinkle the paprika. Bake in the oven till it becomes bubbly.

Nutrition: Calories 57, Carbohydrates 12g, Total Fat 0g, Protein 4g, Fiber 5g, Sodium 91mg, Sugars 5g

72) Quinoa Porridge Recipe 2

Ingredients:

- 1 cup dry quinoa, rinsed
- 1½ cups unsweetened almond milk
- 1 teaspoon vanilla extract
- 1 teaspoon ground cinnamon
- 2 tablespoons maple syrup
- 4 tablespoons peanut butter
- ¼ cup fresh strawberries, hulled and chopped
- ¼ cup fresh blueberries

Direction: Servings: 2 Cooking Time: 20 Minutes

- ✓ In a small pan, place quinoa, almond milk, vanilla extract, and cinnamon over medium heat and bring to a boil.
- ✓ Now, adjust the heat to low and simmer, covered for about 15 minutes or until all the liquid is absorbed.
- ✓ Remove the pan of quinoa from heat and stir in maple syrup and peanut butter.
- ✓ Serve warm with the topping of berries.

Nutrition: Calories 608 Total Fat 24 g Saturated Fat 4.2 g Cholesterol 0 mg Sodium 289 mg Total Carbs 81 g Fiber 10 g Sugar 17.9 g Protein 21.1 g

73) Vanilla Mixed Berry Smoothie

Ingredients:

- 1 cup fat-free milk
- ½ cup nonfat Greek yogurt, plain
- ½ cup frozen blueberries
- ¼ cup frozen strawberries
- 3 to 4 ice cubes
- 1 teaspoon fresh lemon juice
- Liquid stevia extract, to taste

Direction: Servings: 1 Cooking Time: None

- ✓ Combine the ingredients in a blender.
- ✓ Pulse the mixture several times to chop the ingredients.
- ✓ Blend for 30 to 60 seconds until smooth and well combined.
- ✓ Sweeten to taste with liquid stevia extract, if desired.
- ✓ Pour into a glass and serve immediately.

Nutrition: : Calories 220, Total Fat 0.3g, Saturated Fat 0g, Total Carbs 31.6g, Net Carbs 28.3g, Protein 21.6g, Sugar 27.3g, Fiber 3.3g, Sodium 204mg

74) Granola With Fruits

Ingredients:

- 3 cups quick cooking oats
- 1 cup almonds, sliced
- ½ cup wheat germ
- 3 tablespoons butter
- 1 teaspoon ground cinnamon
- 1 cup honey
- 3 cups whole grain cereal flakes
- ½ cup raisins
- ½ cup dried cranberries
- ½ cup dates, pitted and chopped

Direction: Servings: 6 Cooking Time: 35 Minutes

- Preheat your oven to 325 degrees F.
- Place the almonds on a baking sheet.
- Bake for 15 minutes.
- Mix the wheat germ, butter, cinnamon and honey in a bowl.
- Add the toasted almonds and oats. Mix well.
- Spread on the baking sheet.
- Bake for 20 minutes.
- Mix with the rest of the ingredients. Let cool and serve.

Nutrition: Calories 210 Total Fat 7 g Saturated Fat 2 g Cholesterol 5 mg Sodium 58 mg Total Carbohydrate 36 g Dietary Fiber 4 g Total Sugars 2 g Protein 5 g Potassium 250 mg

75) Egg Muffins

Ingredients:

- 1 tbsp green pesto
- 3 oz/75g shredded cheese
- 5 oz/150g cooked bacon
- 1 scallion, chopped
- 6 eggs

Direction: Servings: 6 Cooking Time: 20 Minutes

- You should set your oven to 350°F/175°C.
- Place liners in a regular cupcake tin.
- This will help with easy removal and storage.
- Beat the eggs with pepper, salt, and the pesto.
- Mix in the cheese.
- Pour the eggs into the cupcake tin and top with the bacon and scallion.
- Cook for 15-20 minutes

Nutrition: 190 cal.15g fat 7g protein 4g carbs.

76) Eggs On The Go

Ingredients:

- 4 oz/110g bacon, cooked
- Pepper Salt
- 12 eggs

Direction: Servings: 4 Cooking Time: 5 Minutes

- You should set your oven to 200°C.
- Place liners in a regular cupcake tin.
- This will help with easy removal and storage.
- Crack an egg into each of the cups and sprinkle some bacon onto each of them.
- Season with some pepper and salt.
- Bake for 15 minutes, or until the eggs are set.

Nutrition: 75 cal. 6g fat 8g protein 1g carbs.

77) Breakfast Mix

Ingredients:

- 5 tbsp coconut flakes, unsweetened
- 7 tbsp hemp seeds
- 5 tbsp flaxseed, ground
- 2 tbsp sesame, ground
- 2 tbsp cocoa, dark, unsweetened

Direction: Servings: 1 Cooking Time: 5 Minutes

- Grind the sesame and flaxseed. only grind the sesame seeds for a small period.
- Mix all ingredients in a jar and shake it well. Keep refrigerated until ready to eat.
- Serve softened with black coffee or even with still water and add coconut oil if you want to increase the fat content.
- It also blends well with cream or with mascarpone cheese.

Nutrition: 150 cal.9g fat 8g protein 4g carbs.

78) Vegetable Omelet

Ingredients:

- ½ cup yellow summer squash, chopped
- ½ cup canned diced tomatoes with herbs, drained
- ½ ripe avocado, pitted and chopped
- ½ cup cucumber, chopped
- 2 eggs
- 2 tablespoons water
- Salt and pepper to taste
- 1 teaspoon dried basil, crushed
- Cooking spray ¼ cup low-fat
- Monterey Jack cheese, shredded
- Chives, chopped

Direction: Servings: 4 Cooking Time: 25 Minutes

- In a bowl, mix the squash, tomatoes, avocado and cucumber.
- In another bowl, mix the eggs, water, salt, pepper and basil.
- Spray oil on a pan over medium heat.
- Pour egg mixture on the pan. Put the vegetable mixture on top of the egg.
- Lift and fold.
- Cook until the egg has set.
- Sprinkle cheese and chives on top.

Nutrition: Calories 128 Total Fat 6 g Saturated Fat 2 g Cholesterol 97 mg Sodium 357 mg Total Carbohydrate 7 g Dietary Fiber 3 g Total Sugars 4 g Protein 12 g Potassium 341 mg

79) Vegetable Frittata

Ingredients:

- 1 cup mushrooms, sliced
- 4 eggs, beaten lightly
- 2 tablespoons onion, chopped
- ½ cup broccoli, chopped
- ¼ cup cheddar cheese, shredded, low-fat

What you will need from the store cupboard:

- 2 tablespoons green pepper, chopped
- Dash of pepper
- 1/8 teaspoon of salt
- Cooking spray

Direction: Servings: 2 Cooking Time: 20 Minutes

- Bring together all the ingredients in your bowl.
- Coat your baking dish with cooking spray and pour everything into it.
- Bake for 20 minutes and serve immediately.

Nutrition: Calories 230, Carbohydrates 6g, Fiber 1g, Sugar 0.2g, Cholesterol 386mg, Total Fat 14g, Protein 20g

80) Egg-veggie Scramble

Ingredients:

- ¼ tsp salt
- 1 tbsp unsalted butter
- 1/8 tsp ground black pepper
- 3 eggs, beaten
- 4 oz spinach

Direction: Servings: 2 Cooking Time: 3 Minutes

- ✓ Bring out a frying pan, put it over medium heat, add butter and when it melts, add spinach and cook for 5 minutes until leaves have wilted.
- ✓ Then pour in eggs, season with salt and black pepper, and cook for 3 minutes until eggs have scramble to the desired level.

Nutrition: 90 Cal 7 g Fats 5.6 g Protein; 0.7 g Net Carb 0.6 g Fiber

81) Veggie Fritters

Ingredients:

- ½ tsp nutritional yeast
- 1 oz chopped broccoli
- 1 zucchini, grated, squeezed
- 2 eggs
- 2 tbsp almond flour

Direction: Servings: 2 Cooking Time: 3 Minutes

- ✓ Wrap grated zucchini in a cheesecloth, twist it well to remove excess moisture, and then
- ✓ Put zucchini in a bowl.
- ✓ Add remaining ingredients, except for oil, and then whisk well until combined.
- ✓ Bring out a skillet pan, put it over medium heat, add oil and when hot, drop zucchini mixture in four portions, shape them into flat patties and cook for 4 minutes per side until thoroughly cooked.

Nutrition: 191 Cal 16.6 g Fats 9.6 g Protein 0.8 g Net Carb 0.2 g Fiber

82) Millet Porridge

Ingredients:

- 1 cup millet, rinsed and drained
- Pinch of salt
- 3 cups water 2 tablespoons almonds, chopped finely
- 6-8 drops liquid stevia
- 1 cup unsweetened almond milk
- 2 tablespoons fresh blueberries

Direction: Servings: 4 Cooking Time: 25 Minutes

- ✓ In a nonstick pan, add the millet over medium-low heat and cook for about 3 minutes, stirring continuously.
- ✓ Add the salt and water and stir to combine
- ✓ Increase the heat to medium and bring to a boil. Cook for about 15 minutes.
- ✓ Stir in the almonds, stevia and almond milk and cook for 5 minutes.
- ✓ Top with the blueberries and serve.

Nutrition: Calories 219 Total Fat 4.5 g Saturated Fat 0.6 g Cholesterol 0 mg Total Carbs 38.2 g Sugar 0.6 g Fiber 5 g Sodium 92 mg Potassium 1721 mg Protein 6.4 g

83) Tofu & Zucchini Muffins

Ingredients:

- 12 ounces extra-firm silken tofu, drained and pressed
- ¾ cup unsweetened soy milk
- 2 tablespoons canola oil
- 1 tablespoon apple cider vinegar
- 1 cup whole-wheat pastry flour
- ½ cup chickpea flour
- 1 teaspoon baking powder
- ½ teaspoon baking soda
- 1 teaspoon smoked paprika
- 1 teaspoon onion powder
- 1 teaspoon salt
- ½ cup zucchini, chopped
- ¼ cup fresh chives, minced

Direction: Servings: 6 Cooking Time: 40 Minutes

- ✓ Preheat your oven to 400°F. Line a 12-cup muffin tin with paper liners.
- ✓ In a bowl, place tofu and with a fork, mash until smooth. In the bowl of tofu, add almond milk, oil, and vinegar, and mix until slightly smooth.
- ✓ In a separate large bowl, add flours, baking powder, baking soda, spices, and salt, and mix well.
- ✓ Transfer the mixture into muffin cups evenly.
- ✓ Bake for approximately 35–40 minutes or until a toothpick inserted in the center comes out clean.
- ✓ Remove the muffin tin from oven and place onto a wire rack to cool for about 10 minutes.
- ✓ Carefully invert the muffins onto a platter and serve warm.

Nutrition: Calories 237 Total Fat 9 g Saturated Fat 1 g Cholesterol 0 mg Sodium 520 mg Total Carbs 2293.3 g Fiber 5.9 g Sugar 3.7 g Protein 11.1 g

84) Savory Keto Pancake

Ingredients:

- ¼ cup almond flour
- 1 ½ tbsp unsalted butter
- 2 eggs
- 2 oz cream cheese, softened

Direction: Servings: 2 Cooking Time: 2 Minutes

- ✓ Bring out a bowl, crack eggs in it, whisk well until fluffy, and then whisk in flour and cream cheese until well combined.
- ✓ Bring out a skillet pan, put it over medium heat, add butter and when it melts, drop pancake batter in four sections, spread it evenly, and cook for 2 minutes per side until brown.

Nutrition: 166.8 Cal 15 g Fats 5.8 g Protein 1.8 g Net Car 0.8 g Fiber

85) Buckwheat Porridge

Ingredients:

- 1½ cups water
- 1 cup buckwheat groats, rinsed
- ¾ teaspoon vanilla extract
- ½ teaspoon ground cinnamon
- ¼ teaspoon salt
- 2 tablespoons maple syrup
- 1 ripe banana, peeled and mashed
- 1½ cups unsweetened soy milk
- 1 tablespoon peanut butter
- 1/3 cup fresh strawberries, hulled and chopped

Direction: Servings: 2 Cooking Time: 15 Minutes

- ✓ Place the water, buckwheat, vanilla extract, cinnamon, and salt in a pan and bring to a boil.
- ✓ Now, adjust the heat to medium-low and simmer for about 6 minutes, stirring occasionally.
- ✓ Stir in maple syrup, banana, and soy milk, and simmer, covered for about 6 minutes.
- ✓ Remove the pan of porridge from heat and stir in peanut butter. Serve warm with the topping of strawberry pieces.

Nutrition: Calories 453 Total Fat 9.4 g Saturated Fat 1.7 g Cholesterol 0 mg Sodium 374 mg Total Carbs 82.8 g Fiber 9.4 g Sugar 28.8 g Protein 16.2 g

86) Breakfast Sandwich

Ingredients:

- 2 oz/60g cheddar cheese
- 2 tbsp butter 4 eggs
- 1/6 oz/30g smoked ham

Direction: Servings: 2 Cooking Time: 0 Minutes

- ✓ Fry all the eggs and sprinkle the pepper and salt on them.
- ✓ Place an egg down as the sandwich base.
- ✓ Top with the ham and cheese and a drop or two of Tabasco.
- ✓ Place the other egg on top and enjoy.

Nutrition: 600 cal.50g fat 12g protein 7g carbs.

87) Eggplant Omelet

Ingredients:

- 1 large eggplant
- 1 tbsp coconut oil, melted
- 1 tsp unsalted butter
- 2 eggs
- 2 tbsp chopped green onions

Direction: Servings: 2 Cooking Time: 5 Minutes

- ✓ Set the grill and let it preheat at the high setting.
- ✓ In the meantime, prepare the eggplant, and for this, cut two slices from eggplant, about 1-inch thick, and reserve the remaining eggplant for later use.
- ✓ Brush slices of eggplant with oil, season with salt on both sides, then put the slices on grill and cook for 3 to 4 minutes per side.
- ✓ Move grilled eggplant to a cutting board, let it cool for 5 minutes and then make a home in the center of each slice by using a cookie cutter.
- ✓ Bring out a frying pan, put it over medium heat, add butter and when it melts, add eggplant slices in it and crack an egg into its each hole.
- ✓ Let the eggs cook, then carefully flip the eggplant slice and continue cooking for 3 minutes until the egg has thoroughly cooked Season egg with salt and black pepper, move them to a plate, then garnish with green onions and serve.

Nutrition: 184 Cal 14.1 g Fats 7.8 g Protein 3 g Net Carb 3.5 g Fiber

88) Breakfast Muffins

Ingredients:

- 1 medium egg
- ¼ cup heavy cream
- 1 slice cooked bacon (cured, pan-fried, cooked)
- 1 oz cheddar cheese
- Salt and black pepper (to taste)

Direction: Servings: 1 Cooking Time: 5 Minutes

- ✓ Preheat the oven to 350°F.
- ✓ In a bowl, mix the eggs with the cream, salt and pepper.
- ✓ Spread into muffin tins and fill the cups half full.
- ✓ Place 1 slice of bacon into each muffin hole and half ounce of cheese on top of each muffin.
- ✓ Bake for around 15-20 minutes or until lightly browned. Add another ½ oz of cheese onto each muffin and broil until the cheese is slightly browned.
- ✓ Serve!

Nutrition: 150 cal 11g fat 7g protein 2g carbs

LUNCH

89) Sweet Potato, Kale, and White Bean Stew

Ingredients:

- 1 (15-ounce) can low-sodium cannellini beans, rinsed and drained, divided
- 1 tablespoon olive oil
- 1 medium onion, chopped
- 2 garlic cloves, minced
- 2 celery stalks, chopped
- 3 medium carrots, chopped
- 2 cups low-sodium vegetable broth
- 1 teaspoon apple cider vinegar
- 2 medium sweet potatoes (about 1¼ pounds)
- 2 cups chopped kale
- 1 cup shelled edamame
- ¼ cup quinoa
- 1 teaspoon dried thyme
- 1/2 teaspoon cayenne pepper
- 1/2 teaspoon salt
- ¼ teaspoon freshly ground black pepper

Direction: Preparation time: 15 minutes Cooking time: 25 minutes Servings: 4

- ✓ Put half the beans into a blender and blend until smooth. Set aside.
- ✓ In a large soup pot over medium heat, heat the oil. When the oil is shining, include the onion and garlic, and cook until the onion softens and the garlic is sweet, about 3 minutes. Add the celery and carrots, and continue cooking until the vegetables soften, about 5 minutes.
- ✓ Add the broth, vinegar, sweet potatoes, unblended beans, kale, edamame, and quinoa, and bring the mixture to a boil. Reduce the heat and simmer until the vegetables soften, about 10 minutes.
- ✓ Add the blended beans, thyme, cayenne, salt, and black pepper, increase the heat to medium-high, and bring the mixture to a boil. Reduce the heat and simmer, uncovered, until the flavors combine, about 5 minutes.
- ✓ Into each of 4 containers, scoop 1¾ cups of stew.

Nutrition: calories: 373; total fat: 7g; saturated fat: 1g; protein: 15g; total carbs: 65g; fiber: 15g; sugar: 13g; sodium: 540mg

90) Slow Cooker Two-Bean Sloppy Joes

Ingredients:

- 1 (15-ounce) can low-sodium black beans
- 1 (15-ounce) can low-sodium pinto beans
- 1 (15-ounce) can no-salt-added diced tomatoes
- 1 medium green bell pepper, cored, seeded, and chopped
- 1 medium yellow onion, chopped
- ¼ cup low-sodium vegetable broth
- 2 garlic cloves, minced
- 2 servings (¼ cup) meal prep barbecue sauce or bottled barbecue sauce
- ¼ teaspoon salt
- ¼ teaspoon freshly ground black pepper
- 4 whole-wheat buns

Direction: Preparation time: 10 minutes
Cooking time: 6 hours Servings: 4

- ✓ In a slow cooker, combine the black beans, pinto beans, diced tomatoes, bell pepper, onion, broth, garlic, meal prep barbecue sauce, salt, and black pepper. Stir the ingredients, then cover and cook on low for 6 hours.
- ✓ Into each of 4 containers, spoon 1¼ cups of sloppy sloppy joe mix. Serve with 1 whole-wheat bun.
- ✓ Storage: place airtight containers in the refrigerator for up to 1 week. To freeze, place freezer-safe containers in the freezer for up to 2 months. To defrost, refrigerate overnight.
- Alternatively, reheat the entire dish in a saucepan on the stove top. Bring the sloppy joes to a boil, then reduce the heat and simmer until heated through, 10 to 15 minutes. Serve with a whole-wheat bun.
- ✓ . To reheat individual portions, microwave uncovered on high for 2 to 2 1/2 minutes

Nutrition: calories: 392; total fat: 3g; saturated fat: 0g; protein: 17g; total carbs: 79g; fiber: 19g; sugar: 15g; sodium: 759mg

91) Lighter Eggplant Parmesan

Ingredients:

- Nonstick cooking spray
- 3 eggs, beaten, 1 tablespoon dried parsley
- 2 teaspoons ground oregano
- 1/8 teaspoon freshly ground black pepper
- 1 cup panko bread crumbs, preferably whole-wheat
- 1 large eggplant (about 2 pounds)
- 5 servings (2 1/2 cups) chunky tomato sauce or jarred low-sodium tomato sauce
- 1 cup part-skim mozzarella cheese
- ¼ cup grated parmesan cheese

Direction: Preparation time: 15 minutes
Cooking time: 35 minutes Servings: 4

- ✓ Preheat the oven to 450f. Coat a baking sheet with cooking spray.
- ✓ In a medium bowl, whisk together the eggs, parsley, oregano, and pepper.
- ✓ Pour the panko into a separate medium bowl.
- ✓ Slice the eggplant into ¼-inch-thick slices. Dip each slice of eggplant into the egg mixture, shaking off the excess. Then dredge both sides of the eggplant in the panko bread crumbs. Place the coated eggplant on the prepared baking sheet, leaving a 1/2-inch space between each slice.
- ✓ Bake for about 15 minutes until soft and golden brown. Remove from the oven and set aside to slightly cool.
- ✓ Pour 1/2 cup of chunky tomato sauce on the bottom of an 8-by-15-inch baking dish. Using a spatula or the back of a spoon spread the tomato sauce evenly. Place half the slices of cooked eggplant, slightly overlapping, in the dish, and top with 1 cup of chunky tomato sauce, 1/2 cup of mozzarella and 2 tablespoons of grated parmesan. Repeat the layer, ending with the cheese.
- ✓ Bake uncovered for 20 minutes until the cheese is bubbling and slightly browned.
- ✓ Remove from the oven and allow cooling for 15 minutes before dividing the eggplant equally into 4 separate containers.

Nutrition: calories: 333; total fat: 14g; saturated fat: 6g; protein: 20g; total carbs: 35g; fiber: 11g; sugar: 15g

92) Coconut-Lentil Curry

Ingredients:

- 1 tablespoon olive oil
- 1 medium yellow onion, chopped, 1 garlic clove, minced
- 1 medium red bell pepper, diced
- 1 (15-ounce) can green or brown lentils, rinsed and drained
- 2 medium sweet potatoes, washed, peeled, and cut into bite-size chunks (about 1¼ pounds)
- 1 (15-ounce) can no-salt-added diced tomatoes
- 2 tablespoons tomato paste
- 4 teaspoons curry powder
- 1/8 teaspoon ground cloves
- 1 (15-ounce) can light coconut milk
- ¼ teaspoon salt
- 2 pieces whole-wheat naan bread, halved, or 4 slices crusty bread

Direction: Preparation time: 15 minutes Cooking time: 35 minutes Servings: 4

- ✓ In a large saucepan over medium heat, heat the olive oil. When the oil is shimmering, add both the onion and garlic and cook until the onion softens and the garlic is sweet, for about 3 minutes.
- ✓ Add the bell pepper and continue cooking until it softens, about 5 minutes more. Add the lentils, sweet potatoes, tomatoes, tomato paste, curry powder, and cloves, and bring the mixture to a boil. are softened, about 20 minutes.
- ✓ Reduce the heat to medium-low, cover, and simmer until the potatoes
- ✓ Add the coconut milk and salt, and return to a boil. Reduce the heat and simmer until the flavors combine, about 5 minutes.
- ✓ Into each of 4 containers, spoon 2 cups of curry.
- ✓ Enjoy each serving with half of a piece of naan bread or 1 slice of crusty bread.

Nutrition: calories: 559; total fat: 16g; saturated fat: 7g; protein: 16g; total carbs: 86g; fiber: 16g; sugar: 18g; sodium: 819mg

93) Stuffed Portobello with Cheese

Ingredients:

- 4 Portobello mushroom caps
- 1 tablespoon olive oil
- 1/2 teaspoon salt, divided
- 1/4 teaspoon freshly ground black pepper, divided
- 1 cup baby spinach, chopped
- 1 1/2 cups part-skim ricotta cheese
- 1/2 cup part-skim shredded mozzarella cheese
- 1/4 cup grated parmesan cheese
- 1 garlic clove, minced
- 1 tablespoon dried parsley
- 2 teaspoons dried oregano
- 4 teaspoons unseasoned bread crumbs, divided
- 4 servings (4 cups) roasted broccoli with shallots

Direction: Preparation time: 15 minutes
Cooking time: 25 minutes Servings: 4

- ✓ Preheat the oven to 375f. Line a baking sheet with aluminum foil.
- ✓ Brush the mushroom caps with the olive oil, and sprinkle with ¼ teaspoon salt and 1/8 teaspoon pepper. Put the mushroom caps on the prepared baking sheet and bake until soft, about 12 minutes.
- ✓ In a medium bowl, mix together the spinach, ricotta, mozzarella, parmesan, garlic, parsley, oregano, and the remaining ¼ teaspoon of salt and 1/8 teaspoon of pepper.
- ✓ Spoon 1/2 cup of cheese mixture into each mushroom cap, and sprinkle each with 1 teaspoon of bread crumbs. Return the mushrooms to the oven for an additional 8 to 10 minutes until warmed through.
- ✓ Remove from the oven and allow the mushrooms to cool for about 10 minutes before placing each in an individual container. Add 1 cup of roasted broccoli with shallots to each container.

Nutrition: calories: 419; total fat: 30g; saturated fat: 10g; protein: 23g; total carbs: 19g; fiber: 2g; sugar: 3g; sodium: 790mg

94) Lighter Shrimp Scampi

Ingredients:

- 1 1/2 pounds large peeled and deveined shrimp
- ¼ teaspoon salt
- 1/8 teaspoon freshly ground black pepper
- 2 tablespoons olive oil
- 1 shallot, chopped
- 2 garlic cloves, minced
- ¼ cup cooking white wine
- Juice of 1/2 lemon (1 tablespoon)
- 1/2 teaspoon sriracha
- 2 tablespoons unsalted butter, at room temperature
- ¼ cup chopped fresh parsley
- 4 servings (6 cups) zucchini noodles with lemon vinaigrette

Direction: Preparation time: 15 minutes
Cooking time: 15 minutes Servings: 4

- ✓ Season the shrimp with the salt and pepper.
- ✓ In a medium saucepan over medium heat, heat the oil. Add the shallot and garlic, and cook until the shallot softens and the garlic is fragrant, about 3 minutes. Add the shrimp, cover, and cook until opaque, 2 to 3 minutes on each side. Using a slotted spoon, transfer the shrimp to a large plate.
- ✓ Add the wine, lemon juice, and sriracha to the saucepan, and stir to combine. Bring the mixture to a boil, then reduce the heat and simmer until the liquid is reduced by about half, 3 minutes. Add the butter and stir until melted, about 3 minutes. Return the shrimp to the saucepan and toss to coat. Add the parsley and stir to combine.
- ✓ Into each of 4 containers, place 1 1/2 cups of zucchini noodles with lemon vinaigrette, and top with ¾ cup of scampi.

Nutrition: calories: 364; total fat: 21g; saturated fat: 6g; protein: 37g; total carbs: 10g; fiber: 2g; sugar: 6g; sodium: 557mg

95) Maple-Mustard Salmon

Ingredients:

- Nonstick cooking spray
- 1/2 cup 100% maple syrup
- 2 tablespoons Dijon mustard
- ¼ teaspoon salt
- 4 (5-ounce) salmon fillets
- 4 servings (4 cups) roasted broccoli with shallots
- 4 servings (2 cups) parsleyed whole-wheat couscous

Direction: Preparation time: 10 minutes, plus 30 minutes marinating time Cooking time: 20 minutes Servings: 4

- ✓ Preheat the oven to 400f. Line a baking sheet with aluminum foil and coat with cooking spray.
- ✓ In a medium bowl, whisk together the maple syrup, mustard, and salt until smooth.
- ✓ Put the salmon fillets into the bowl and toss to coat. Cover and place in the refrigerator to marinate for at least 30 minutes and up to overnight.
- ✓ Shake off excess marinade from the salmon fillets and place them on the prepared baking sheet, leaving a 1-inch space between each fillet. Discard the extra marinade.
- ✓ Bake for about 20 minutes until the salmon is opaque and a thermometer inserted in the thickest part of a fillet reads 145f.
- ✓ Into each of 4 resealable containers, place 1 salmon fillet, 1 cup of roasted broccoli with shallots, and 1/2 cup of parsleyed whole-wheat couscous.

Nutrition: calories: 601; total fat: 29g; saturated fat: 4g; protein: 36g; total carbs: 51g; fiber: 3g; sugar: 23g; sodium: 610mg

96) Chicken Salad with Grapes and Pecans

Ingredients:

- 1/3 cup unsalted pecans, chopped
- 10 ounces cooked skinless, boneless chicken breast or rotisserie chicken, finely chopped
- 1/2 medium yellow onion, finely chopped
- 1 celery stalk, finely chopped
- ¾ cup red or green seedless grapes, halved
- ¼ cup light mayonnaise
- ¼ cup nonfat plain Greek yogurt
- 1 tablespoon Dijon mustard
- 1 tablespoon dried parsley
- ¼ teaspoon salt
- 1/8 teaspoon freshly ground black pepper
- 1 cup shredded romaine lettuce
- 4 (8-inch) whole-wheat pitas

Direction: Preparation Time: 15 Minutes
Cooking Time: 5 Minutes Servings: 4

- ✓ Heat a small skillet over medium-low heat to toast the pecans. Cook the pecans until fragrant, about 3 minutes. Remove from the heat and set aside to cool.
- ✓ In a medium bowl, mix the chicken, onion, celery, pecans, and grapes.
- ✓ In a small bowl, whisk together the mayonnaise, yogurt, mustard, parsley, salt, and pepper. Spoon the sauce over the chicken mixture and stir until well combined.
- ✓ Into each of 4 containers, place ¼ cup of lettuce and top with 1 cup of chicken salad. Store the pitas separately until ready to serve.
- ✓ When ready to eat, stuff the serving of salad and lettuce into 1 pita.

Nutrition: Calories: 418; Total Fat: 14g; Saturated Fat: 2g; Protein: 31g; Total Carbs: 43g; Fiber: 6g;

97) Lemony Salmon Burgers

Ingredients:

- 2 (3-oz) cans boneless, skinless pink salmon
- 1/4 cup panko breadcrumbs
- 4 tsp. lemon juice
- 1/4 cup red bell pepper
- 1/4 cup sugar-free yogurt
- 1 egg
- 2 (1.5-oz) whole wheat hamburger toasted buns

Direction: Preparation Time: 10 Minutes
Cooking Time: 10 Minutes Servings: 4

- ✓ Mix drained and flaked salmon, finely-chopped bell pepper, panko breadcrumbs.
- ✓ Combine 2 tbsp. cup sugar-free yogurt, 3 tsp. fresh lemon juice, and egg in a bowl. Shape mixture into 2 (3-inch) patties, bake on the skillet over medium heat 4 to 5 Minutes per side.
- ✓ Stir together 2 tbsp. sugar-free yogurt and 1 tsp. lemon juice; spread over bottom halves of buns.
- ✓ Top each with 1 patty, and cover with bun tops. This dish is very mouth-watering!

Nutrition: Calories 131 / Protein 12 g / Fat 1 g / Carbs 19 g

98) Caprese Turkey Burgers

Ingredients:

- 1/2 lb. 93% lean ground turkey
- 2 (1.5-oz) whole wheat hamburger buns (toasted)
- 1/4 cup shredded mozzarella cheese (part-skim)
- 1 egg
- 1 small clove garlic
- 4 large basil leaves
- 1/8 tsp. salt
- 1/8 tsp. pepper
- 1 big tomato

Direction: •Preparation Time 10 Minutes
Cooking Time: 10 Minutes Servings: 4

- ✓ Combine turkey, white egg, Minced garlic, salt, and pepper (mix until combined);
- ✓ Shape into 2 cutlets. Put cutlets into a skillet; cook 5 to 7 Minutes per side.
- ✓ Top cutlets properly with cheese and sliced tomato at the end of cooking.
- ✓ Put 1 cutlet on the bottom of each bun.
- ✓ Top each patty with 2 basil leaves. Cover with bun tops.

Nutrition: Calories 180 / Protein 7 g / Fat 4 g / Carbs 20 g

99) Pasta Salad

Ingredients:

- 8 oz. whole-wheat pasta
- 2 tomatoes
- 1 (5-oz) pkg spring mix
- 9 slices bacon
- 1/3 cup mayonnaise (reduced-fat)
- 1 tbsp. Dijon mustard
- 3 tbsp. apple cider vinegar
- 1/4 tsp. salt
- 1/2 tsp. pepper

Direction: Preparation Time: 15 Minutes
Cooking Time: 15 Minutes Servings: 4

- ✓ Cook pasta.
- ✓ Chilled pasta, chopped tomatoes and spring mix in a bowl.
- ✓ Crumble cooked bacon over pasta.
- ✓ Combine mayonnaise, mustard, vinegar, salt and pepper in a small bowl.
- ✓ Pour dressing over pasta, stirring to coat.

Nutrition: Calories 200 / Protein 15 g / Fat 3 g / Carbs 6 g

100) Chicken, Strawberry, And Avocado Salad

Ingredients:

- 1,5 cups chicken (skin removed)
- 1/4 cup almonds
- 2 (5-oz) pkg salad greens
- 1 (16-oz) pkg strawberries
- 1 avocado
- 1/4 cup green onion
- 1/4 cup lime juice
- 3 tbsp. extra virgin olive oil
- 2 tbsp. honey
- 1/4 tsp. salt
- 1/4 tsp. pepper

Direction: Preparation Time: 10 Minutes
Cooking Time: 5 Minutes

- ✓ Toast almonds until golden and fragrant.
- ✓ Mix lime juice, oil, honey, salt, and pepper.
- ✓ Mix greens, sliced strawberries, chicken, diced avocado, and sliced green onion and sliced almonds; drizzle with dressing. Toss to coat.

Nutrition: Calories 150 / Protein 15 g / Fat 10 g / Carbs 5 g

101) Lemon-Thyme Eggs

Ingredients:

- 7 large eggs
- 1/4 cup mayonnaise (reduced-fat)
- 2 tsp. lemon juice
- 1 tsp. Dijon mustard
- 1 tsp. chopped fresh thyme
- 1/8 tsp. cayenne pepper

Direction: Preparation Time: 10 Minutes
Cooking Time: 5 Minutes Servings: 4

- ✓ Bring eggs to a boil.
- ✓ Peel and cut each egg in half lengthwise.
- ✓ Remove yolks to a bowl. Add mayonnaise, lemon juice, mustard, thyme, and cayenne to egg yolks; mash to blend. Fill egg white halves with yolk mixture.
- ✓ Chill until ready to serve.

Nutrition: Calories 40 / Protein 10 g / Fat 6 g / Carbs 2 g

102) Spinach Salad with Bacon

Ingredients:

- 8 slices center-cut bacon
- 3 tbsp. extra virgin olive oil
- 1 (5-oz) pkg baby spinach
- 1 tbsp. apple cider vinegar
- 1 tsp. Dijon mustard
- 1/2 tsp. honey
- 1/4 tsp. salt
- 1/2 tsp. pepper

Direction: Preparation Time: 15 Minutes
Cooking Time: 0 Minutes Servings: 4

- ✓ Mix vinegar, mustard, honey, salt and pepper in a bowl.
- ✓ Whisk in oil. Place spinach in a serving bowl; drizzle with dressing, and toss to coat.
- ✓ Sprinkle with cooked and crumbled bacon.

Nutrition: Calories 110 / Protein 6 g / Fat 2 g / Carbs 1 g

103) Pea and Collards Soup

Ingredients:

- 1/2 (16-oz) pkg black-eyed peas
- 1 onion
- 2 carrots
- 1,5 cups ham (low-sodium)
- 1 (1-lb) bunch collard greens (trimmed)
- 1 tbsp. extra virgin olive oil
- 2 cloves garlic
- 1/2 tsp. black pepper
- Hot sauce

Direction: Preparation Time: 10 Minutes
Cooking Time: 50 Minutes Servings: 4

- ✓ Cook chopped onion and carrots 10 Minutes.
- ✓ Add peas, diced ham, collards, and Minced garlic. Cook 5 Minutes.
- ✓ Add broth, 3 cups water, and pepper. Bring to a boil; simmer 35 Minutes, adding water if needed.

Nutrition: Calories 86 / Protein 15 g / Fat 2 g / Carbs 9 g

104) Spanish Stew

Ingredients:

- 1.1/2 (12-oz) pkg smoked chicken sausage links
- 1 (5-oz) pkg baby spinach
- 1 (15-oz) can chickpeas
- 1 (14.5-oz) can tomatoes with basil, garlic, and oregano
- 1/2 tsp. smoked paprika
- 1/2 tsp. cumin
- 3/4 cup onions
- 1 tbsp. extra virgin olive oil

Direction: Preparation Time: 10 Minutes
Cooking Time: 25 Minutes Servings: 4

- ✓ Cook sliced the sausage in hot oil until browned. Remove from pot.
- ✓ Add chopped onions; cook until tender.
- ✓ Add sausage, drained and rinsed chickpeas, diced tomatoes, paprika, and ground cumin. Cook 15 Minutes.
- ✓ Add in spinach; cook 1 to 2 Minutes.

Nutrition: Calories 200 / Protein 10 g / Fat 20 g / Carbs 1 g

105) Creamy Taco Soup

Ingredients:

- 3/4 lb. ground sirloin
- 1/2 (8-oz) cream cheese
- 1/2 onion
- 1 clove garlic
- 1 (10-oz) can tomatoes and green chiles
- 1 (14.5-oz) can beef broth
- 1/4 cup heavy cream
- 1,5 tsp. cumin
- 1/2 tsp. chili powder

Direction: Preparation Time: 10 Minutes
Cooking Time: 20 Minutes Servings: 4

- ✓ Cook beef, chopped onion, and Minced garlic until meat is browned and crumbly; drain and return to pot.
- ✓ Add ground cumin, chili powder, and cream cheese cut into small pieces and softened, stirring until cheese is melted.
- ✓ Add diced tomatoes, broth, and cream; bring to a boil, and simmer 10 Minutes. Season with pepper and salt to taste.

Nutrition: Calories 60 / Protein 3 g / Fat 1 g / Carbs 8 g

106) Chicken with Caprese Salsa

Ingredients:

- 3/4 lb. boneless, skinless chicken breasts
- 2 big tomatoes
- 1/2 (8-oz) ball fresh mozzarella cheese
- 1/4 cup red onion
- 2 tbsp. fresh basil
- 1 tbsp. balsamic vinegar
- 2 tbsp. extra virgin olive oil (divided)
- 1/2 tsp. salt (divided)
- 1/4 tsp. pepper (divided)

Direction: Preparation Time: 15 Minutes
Cooking Time: 5 Minutes Servings: 4

- ✓ Sprinkle cut in half lengthwise chicken with 1/4 tsp. salt and 1/8 tsp. pepper.
- ✓ Heat 1 tbsp. olive oil, cook chicken 5 Minutes.
- ✓ Meanwhile, mix chopped tomatoes, diced cheese, finely chopped onion, chopped basil, vinegar, 1 tbsp. oil, and 1/4 tsp. salt and 1/8 tsp. pepper.
- ✓ Spoon salsa over chicken.

Nutrition: Calories 210 / Protein 28 g / Fat 17 g / Carbs 0, 1 g

107) Balsamic-Roasted Broccoli

Ingredients:

- 1 lb. broccoli
- 1 tbsp. extra virgin olive oil
- 1 tbsp. balsamic vinegar
- 1 clove garlic
- 1/8 tsp. salt
- Pepper to taste

Direction: Preparation Time: 10 Minutes
Cooking Time: 15 Minutes Servings: 4

- ✓ Preheat oven to 450F.
- ✓ Combine broccoli, olive oil, vinegar, Minced garlic, salt, and pepper; toss.
- ✓ Spread broccoli on a baking sheet.
- ✓ Bake 12 to 15 Minutes.

Nutrition: Calories 27 / Protein 3 g / Fat 0, 3 g / Carbs 4 g

108) Hearty Beef and Vegetable Soup

Ingredients:

- 1/2 lb. lean ground beef
- 2 cups beef broth
- 1,5 tbsp. vegetable oil (divided)
- 1 cup green bell pepper
- 1/2 cup red onion
- 1 cup green cabbage
- 1 cup frozen mixed vegetables
- 1/2 can tomatoes
- 1,5 tsp. Worcestershire sauce
- 1 small bay leaf
- 1,8 tsp. pepper
- 2 tbsp. ketchup

Direction: Preparation Time: 10 Minutes
Cooking Time: 30 Minutes Servings: 4

- ✓ Cook beef in 1/2 tbsp. hot oil 2 Minutes.
- ✓ Stir in chopped bell pepper and chopped onion; cook 4 Minutes.
- ✓ Add chopped cabbage, mixed vegetables, stewed tomatoes, broth, Worcestershire sauce, bay leaf, and pepper; bring to a boil.
- ✓ Reduce heat to medium; cover, and cook 15 Minutes.
- ✓ Stir in ketchup and 1 tbsp. oil, and remove from heat. Let stand 10 Minutes.

Nutrition: Calories 170 / Protein 17 g / Fat 8 g / Carbs 3 g

109) Cauliflower Muffin

Ingredients:

- 2,5 cup cauliflower
- 2/3 cup ham
- 2,5 cups of cheese
- 2/3 cup champignon
- 1,5 tbsp. flaxseed
- 3 eggs
- 1/4 tsp. salt
- 1/8 tsp. pepper

Direction: Preparation Time: 15 Minutes
Cooking Time: 30 Minutes Servings: 4

- ✓ Preheat oven to 375 F.
- ✓ Put muffin liners in a 12-muffin tin.
- ✓ Combine diced cauliflower, ground flaxseed, beaten eggs, cup diced ham, grated cheese, and diced mushrooms, salt, pepper.
- ✓ Divide mixture rightly between muffin liners.
- ✓ Bake 30 Minutes.

Nutrition: Calories 116 / Protein 10 g / Fat 7 g / Carbs 3 g

110) Ham and Egg Cups

Ingredients:

- 5 slices ham
- 4 tbsp. cheese
- 1,5 tbsp. cream
- 3 egg whites
- 1,5 tbsp. pepper (green)
- 1 tsp. salt
- pepper to taste

Direction: Preparation Time: 10 Minutes
Cooking Time: 15 Minutes Servings: 4

- ✓ Preheat oven to 350 F.
- ✓ Arrange each slice of thinly sliced ham into 4 muffin tin.
- ✓ Put 1/4 of grated cheese into ham cup.
- ✓ Mix eggs, cream, salt and pepper and divide it into 2 tins.
- ✓ Bake in oven 15 Minutes; after baking, sprinkle with green onions.

Nutrition: Calories 180 / Protein 13 g / Fat 13 g / Carbs 2 g

111) Cauliflower Rice with Chicken

Ingredients:

- 1/2 large cauliflower
- 3/4 cup cooked meat
- 1/2 bell pepper
- 1 carrot
- 2 ribs celery
- 1 tbsp. stir fry sauce (low carb)
- 1 tbsp. extra virgin olive oil
- Salt and pepper to taste

Direction: Preparation Time: 15 Minutes
Cooking Time: 15 Minutes Servings: 4

- ✓ Chop cauliflower in a processor to "rice." Place in a bowl.
- ✓ Properly chop all vegetables in a food processor into thin slices.
- ✓ Chop cauliflower in a processor to "rice." Place in a bowl.
- ✓ Properly chop all vegetables in a food processor into thin slices.
- ✓ Add cauliflower and other plants to WOK with heated oil. Fry until all veggies are tender.
- ✓ Add chopped meat and sauce to the wok and fry 10 Minutes and Serve. This dish is very mouth-watering!

Nutrition: Calories 200 / Protein 10 g / Fat 12 g /Carbs 10 g

112) Turkey with Fried Eggs

Ingredients:

- 4 large potatoes
- 1 cooked turkey thigh
- 1 large onion (about 2 cups diced)
- butter
- Chile flakes
- 4 eggs
- salt to taste
- pepper to taste

Direction: Preparation Time: 10 Minutes
Cooking Time: 20 Minutes Servings: 4

- ✓ Rub the cold boiled potatoes on the coarsest holes of a box grater. Dice the turkey.
- ✓ Cook the onion in as much unsalted butter as you feel comfortable with until it's just fragrant and translucent.
- ✓ Add the rubbed potatoes and a cup of diced cooked turkey, salt and pepper to taste, and cook 20 Minutes.

Nutrition: Calories 170 / Protein 19 g / Fat 7 g / Carbs 6 g

Lory Ramos

DINNER

113) Salmon with Asparagus

Ingredients:
- 1 lb. Salmon, sliced into fillets
- 1 tbsp. Olive Oil
- Salt & Pepper, as needed
- 1 bunch of Asparagus, trimmed
- 2 cloves of Garlic, minced
- Zest & Juice of 1/2 Lemon
- 1 tbsp. Butter, salted

Direction: Preparation Time: 5 Minutes
Cooking Time: 10 Minutes Servings: 3

- ✓ Spoon in the butter and olive oil into a large pan and heat it over medium-high heat.
- ✓ Once it becomes hot, place the salmon and season it with salt and pepper.
- ✓ Cook for 4 minutes per side and then cook the other side.
- ✓ Stir in the garlic and lemon zest to it.
- ✓ Cook for further 2 minutes or until lightly browned.
- ✓ Off the heat and squeeze the lemon juice over it.
- ✓ Serve it hot.

Nutrition: Calories: 409Kcal; Carbohydrates: 2.7g; Proteins: 32.8g; Fat: 28.8g; Sodium: 497mg

114) Shrimp in Garlic Butter

Ingredients:
- 1 lb. Shrimp, peeled & deveined
- ¼ tsp. Red Pepper Flakes
- 6 tbsp. Butter, divided
- 1/2 cup Chicken Stock
- Salt & Pepper, as needed
- 2 tbsp. Parsley, minced
- 5 cloves of Garlic, minced
- 2 tbsp. Lemon Juice

Direction: Preparation Time: 5 Minutes
Cooking Time: 20 Minutes Servings: 4

- ✓ Heat a large bottomed skillet over medium-high heat.
- ✓ Spoon in two tablespoons of the butter and melt it. Add the shrimp.
- ✓ Season it with salt and pepper. Sear for 4 minutes or until shrimp gets cooked.
- ✓ Transfer the shrimp to a plate and stir in the garlic.
- ✓ Sauté for 30 seconds or until aromatic.
- ✓ Pour the chicken stock and whisk it well. Allow it to simmer for 5 to 10 minutes or until it has reduced to half.
- ✓ Spoon the remaining butter, red pepper, and lemon juice to the sauce. Mix.
- ✓ Continue cooking for another 2 minutes.
- ✓ Take off the pan from the heat and add the cooked shrimp to it.
- ✓ Garnish with parsley and transfer to the serving bowl.

Nutrition: Calories: 307Kcal; Carbs: 3g; Proteins: 27g; Fat: 20g; Sodium: 522mg

115) Cobb Salad

Ingredients:
- 4 Cherry Tomatoes, chopped
- ¼ cup Bacon, cooked & crumbled
- 1/2 of 1 Avocado, chopped
- 2 oz. Chicken Breast, shredded
- 1 Egg, hardboiled
- 2 cups Mixed Green salad
- 1 oz. Feta Cheese, crumbled

Direction: Preparation Time: 5 Minutes
Cooking Time: 5 Minutes Servings: 1

- ✓ Toss all the ingredients for the Cobb salad in a large mixing bowl and toss well.
- ✓ Serve and enjoy it.

Nutrition: Calories: 307Kcal; Carbs: 3g; Proteins: 27g; Fat: 20g; Sodium: 522mg

116) Seared Tuna Steak

Ingredients:
- 1 tsp. Sesame Seeds
- 1 tbsp. Sesame Oil
- 2 tbsp. Soya Sauce
- Salt & Pepper, to taste
- 2 × 6 oz. Ahi Tuna Steaks

Direction: Preparation Time: 10 Minutes
Cooking Time: 10 Minutes Serving Size: 2

- ✓ Seasoning the tuna steaks with salt and pepper. Keep it aside on a shallow bowl.
- ✓ In another bowl, mix soya sauce and sesame oil.
- ✓ pour the sauce over the salmon and coat them generously with the sauce.
- ✓ Keep it aside for 10 to 15 minutes and then heat a large skillet over medium heat.
- ✓ Once hot, keep the tuna steaks and cook them for 3 minutes or until seared underneath.
- ✓ Flip the fillets and cook them for a further 3 minutes.
- ✓ Transfer the seared tuna steaks to the serving plate and slice them into 1/2 inch slices. Top with sesame seeds.

Nutrition: Calories: 255Kcal; Fat: 9g; Carbs: 1g; Proteins: 40.5g; Sodium: 293mg

117) Beef Chili

Ingredients:
- 1/2 tsp. Garlic Powder
- 1 tsp. Coriander, grounded
- 1 lb. Beef, grounded
- 1/2 tsp. Sea Salt
- 1/2 tsp. Cayenne Pepper
- 1 tsp. Cumin, grounded
- 1/2 tsp. Pepper, grounded
- 1/2 cup Salsa, low-carb & no-sugar

Direction: Preparation Time: 10 Minutes
Cooking Time: 20 Minutes Serving Size: 4

- ✓ Heat a large-sized pan over medium-high heat and cook the beef in it until browned.
- ✓ Stir in all the spices and cook them for 7 minutes or until everything is combined.
- ✓ When the beef gets cooked, spoon in the salsa.
- ✓ Bring the mixture to a simmer and cook for another 8 minutes or until everything comes together.
- ✓ Take it from heat and transfer to a serving bowl

Nutrition: Calories: 229Kcal; Fat: 10g; Carbs: 2g; Proteins: 33g; Sodium: 675mg

118) Greek Broccoli Salad

Ingredients:
- 1 ¼ lb. Broccoli, sliced into small bites
- ¼ cup Almonds, sliced
- 1/3 cup Sun-dried Tomatoes
- ¼ cup Feta Cheese, crumbled
- ¼ cup Red Onion, sliced

For the dressing:
- 1/4 cup Olive Oil
- Dash of Red Pepper Flakes
- 1 Garlic clove, minced
- ¼ tsp. Salt
- 2 tbsp. Lemon Juice
- 1/2 tsp. Dijon Mustard
- 1 tsp. Low Carb Sweetener Syrup
- 1/2 tsp. Oregano, dried

Direction: Preparation Time: 10 Minutes
Cooking Time: 15 Minutes Servings: 4

- ✓ Mix broccoli, onion, almonds and sun-dried tomatoes in a large mixing bowl.
- ✓ In another small-sized bowl, combine all the dressing ingredients until emulsified.
- ✓ Spoon the dressing over the broccoli salad.
- ✓ Allow the salad to rest for half an hour before serving.

Nutrition: Calories: 272Kcal; Carbohydrates: 11.9g; Proteins: 8g

119) Cheesy Cauliflower Gratin

Ingredients:
- 6 deli slices Pepper Jack Cheese
- 4 cups Cauliflower florets
- Salt and Pepper, as needed
- 4 tbsp. Butter
- 1/3 cup Heavy Whipping Cream

Direction: Preparation Time: 5 Minutes
Cooking Time: 25 Minutes **Servings:** 6

- ✓ Mix the cauliflower, cream, butter, salt, and pepper in a safe microwave bowl and combine well.
- ✓ Microwave the cauliflower mixture for 25 minutes on high until it becomes soft and tender.
- ✓ Remove the ingredients from the bowl and mash with the help of a fork.
- ✓ Taste for seasonings and spoon in salt and pepper as required.
- ✓ Arrange the slices of pepper jack cheese on top of the cauliflower mixture and microwave for 3 minutes until the cheese starts melting.
- ✓ Serve warm.

Nutrition: Calories: 421Kcal; Carbs: 3g; Proteins: 19g; Fat: 37g; Sodium: 111mg

120) Strawberry Spinach Salad

Ingredients:
- 4 oz. Feta Cheese, crumbled
- 8 Strawberries, sliced
- 2 oz. Almonds
- 6 Slices Bacon, thick-cut, crispy and crumbled
- 10 oz. Spinach leaves, fresh
- 2 Roma Tomatoes, diced
- 2 oz. Red Onion, sliced thinly

Direction: Preparation Time: 5 Minutes
Cooking Time: 10 Minutes **Servings:** 4

- ✓ For making this healthy salad, mix all the ingredients needed to make the salad in a large-sized bowl and toss them well.
- ✓ Enjoy

Nutrition: Calories – 255kcal; Fat – 16g; Carbs – 8g; Proteins – 14g; Sodium: 27mg

121) Cauliflower Mac & Cheese

Ingredients:
- 1 Cauliflower Head, torn into florets
- Salt & Black Pepper, as needed
- 1/4 cup Almond Milk, unsweetened
- 1/4 cup Heavy Cream
- 3 tbsp. Butter, preferably grass-fed
- 1 cup Cheddar Cheese, shredded

Direction: Preparation Time: 5 Minutes
Cooking Time: 25 Minutes **Serving Size:** 4

- ✓ Preheat the oven to 450 F.
- ✓ Melt the butter in a small microwave-safe bowl and heat it for 30 seconds.
- ✓ Pour the melted butter over the cauliflower florets along with salt and pepper. Toss them well.
- ✓ Place the cauliflower florets in a parchment paper-covered large baking sheet.
- ✓ Bake them for 15 minutes or until the cauliflower is crisp-tender.
- ✓ Once baked, mix the heavy cream, cheddar cheese, almond milk, and the remaining butter in a large microwave-safe bowl and heat it on high heat for 2 minutes or until the cheese mixture is smooth. Repeat the procedure until the cheese has melted.
- ✓ Finally, stir in the cauliflower to the sauce mixture and coat well.

Nutrition: Calories: 294Kcal; Fat: 23g; Carbohydrates: 7g; Proteins: 11g

122) Easy Egg Salad

Ingredients:
- 6 Eggs, preferably free-range
- 1/4 tsp. Salt
- 2 tbsp. Mayonnaise
- 1 tsp. Lemon juice
- 1 tsp. Dijon mustard
- Pepper, to taste
- Lettuce leaves, to serve

Direction: Preparation Time: 5 Minutes
Cooking Time: 15 to 20 Minutes **Servings:** 4

- ✓ Keep the eggs in a saucepan of water and pour cold water until it covers the egg by another 1 inch.
- ✓ Bring to a boil and then remove the eggs from heat.
- ✓ Peel the eggs under cold running water.
- ✓ Transfer the cooked eggs into a food processor and pulse them until chopped.
- ✓ Stir in the mayonnaise, lemon juice, salt, Dijon mustard, and pepper and mix them well.
- ✓ Taste for seasoning and add more if required.
- ✓ Serve in the lettuce leaves.

Nutrition: Calories – 166kcal; Fat – 14g; Carbs – 0.85g; Proteins – 10g; Sodium 132mg

123) Baked Chicken Legs

Ingredients:
- 6 Chicken Legs
- 1/4 tsp. Black Pepper
- 1/4 cup Butter
- 1/2 tsp. Sea Salt
- 1/2 tsp. Smoked Paprika
- 1/2 tsp. Garlic Powder

Direction: Preparation Time: 10 Minutes
Cooking Time: 40 Minutes **Servings:** 6

- ✓ Preheat the oven to 425 F.
- ✓ Pat the chicken legs with a paper towel to absorb any excess moisture.
- ✓ Marinate the chicken pieces by first applying the butter over them and then with the seasoning. Set it aside for a few minutes.
- ✓ Bake them for 25 minutes. Turnover and bake for further 10 minutes or until the internal temperature reaches 165 F.
- ✓ Serve them hot.

Nutrition: Calories – 236kL; Fat – 16g; Carbs – 0g; Protein – 22g; Sodium – 314mg

124) Creamed Spinach

Ingredients:
- 3 tbsp. Butter
- 1/4 tsp. Black Pepper
- 4 cloves of Garlic, minced
- 1/4 tsp. Sea Salt
- 10 oz. Baby Spinach, chopped
- 1 tsp. Italian Seasoning
- 1/2 cup Heavy Cream
- 3 oz. Cream Cheese

Direction: Preparation Time: 5 Minutes
Cooking Time: 10 Minutes **Servings:** 4

- ✓ Melt butter in a large sauté pan over medium heat.
- ✓ Once the butter has melted, spoon in the garlic and sauté for 30 seconds or until aromatic.
- ✓ Spoon in the spinach and cook for 3 to 4 minutes or until wilted.
- ✓ Add all the remaining ingredients to it and continuously stir until the cream cheese melts and the mixture gets thickened.
- ✓ Serve hot

Nutrition: Calories – 274kL; Fat – 27g; Carbs – 4g; Protein – 4g; Sodium – 114mg

125) Stuffed Mushrooms

Ingredients:

- 4 Portobello Mushrooms, large
- 1/2 cup Mozzarella Cheese, shredded
- 1/2 cup Marinara, low-sugar
- Olive Oil Spray

Direction: Preparation Time: 10 Minutes
Cooking Time: 20 Minutes Servings: 4

- ✓ Preheat the oven to 375 F.
- ✓ Take out the dark gills from the mushrooms with the help of a spoon.
- ✓ Keep the mushroom stem upside down and spoon it with two tablespoons of marinara sauce and mozzarella cheese.
- ✓ Bake for 18 minutes or until the cheese is bubbly.

Nutrition: Calories – 113kL; Fat – 6g; Carbs – 4g; Protein – 7g; Sodium – 14mg

126) Vegetable Soup

Ingredients:

- 8 cups Vegetable Broth
- 2 tbsp. Olive Oil
- 1 tbsp. Italian Seasoning
- 1 Onion, large & diced
- 2 Bay Leaves, dried
- 2 Bell Pepper, large & diced
- Sea Salt & Black Pepper, as needed
- 4 cloves of Garlic, minced
- 28 oz. Tomatoes, diced
- 1 Cauliflower head, medium & torn into florets
- 2 cups Green Beans, trimmed & chopped

Direction: Preparation Time: 10 Minutes
Cooking Time: 30 Minutes Servings: 5

- ✓ Heat oil in a Dutch oven over medium heat.
- ✓ Once the oil becomes hot, stir in the onions and pepper.
- ✓ Cook for 10 minutes or until the onion is softened and browned.
- ✓ Spoon in the garlic and sauté for a minute or until fragrant.
- ✓ Add all the remaining ingredients to it. Mix until everything comes together.
- ✓ Bring the mixture to a boil. Lower the heat and cook for further 20 minutes or until the vegetables have softened.
- ✓ Serve hot.

Nutrition: Calories – 79kL; Fat – 2g; Carbs – 8g; Protein – 2g; Sodium – 187mg

127) Misto Quente

Ingredients:

- 4 slices of bread without shell
- 4 slices of turkey breast
- 4 slices of cheese
- 2 tbsp. cream cheese
- 2 spoons of butter

Direction: Preparation time: 5 minutes
Cooking time: 10 minutes Servings: 4

- ✓ Preheat the air fryer. Set the timer of 5 minutes and the temperature to 200C.
- ✓ Pass the butter on one side of the slice of bread, and on the other side of the slice, the cream cheese.
- ✓ Mount the sandwiches placing two slices of turkey breast and two slices cheese between the breads, with the cream cheese inside and the side with butter.
- ✓ Place the sandwiches in the basket of the air fryer. Set the timer of the air fryer for 5 minutes and press the power button.

Nutrition: Calories: 340 Fat: 15g Carbs: 32g Protein: 15g Sugar: 0g Cholesterol: 0mg

128) Garlic Bread

Ingredients: Garlic Bread

- 2 stale French rolls
- 4 tbsp. crushed or crumpled garlic
- 1 cup of mayonnaise
- Powdered grated Parmesan
- 1 tbsp. olive oil

Direction: Preparation time: 10 minutes
Cooking time: 15 minutes Servings: 4-5

- ✓ Preheat the air fryer. Set the time of 5 minutes and the temperature to 2000C.
- ✓ Mix mayonnaise with garlic and set aside.
- ✓ Cut the baguettes into slices, but without separating them completely.
- ✓ Fill the cavities of equals. Brush with olive oil and sprinkle with grated cheese.
- ✓ Place in the basket of the air fryer. Set the timer to 10 minutes, adjust the temperature to 1800C and press the power button.

Nutrition: Calories: 340 Fat: 15g Carbs: 32g Protein: 15g Sugar: 0g Cholesterol: 0mg

129) Bruschetta

Ingredients:

- 4 slices of Italian bread
- 1 cup chopped tomato tea
- 1 cup grated mozzarella tea
- Olive oil
- Oregano, salt, and pepper
- 4 fresh basil leaves

Direction: Preparation time: 5 minutes|
Cooking time: 10 minutes Servings: 2

- ✓ Preheat the air fryer. Set the timer of 5 minutes and the temperature to 2000C.
- ✓ Sprinkle the slices of Italian bread with olive oil. Divide the chopped tomatoes and mozzarella between the slices. Season with salt, pepper, and oregano.
- ✓ Put oil in the filling. Place a basil leaf on top of each slice.
- ✓ Put the bruschetta in the basket of the air fryer being careful not to spill the filling. Set the timer of 5 minutes, set the temperature to 180C, and press the power button.
- ✓ Transfer the bruschetta to a plate and serve.

Nutrition: Calories: 434 Fat: 14g Carbohydrates: 63g Protein: 11g Sugar: 8g Cholesterol: 0mg

130) Cauliflower Potato Mash

Ingredients:

- 2 cups potatoes, peeled and cubed
- 2 tbsp. butter
- ¼ cup milk
- 10 oz. cauliflower florets
- ¾ tsp. salt

Direction: Preparation Time: 30 minutes Servings: 4
Cooking Time: 5 minutes

- ✓ Add water to the saucepan and bring to boil.
- ✓ Reduce heat and simmer for 10 minutes.
- ✓ Drain vegetables well. Transfer vegetables, butter, milk, and salt in a blender and blend until smooth.

Nutrition: Calories 128 Fat 6.2 g, Sugar 3.3 g, Protein 3.2 g, Cholesterol 17 mg

131) Cream Buns with Strawberries

Ingredients:

- 240g all-purpose flour
- 50g granulated sugar
- 8g baking powder
- 1g of salt
- 85g chopped cold butter
- 84g chopped fresh strawberries
- 120 ml whipping cream
- 2 large eggs
- 10 ml vanilla extract
- 5 ml of water

Direction: Preparation time: 10 minutes
Cooking time: 12 minutes Servings: 6

- ✓ Sift flour, sugar, baking powder and salt in a large bowl. Put the butter with the flour with the use of a blender or your hands until the mixture resembles thick crumbs.
- ✓ Mix the strawberries in the flour mixture. Set aside for the mixture to stand. Beat the whipping cream, 1 egg and the vanilla extract in a separate bowl.
- ✓ Put the cream mixture in the flour mixture until they are homogeneous, and then spread the mixture to a thickness of 38 mm.
- ✓ Use a round cookie cutter to cut the buns. Spread the buns with a combination of egg and water. Set aside
- ✓ Preheat the air fryer, set it to 180C.
- ✓ Place baking paper in the preheated inner basket.
- ✓ Place the buns on top of the baking paper and cook for 12 minutes at 180C, until golden brown.

Nutrition: Calories: 150 Fat: 14g Carbs: 3g Protein: 11g Sugar: 8g Cholesterol: 0mg

132) Blueberry Buns

Ingredients:

- 240g all-purpose flour
- 50g granulated sugar
- 8g baking powder
- 2g of salt
- 85g chopped cold butter
- 85g of fresh blueberries
- 3g grated fresh ginger
- 113 ml whipping cream
- 2 large eggs
- 4 ml vanilla extract
- 5 ml of water

Direction: Preparation time: 10 minutes
Cooking time: 12 minutes Servings: 6

- ✓ Put sugar, flour, baking powder and salt in a large bowl.
- ✓ Put the butter with the flour using a blender or your hands until the mixture resembles thick crumbs.
- ✓ Mix the blueberries and ginger in the flour mixture and set aside
- ✓ Mix the whipping cream, 1 egg and the vanilla extract in a different container.
- ✓ Put the cream mixture with the flour mixture until combined.
- ✓ Shape the dough until it reaches a thickness of approximately 38 mm and cut it into eighths.
- ✓ Spread the buns with a combination of egg and water. Set aside Preheat the air fryer set it to 180C.
- ✓ Place baking paper in the preheated inner basket and place the buns on top of the paper. Cook for 12 minutes at 180C, until golden brown

Nutrition: Calories: 105 Fat: 1.64g Carbs: 20.0g Protein: 2.43g Sugar: 2.1g Cholesterol: 0mg

133) French toast in Sticks

Ingredients:

- 4 slices of white bread, 38 mm thick, preferably hard
- 2 eggs
- 60 ml of milk
- 15 ml maple sauce
- 2 ml vanilla extract
- Nonstick Spray Oil
- 38g of sugar
- 3g ground cinnamon
- Maple syrup, to serve
- Sugar to sprinkle

Direction: Preparation time: 5 minutes
Cooking time: 10 minutes Servings: 4

- ✓ Cut each slice of bread into thirds making 12 pieces. Place sideways
- ✓ Beat the eggs, milk, maple syrup and vanilla.
- ✓ Preheat the air fryer, set it to 175C.
- ✓ Dip the sliced bread in the egg mixture and place it in the preheated air fryer. Sprinkle French toast generously with oil spray.
- ✓ Cook French toast for 10 minutes at 175C. Turn the toast halfway through cooking.
- ✓ Mix the sugar and cinnamon in a bowl.
- ✓ Cover the French toast with the sugar and cinnamon mixture when you have finished cooking.
- ✓ Serve with Maple syrup and sprinkle with powdered sugar

Nutrition: : Calories 128, Fat 6.2 g, Carbs 16.3 g, Sugar 3.3 g, Protein 3.2 g   Cholesterol 17 mg

134) Muffins Sandwich

Ingredients:

- Nonstick Spray Oil
- 1 slice of white cheddar cheese
- 1 slice of Canadian bacon
- 1 English muffin, divided
- 15 ml hot water
- 1 large egg
- Salt and pepper to taste

Direction: Preparation time: 2 minutes
Cooking time: 10 minutes Servings: 1

- ✓ Spray the inside of an 85g mold with oil spray and place it in the air fryer.
- ✓ Preheat the air fryer, set it to 160C.
- ✓ Add the Canadian cheese and bacon in the preheated air fryer.
- ✓ Pour the hot water and the egg into the hot pan and season with salt and pepper.
- ✓ Select Bread, set to 10 minutes.
- ✓ Take out the English muffins after 7 minutes, leaving the egg for the full time.
- ✓ Build your sandwich by placing the cooked egg on top of the English muffins and serve

Nutrition: Calories 400 Fat 26g, Carbs 26g, Sugar 15 g, Protein 3 g, Cholesterol 155 mg

135) Bacon BBQ

Ingredients:

- 13g dark brown sugar
- 5g chili powder
- 1g ground cumin
- 1g cayenne pepper
- 4 slices of bacon, cut in half

Direction: Preparation time: 2 minutes Cooking time: 8 minutes
Servings: 2

- ✓ Mix seasonings until well combined.
- ✓ Dip the bacon in the dressing until it is completely covered. Leave aside.
- ✓ Preheat the air fryer, set it to 160C.
- ✓ Place the bacon in the preheated air fryer
- ✓ Select Bacon and press Start/Pause.

Nutrition: Calories: 1124 Fat: 72g Carbs: 59g Protein: 49g Sugar: 11g Cholesterol 77mg

136) Stuffed French toast

Ingredients:

- 1 slice of brioche bread,
- 64 mm thick, preferably rancid
- 113g cream cheese
- 2 eggs
- 15 ml of milk
- 30 ml whipping cream
- 38g of sugar
- 3g cinnamon
- 2 ml vanilla extract
- Nonstick Spray Oil
- Pistachios chopped to cover
- Maple syrup, to serve

Direction: Preparation time: 4 minutes
Cooking time: 10 minutes **Servings:** 1

- Preheat the air fryer, set it to 175C.
- Cut a slit in the middle of the muffin.
- Fill the inside of the slit with cream cheese. Leave aside.
- Mix the eggs, milk, whipping cream, sugar, cinnamon, and vanilla extract.
- Moisten the stuffed French toast in the egg mixture for 10 seconds on each side.
- Sprinkle each side of French toast with oil spray.
- Place the French toast in the preheated air fryer and cook for 10 minutes at 175C
- Stir the French toast carefully with a spatula when you finish cooking.
- Serve topped with chopped pistachios and acrid syrup.

Nutrition: Calories: 159 Fat: 7.5g Carbs: 25.2g Protein: 14g Sugar: 0g Cholesterol 90mg

137) Scallion Sandwich

Ingredients:

- 2 slices wheat bread
- 2 teaspoons butter, low fat
- 2 scallions, sliced thinly
- 1 tablespoon of parmesan cheese, grated
- 3/4 cup of cheddar cheese, reduced fat, grated

Direction: Preparation Time: 10 minutes
Cooking Time: 10 minutes **Servings:** 1

- Preheat the Air fryer to 356 degrees.
- Spread butter on a slice of bread. Place inside the cooking basket with the butter side facing down.
- Place cheese and scallions on top. Spread the rest of the butter on the other slice of bread Put it on top of the sandwich and sprinkle with parmesan cheese.
- Cook for 10 minutes.

Nutrition: Calorie: 154 Carbohydrate: 9g Fat: 2.5g Protein: 8.6g Fiber: 2.4g

138) Lean Lamb and Turkey Meatballs with Yogurt

Ingredients:

- 1 egg white
- 4 ounces ground lean turkey
- 1 pound of ground lean lamb
- 1 teaspoon each of cayenne pepper, ground coriander, red chili paste, salt, and ground cumin
- 2 garlic cloves, minced
- 1 1/2 tablespoons parsley, chopped
- 1/4 cup of olive oil
- 1 tablespoon mint, chopped, For the yogurt
- 2 tablespoons of buttermilk
- 1 garlic clove, minced
- 1/4 cup mint, chopped
- 1/2 cup of Greek yogurt, non-fat
- Salt to taste

Direction: Preparation Time: 10 minutes
Servings: 4 **Cooking Time:** 8 minutes

- Set the Air Fryer to 390 degrees.
- Mix all the ingredients for the meatballs in a bowl. Roll and mold them into golf-size round pieces. Arrange in the cooking basket. Cook for 8 minutes.
- While waiting, combine all the ingredients for the mint yogurt in a bowl. Mix well.
- Serve the meatballs with the mint yogurt. Top with olives and fresh mint.

Nutrition: Calorie: 154 Carbohydrate: 9g Fat: 2.5g Protein: 8.6g Fiber: 2.4g

139) Air Fried Section and Tomato

Ingredients:

- 1 aubergine, sliced thickly into 4 disks
- 1 tomato, sliced into 2 thick disks
- 2 tsp. feta cheese, reduced fat
- 2 fresh basil leaves, minced
- 2 balls, small buffalo mozzarella, reduced fat, roughly torn
- Pinch of salt
- Pinch of black pepper

Direction: Preparation Time: 10 minutes
Cooking Time: 5 minutes **Servings:** 2

- Preheat Air Fryer to 330 degrees F.
- Spray small amount of oil into the Air fryer basket. Fry aubergine slices for 5 minutes or until golden brown on both sides. Transfer to a plate.
- Fry tomato slices in batches for 5 minutes or until seared on both sides.
- To serve, stack salad starting with an aborigine base, buffalo mozzarella, basil leaves, tomato slice, and 1/2-teaspoon feta cheese.
- Top of with another slice of aborigine and 1/2 tsp. feta cheese. Serve.

Nutrition: Calorie: 140.3 Carbohydrate: 26.6 Fat: 3.4g Protein: 4.2g Fiber: 7.3g

140) Cheesy Salmon Fillets

Ingredients:

Ingredients: For the salmon fillets

- 2 pieces, 4 oz. each salmon fillets, choose even cuts
- 1/2 cup sour cream, reduced fat
- ¼ cup cottage cheese, reduced fat
- ¼ cup Parmigiano-Reggiano cheese, freshly grated

Garnish:

- Spanish paprika
- 1/2 piece lemon, cut into wedges

Direction: Preparation Time: 15 minutes
Cooking Time: 20 minutes Servings: 2-3

- ✓ Preheat Air Fryer to 330 degrees F.
- ✓ To make the salmon fillets, mix sour cream, cottage cheese, and Parmigiano-Reggiano cheese in a bowl.
- ✓ Layer salmon fillets in the Air fryer basket. Fry for 20 minutes or until cheese turns golden brown.
- ✓ To assemble, place a salmon fillet and sprinkle paprika. Garnish with lemon wedges and squeeze lemon juice on top. Serve.

Nutrition: Calorie: 274 Carbohydrate: 1g Fat: 19g Protein: 24g Fiber: 0.5g

SALAD

141) Tuna Salad Recipe 1

Ingredients:

- 1 can tuna (6 oz.)
- 1/3 cup fresh cucumber, chopped
- 1/3 cup fresh tomato, chopped
- 1/3 cup avocado, chopped
- 1/3 cup celery, chopped
- 2 garlic cloves, minced
- 4 tsp. olive oil
- 2 tbsp. lime juice
- Pinch of black pepper

Direction: Preparation Time: 10 minutes
Cooking time: none Servings: 3

- ✓ Prepare the dressing by combining olive oil, lime juice, minced garlic and black pepper.
- ✓ Mix the salad ingredients in a salad bowl and drizzle with the dressing.

Nutrition: Carbohydrates: 4.8 g Protein: 14.3 g Total sugars: 1.1 g Calories: 212 g

142) Roasted Portobello Salad

Ingredients:

- 1 1/2 lb. Portobello mushrooms, stems trimmed
- 3 heads Belgian endive, sliced
- 1 small red onion, sliced
- 4 oz. blue cheese
- 8 oz. mixed salad greens

Dressing:

- 3 tbsp. red wine vinegar
- 1 tbsp. Dijon mustard
- 2/3 cup olive oil
- Salt and pepper to taste

Direction: Preparation Time: 10 minutes
Cooking time: none Servings: 4

- ✓ Preheat the oven to 450F.
- ✓ Prepare the dressing by whisking together vinegar, mustard, salt and pepper. Slowly add olive oil while whisking.
- ✓ Cut the mushrooms and arrange them on a baking sheet, stem-side up. Coat the mushrooms with some dressing and bake for 15 minutes.
- ✓ In a salad bowl toss the salad greens with onion, endive and cheese. Sprinkle with the dressing.
- ✓ Add mushrooms to the salad bowl.

Nutrition: Carbohydrates: 22.3 g Protein: 14.9 g Total sugars: 2.1 g Calories: 501

143) Shredded Chicken Salad

Ingredients:

- 2 chicken breasts, boneless, skinless
- 1 head iceberg lettuce, cut into strips
- 2 bell peppers, cut into strips
- 1 fresh cucumber, quartered, sliced
- 3 scallions, sliced
- 2 tbsp. chopped peanuts
- 1 tbsp. peanut vinaigrette
- Salt to taste
- 1 cup water

Direction: Preparation Time: 5 minutes
Cooking time: 10 minutes Servings: 6

- ✓ In a skillet simmer one cup of salted water.
- ✓ Add the chicken breasts, cover and cook on low for 5 minutes. Remove the cover. Then remove the chicken from the skillet and shred with a fork.
- ✓ In a salad bowl mix the vegetables with the cooled chicken, season with salt and sprinkle with peanut vinaigrette and chopped peanuts.

Nutrition: Carbohydrates: 9 g Protein: 11.6 g Total sugars: 4.2 g Calories: 117

144) Broccoli Salad 1

Ingredients:

- 1 medium head broccoli, raw, florets only
- 1/2 cup red onion, chopped
- 12 oz. turkey bacon, chopped, fried until crisp
- 1/2 cup cherry tomatoes, halved
- ¼ cup sunflower kernels
- ¾ cup raisins
- ¾ cup mayonnaise
- 2 tbsp. white vinegar

Direction: Preparation Time: 10 minutes
Cooking time: none Servings: 6

- ✓ In a salad bowl combine the broccoli, tomatoes and onion.
- ✓ Mix mayo with vinegar and sprinkle over the broccoli.
- ✓ Add the sunflower kernels, raisins and bacon and toss well.

Nutrition: Carbohydrates: 17.3 g Protein: 11 g Total sugars: 10 g Calories: 220

145) Cherry Tomato Salad

Ingredients:

- 40 cherry tomatoes, halved
- 1 cup mozzarella balls, halved
- 1 cup green olives, sliced
- 1 can (6 oz.) black olives, sliced
- 2 green onions, chopped
- 3 oz. roasted pine nuts

Dressing:

- 1/2 cup olive oil
- 2 tbsp. red wine vinegar
- 1 tsp. dried oregano
- Salt and pepper to taste

Direction: Preparation Time: 10 minutes
Cooking time: none Servings: 6

- ✓ In a salad bowl, combine the tomatoes, olives and onions.
- ✓ Prepare the dressing by combining olive oil with red wine vinegar, dried oregano, salt and pepper.
- ✓ Sprinkle with the dressing and add the nuts.
- ✓ Let marinate in the fridge for 1 hour.

Nutrition: Carbohydrates: 10.7 g Protein: 2.4 g Total sugars: 3.6 g

146) Ground Turkey Salad

Ingredients:

- 1 lb. lean ground turkey
- 1/2 inch ginger, minced
- 2 garlic cloves, minced
- 1 onion, chopped
- 1 tbsp. olive oil
- 1 bag lettuce leaves (for serving)
- ¼ cup fresh cilantro, chopped
- 2 tsp. coriander powder
- 1 tsp. red chili powder
- 1 tsp. turmeric powder
- Salt to taste
- 4 cups water
- Dressing:
- 2 tbsp. fat free yogurt
- 1 tbsp. sour cream, non-fat
- 1 tbsp. low fat mayonnaise
- 1 lemon, juiced
- 1 tsp. red chili flakes
- Salt and pepper to taste

Direction: Preparation Time: 10 minutes
Cooking time: 35 minutes **Servings:** 6

- ✓ In a skillet sauté the garlic and ginger in olive oil for 1 minute. Add onion and season with salt. Cook for 10 minutes over medium heat.
- ✓ Add the ground turkey and sauté for 3 more minutes. Add the spices (turmeric, red chili powder and coriander powder).
- ✓ Add 4 cups water and cook for 30 minutes, covered.
- ✓ Prepare the dressing by combining yogurt, sour cream, mayo, lemon juice, chili flakes, salt and pepper.
- ✓ To serve arrange the salad leaves on serving plates and place the cooked ground turkey on them. Top with dressing.

Nutrition: Carbohydrates: 9.1 g Protein: 17.8 g Total sugars: 2.5 g
Calories: 176

147) Asian Cucumber Salad

Ingredients:

- 1 lb. cucumbers, sliced
- 2 scallions, sliced
- 2 tbsp. sliced pickled ginger, chopped
- ¼ cup cilantro
- 1/2 red jalapeño, chopped
- 3 tbsp. rice wine vinegar
- 1 tbsp. sesame oil
- 1 tbsp. sesame seeds

Direction: Preparation Time: 10 minutes
Cooking time: none **Servings:** 6

- ✓ In a salad bowl combine all ingredients and toss together.
- ✓ Enjoy!

Nutrition: Carbohydrates: 5.7 g Protein: 1 g Total sugars: 3.1 g
Calories: 52

148) Cauliflower Tofu Salad

Ingredients:

- 2 cups cauliflower florets, blended
- 1 fresh cucumber, diced
- 1/2 cup green olives, diced
- 1/3 cup red onion, diced
- 2 tbsp. toasted pine nuts
- 2 tbsp. raisins
- 1/3 cup feta, crumbled
- 1/2 cup pomegranate seeds
- 2 lemons (juiced, zest grated)
- 8 oz. tofu
- 2 tsp. oregano
- 2 garlic cloves, minced
- 1/2 tsp. red chili flakes
- 3 tbsp. olive oil
- Salt and pepper to taste

Direction: Preparation time: 10 minutes
Cooking time: 15 minutes **Servings:** 4

- ✓ Season the processed cauliflower with salt and transfer to a strainer to drain.
- ✓ Prepare the marinade for tofu by combining 2 tbsp. lemon juice, 1.5 tbsp. olive oil, minced garlic, chili flakes, oregano, salt and pepper. Coat tofu in the marinade and set aside.
- ✓ Preheat the oven to 450F.
- ✓ Bake tofu on a baking sheet for 12 minutes.
- ✓ In a salad bowl mix the remaining marinade with onions, cucumber, cauliflower, olives and raisins. Add in the remaining olive oil and grated lemon zest.
- ✓ Top with tofu, pine nuts, and feta and pomegranate seeds.

Nutrition: Carbohydrates: 34.1 g Protein: 11.1 g Total sugars: 11.5 g
Calories: 328

149) Scallop Caesar Salad

Ingredients:

- 8 sea scallops
- 4 cups romaine lettuce
- 2 tsp. olive oil
- 3 tbsp. Caesar Salad Dressing
- 1 tsp. lemon juice
- Salt and pepper to taste

Direction: Preparation Time: 5 minutes
Cooking Time: 2 minutes **Servings:** 2

- ✓ In a frying pan heat olive oil and cook the scallops in one layer no longer than 2 minutes per both sides. Season with salt and pepper to taste.
- ✓ Arrange lettuce on plates and place scallops on top.
- ✓ Pour over the Caesar dressing and lemon juice.

Nutrition: Carbohydrates: 14 g Protein: 30.7 g Total sugars: 2.2 g
Calories: 340 g

150) Chicken Avocado Salad

Ingredients:

- 1 lb. chicken breast, cooked, shredded
- 1 avocado, pitted, peeled, sliced
- 2 tomatoes, diced
- 1 cucumber, peeled, sliced
- 1 head lettuce, chopped
- 3 tbsp. olive oil
- 2 tbsp. lime juice
- 1 tbsp. cilantro, chopped
- Salt and pepper to taste

Direction: Preparation Time: 30 minutes
Cooking time: 15 minutes **Servings:** 4

- ✓ In a bowl whisk together oil, lime juice, cilantro, salt, and a pinch of pepper.
- ✓ Combine lettuce, tomatoes, cucumber in a salad bowl and toss with half of the dressing.
- ✓ Toss chicken with the remaining dressing and combine with vegetable mixture.
- ✓ Top with avocado.

Nutrition: Carbohydrates: 10 g Protein: 38 g Total sugars: 11.5 g
Calories: 380

151) California Wraps

Ingredients:

- 4 slices turkey breast, cooked
- 4 slices ham, cooked
- 4 lettuce leaves
- 4 slices tomato
- 4 slices avocado
- 1 tsp. lime juice
- A handful watercress leaves
- 4 tbsp. Ranch dressing, sugar free

Direction: Preparation Time: 5 minutes
Cooking Time: 15 minutes Servings: 4

- ✓ Top a lettuce leaf with turkey slice, ham slice and tomato.
- ✓ In a bowl combine avocado and lime juice and place on top of tomatoes. Top with water cress and dressing.
- ✓ Repeat with the remaining ingredients for 4. Topping each lettuce leaf with a turkey slice, ham slice, tomato and dressing.

Nutrition: Carbohydrates: 4 g Protein: 9 g Total sugars: 0.5 g Calories: 140

152) Chicken Breast Salad

Ingredients:

- 1/2 chicken breast, skinless, boiled and shredded
- 2 long cucumbers, cut into 8 thick rounds each, scooped out (won't use in a).
- 1 tsp. ginger, minced
- 1 tsp. lime zest, grated
- 4 tsp. olive oil
- 1 tsp. sesame oil
- 1 tsp. lime juice
- Salt and pepper to taste

Direction: Preparation Time: 5 minutes
Cooking Time: 15 minutes Servings: 4

- ✓ In a bowl combine lime zest, juice, olive and sesame oils, ginger, and season with salt.
- ✓ Toss the chicken with the dressing and fill the cucumber cups with the salad.

Nutrition: Carbohydrates: 4 g Protein: 12 g Total sugars: 0.5 g Calories: 116 g

153) Sunflower Seeds and Arugula Garden Salad

Ingredients:

- ¼ tsp. black pepper
- ¼ tsp. salt
- 1 tsp. fresh thyme, chopped
- 2 tbsp. sunflower seeds, toasted
- 2 cups red grapes, halved
- 7 cups baby arugula, loosely packed
- 1 tbsp. coconut oil
- 2 tsp. honey
- 3 tbsp. red wine vinegar
- 1/2 tsp. stone-ground mustard

Direction: Preparation time: 5 minutes
Cooking time: 10 minutes   Servings: 6

- ✓ In a small bowl, whisk together mustard, honey and vinegar. Slowly pour oil as you whisk.
- ✓ In a large salad bowl, mix thyme, seeds, grapes and arugula.
- ✓ Drizzle with dressing and serve.

Nutrition: Calories: 86.7g Protein: 1.6g Carbs: 13.1g Fat: 3.1g.

154) Supreme Caesar Salad

Ingredients:

- ¼ cup olive oil
- ¾ cup mayonnaise
- 1 head romaine lettuce, torn into bite sized pieces
- 1 tbsp. lemon juice
- 1 tsp. Dijon mustard
- 1 tsp. Worcestershire sauce
- 3 cloves garlic, peeled and minced
- 3 cloves garlic, peeled and quartered
- 4 cups day old bread, cubed
- 5 anchovy filets, minced
- 6 tbsp. grated parmesan cheese, divided
- Ground black pepper to taste
- Salt to taste

Direction: Preparation time: 5 minutes
Cooking time: 10 minutes Servings: 4

- ✓ In a small bowl, whisk well lemon juice, mustard, Worcestershire sauce, 2 tbsp. parmesan cheese, anchovies, mayonnaise, and minced garlic. Season with pepper and salt to taste. Set aside in the ref.
- ✓ On medium fire, place a large nonstick saucepan and heat oil.
- ✓ Sauté quartered garlic until browned around a minute or two. Remove and discard.
- ✓ Add bread cubes in same pan, sauté until lightly browned. Season with pepper and salt. Transfer to a plate.
- ✓ In large bowl, place lettuce and pour in dressing. Toss well to coat. Top with remaining parmesan cheese.
- ✓ Garnish with bread cubes, serve, and enjoy.

Nutrition: Calories: 443.3g Fat: 32.1g Protein: 11.6g Carbs: 27g

155) Tabbouleh- Arabian Salad

Ingredients:

- ¼ cup chopped fresh mint
- 1 2/3 cups boiling water
- 1 cucumber, peeled, seeded and chopped
- 1 cup bulgur
- 1 cup chopped fresh parsley
- 1 cup chopped green onions
- 1 tsp. salt
- 1/3 cup lemon juice
- 1/3 cup olive oil
- 3 tomatoes, chopped
- Ground black pepper to taste

Direction: Preparation time: 5 minutes
Cooking time: 10 minutes   Servings: 6

- ✓ In a large bowl, mix together boiling water and bulgur. Let soak and set aside for an hour while covered.
- ✓ After one hour, toss in cucumber, tomatoes, mint, parsley, onions, lemon juice and oil. Then season with black pepper and salt to taste. Toss well and refrigerate for another hour while covered before serving.

Nutrition: Calories: 185.5g fat: 13.1g Protein: 4.1g Carbs: 12.8g

APPETIZERS AND

156) Broccoli Salad 2

Ingredients:

- 8 cups broccoli florets
- 3 strips of bacon, cooked and crumbled
- ¼ cup sunflower kernels
- 1 bunch of green onion, sliced

What you will need from the store cupboard:

- 3 tablespoons seasoned rice vinegar
- 3 tablespoons canola oil
- 1/2 cup dried cranberries

Direction: Preparation Time: 10 minutes, Cooking Time: 10 minutes; Servings: 10

- ✓ Combine the green onion, cranberries, and broccoli in a bowl.
- ✓ Whisk the vinegar, and oil in another bowl. Blend well.
- ✓ Now drizzle over the broccoli mix.
- ✓ Coat well by tossing.
- ✓ Sprinkle bacon and sunflower kernels before serving.

Nutrition: Calories 121, Carbs 14g, Cholesterol 2mg, Fiber 3g, Sugar 1g, Fat 7g, Protein 3g, Sodium 233mg

157) Tenderloin Grilled Salad

Ingredients:

- 1 lb. pork tenderloin
- 10 cups mixed salad greens
- 2 oranges, seedless, cut into bite-sized pieces
- 1 tablespoon orange zest, grated

What you will need from the store cupboard:

- 2 tablespoons of cider vinegar
- 2 tablespoons olive oil
- 2 teaspoons Dijon mustard
- 1/2 cup juice of an orange
- 2 teaspoons honey
- 1/2 teaspoon ground pepper

Direction:

- ✓ Bring together all the dressing ingredients in a bowl.
- ✓ Grill each side of the pork covered over medium heat for 9 minutes.
- ✓ Slice after 5 minutes.
- ✓ Slice the tenderloin thinly.
- ✓ Keep the greens on your serving plate.
- ✓ Top with the pork and oranges.
- ✓ Sprinkle nuts (optional).

Nutrition: Calories 211, Carbs 13g, Cholesterol 51mg, Fiber 3g, Sugar 0.8g, Fat 9g, Protein 20g, Sodium 113mg

158) Barley Veggie Salad

Ingredients:

- 1 tomato, seeded and chopped
- 2 tablespoons parsley, minced
- 1 yellow pepper, chopped
- 1 tablespoon basil, minced
- ¼ cup almonds, toasted

What you will need from the store cupboard:

- 1-1/4 cups vegetable broth
- 1 cup barley
- 1 tablespoon lemon juice
- 2 tablespoons of white wine vinegar
- 3 tablespoons olive oil
- ¼ teaspoon pepper
- 1/2 teaspoon salt
- 1 cup of water

Direction: Preparation Time: 10 minutes, Cooking Time: 20 minutes; Servings: 6

- ✓ Boil the broth, barley, and water in a saucepan.
- ✓ Reduce heat. Cover and let it simmer for 10 minutes.
- ✓ Take out from the heat.
- ✓ In the meantime, bring together the parsley, yellow pepper, and tomato in a bowl.
- ✓ Stir the barley in.
- ✓ Whisk the vinegar, oil, basil, lemon juice, water, pepper and salt in a bowl.
- ✓ Pour this over your barley mix. Toss to coat well.
- ✓ Stir the almonds in before serving.

Nutrition: Calories 211, Carbs 27g, Cholesterol 0mg, Fiber 7g, Sugar 0g, Fat 10g, Protein 6g, Sodium 334mg

159) Spinach Shrimp Salad

Ingredients:

- 1 lb. uncooked shrimp, peeled and deveined
- 2 tablespoons parsley, minced
- ¾ cup halved cherry tomatoes
- 1 medium lemon
- 4 cups baby spinach

What you will need from the store cupboard:

- 2 tablespoons butter
- 3 minced garlic cloves
- ¼ teaspoon pepper
- ¼ teaspoon salt

Direction:

- ✓ Melt the butter over medium temperature in a nonstick skillet.
- ✓ Add the shrimp.
- ✓ Now cook the shrimp for 3 minutes until your shrimp becomes pink.
- ✓ Add the parsley and garlic.
- ✓ Cook for another minute. Take out from the heat.
- ✓ Keep the spinach in your salad bowl.
- ✓ Top with the shrimp mix and tomatoes.
- ✓ Drizzle lemon juice on the salad.
- ✓ Sprinkle pepper and salt.

Nutrition: Calories 201, Carbs 6g, Cholesterol 153mg, Fiber 2g, Sugar 0g, Fat 10g, Protein 21g, Sodium 350mg

160) Sweet Potato and Roasted Beet Salad

Ingredients:

- 2 beets
- 1 sweet potato, peeled and cubed
- 1 garlic clove, minced
- 2 tablespoons walnuts, chopped and toasted
- 1 cup fennel bulb, sliced

What you will need from the store cupboard:

- 3 tablespoons balsamic vinegar
- 1 teaspoon Dijon mustard
- 1 tablespoon honey
- 3 tablespoons olive oil
- ¼ teaspoon pepper
- ¼ teaspoon salt
- 3 tablespoons water

Direction:

- Scrub the beets. Trim the tops to 1 inch.
- Wrap in foil and keep on a baking sheet.
- Bake until tender. Take off the foil.
- Combine water and sweet potato in a bowl.
- Cover. Microwave for 5 minutes. Drain off.
- Now peel the beets. Cut into small wedges.
- Arrange the fennel, sweet potato and beets on 4 salad plates.
- Sprinkle nuts.
- Whisk the honey, mustard, vinegar, water, garlic, pepper and salt.
- Whisk in oil gradually.
- Drizzle over the salad.

Nutrition: Calories 270, Carbs 37g, Cholesterol 0mg, Fiber 6g, Sugar 0.3g, Fat 13g, Protein 5g, Sodium 309mg

161) Potato Calico Salad

Ingredients:

- 4 red potatoes, peeled and cooked
- 1-1/2 cups kernel corn, cooked
- 1/2 cup green pepper, diced
- 1/2 cup red onion, chopped
- 1 cup carrot, shredded

What you will need from the store cupboard:

- 1/2 cup olive oil
- ¼ cup vinegar
- 1-1/2 teaspoons chili powder
- 1 teaspoon salt
- Dash of hot pepper sauce

Direction: Preparation Time: 15 minutes, Cooking Time: 5 minutes; Servings: 14

- Keep all the ingredients together in a jar.
- Close it and shake well.
- Cube the potatoes. Combine with the carrot, onion, and corn in your salad bowl.
- Pour the dressing over.
- Now toss lightly.

Nutrition: Calories 146, Carbs 17g, Cholesterol 0mg, Fiber 0g, Sugar 0g, Fat 9g, Protein 2g, Sodium 212mg

162) Mango and Jicama Salad

Ingredients:

- 1 jicama, peeled
- 1 mango, peeled
- 1 teaspoon ginger root, minced
- 1/3 cup chives, minced
- 1/2 cup cilantro, chopped

What you will need from the store cupboard:

- ¼ cup canola oil
- 1/2 cup white wine vinegar
- 2 tablespoons of lime juice
- ¼ cup honey
- 1/8 teaspoon pepper
- ¼ teaspoon salt

Direction: Preparation Time: 15 minutes, Cooking Time: 5 minutes; Servings: 8

- Whisk together the vinegar, honey, canola oil, gingerroot, paper, and salt.
- Cut the mango and jicama into matchsticks.
- Keep in a bowl.
- Now toss with the lime juice.
- Add the dressing and herbs. Combine well by tossing.

Nutrition: Calories 143, Carbs 20g, Cholesterol 0mg, Fiber 3g, Sugar 1.6g, Fat 7g, Protein 1g, Sodium 78mg

163) Asian Crispy Chicken Salad

Ingredients:

- 2 chicken breast halved, skinless
- 1/2 cup panko bread crumbs
- 4 cups spring mix salad greens
- 4 teaspoons of sesame seeds
- 1/2 cup mushrooms, sliced

What you will need from the store cupboard:

- 1 teaspoon sesame oil
- 2 teaspoons of canola oil
- 2 teaspoons hoisin sauce
- ¼ cup sesame ginger salad dressing

Direction:

- Flatten the chicken breasts to half-inch thickness.
- Mix the sesame oil and hoisin sauce. Brush over the chicken.
- Combine the sesame seeds and panko in a bowl.
- Now dip the chicken mix in it.
- Cook each side of the chicken for 5 minutes.
- In the meantime, divide the salad greens between two plates.
- Top with mushroom.
- Slice the chicken and keep on top. Drizzle the dressing.

Nutrition: Calories 386, Carbs 29g, Cholesterol 63mg, Fiber 6g, Sugar 1g, Fat 17g, Protein 30g, Sodium 620mg

164) Kale, Grape and Bulgur Salad

Ingredients:

- 1 cup bulgur
- 1 cup pecan, toasted and chopped
- ¼ cup scallions, sliced
- 1/2 cup parsley, chopped
- 2 cups California grapes, seedless and halved

What you will need from the store cupboard:

- 2 tablespoons of extra virgin olive oil
- ¼ cup of juice from a lemon
- Pinch of kosher salt
- Pinch of black pepper
- 2 cups of water

Direction:

- Boil 2 cups of water in a saucepan
- Stir the bulgur in and 1/2 teaspoon of salt.
- Take out from the heat.
- Keep covered. Drain.
- Stir in the other ingredients.
- Season with pepper and salt.

Nutrition: Calories 289, Carbohydrates 33g, Fat 17g, Protein 6g,

165) Strawberry Salsa

Ingredients:

- 4 tomatoes, seeded and chopped
- 1-pint strawberry, chopped
- 1 red onion, chopped
- 2 tablespoons of juice from a lime
- 1 jalapeno pepper, minced

Direction:

- ✓ Bring together the strawberries, tomatoes, jalapeno, and onion in the bowl.
- ✓ Stir in the garlic, oil, and lime juice.

What you will need from the store cupboard:

- 1 tablespoon olive oil
- 2 garlic cloves, minced

- ✓ Refrigerate. Serve with separately cooked pork or poultry.

Nutrition: Calories 19, Carbs 3g, Fiber 1g, Sugar 0.2g, Cholesterol 0mg, Total Fat 1g, Protein 0g

166) Garden Wraps

Ingredients:

- 1 cucumber, chopped
- 1 sweet corn
- 1 cabbage, shredded
- 1 tablespoon lettuce, minced
- 1 tomato, chopped

What you will need from the store cupboard:

- 3 tablespoons of rice vinegar
- 2 teaspoons peanut butter
- 1/3 cup onion paste
- 1/3 cup chili sauce
- 2 teaspoons of low-sodium soy sauce

Direction: Preparation Time: 20 minutes, Cooking Time: 10 minutes; Servings: 8

- ✓ Cut corn from the cob. Keep in a bowl.
- ✓ Add the tomato, cabbage, cucumber, and onion paste.
- ✓ Now whisk the vinegar, peanut butter, and chili sauce together.
- ✓ Pour this over the vegetable mix. Toss for coating.

- ✓ Let this stand for 10 minutes.
- ✓ Take your slotted spoon and place 1/2 cup salad in every lettuce leaf.
- ✓ Fold the lettuce over your filling.

Nutrition: Calories 64, Carbs 13g, Fiber 2g, Sugar 1g, Cholesterol 0mg, Total Fat 1g, Protein 2g

167) Party Shrimp

Ingredients:

- 16 oz. uncooked shrimp, peeled and deveined
- 1-1/2 teaspoons of juice from a lemon
- 1/2 teaspoon basil, chopped
- 1 teaspoon coriander, chopped
- 1/2 cup tomato

What you will need from the store cupboard:

- 1 tablespoon of olive oil
- 1/2 teaspoon Italian seasoning
- 1/2 teaspoon paprika
- 1 sliced garlic clove
- 1/4 teaspoon pepper

Direction: Preparation Time: 15 minutes, Cooking Time: 10 minutes; Servings: 30

- ✓ Bring together everything except the shrimp in a dish or bowl.
- ✓ Add the shrimp. Coat well by tossing. Set aside.
- ✓ Drain the shrimp. Discard the marinade.

- ✓ Keep them on a baking sheet. It should not be greased.
- ✓ Broil each side for 4 minutes. The shrimp should become pink.

Nutrition: Calories 14, Carbs 0g, Fiber 0g, Sugar 0g, Cholesterol 18mg

168) Zucchini Mini Pizzas

Ingredients:

- 1 zucchini, cut into ¼ inch slices diagonally
- 1/2 cup pepperoni, small slices
- 1 teaspoon basil, minced
- 1/2 cup onion, chopped
- 1 cup tomatoes

What you will need from the store cupboard:

- 1/8 teaspoon pepper
- 1/8 teaspoon salt
- 3/4 cup mozzarella cheese, shredded
- 1/3 cup pizza sauce

Direction:

- ✓ Preheat your broiler. Keep the zucchini in 1 layer on your greased baking sheet.
- ✓ Add the onion and tomatoes. Broil each side for 1 to 2 minutes till they become tender and crisp.
- ✓ Now sprinkle pepper and salt.

- ✓ Top with cheese, pepperoni, and sauce.
- ✓ Broil for a minute. The cheese should melt.
- ✓ Sprinkle basil on top.

Nutrition: Calories 29, Carbs 1g, Fiber 0g, Sugar 1g, Cholesterol 5mg, Total Fat 2g, Protein 2g

169) Garlic-Sesame Pumpkin Seeds

Ingredients:

- 1 egg white
- 1 teaspoon onion, minced
- 1/2 teaspoon caraway seeds
- 2 cups pumpkin seeds
- 1 teaspoon sesame seeds

What you will need from the store cupboard:

- 1 garlic clove, minced
- 1 tablespoon of canola oil
- ¾ teaspoon of kosher salt

Direction: Preparation Time: 10 minutes

Cooking Time: 20 minutes Servings: 2

- ✓ Preheat your oven to 350 °F.
- ✓ Whisk together the oil and egg white in a bowl.
- ✓ Include pumpkin seeds. Coat well by tossing.
- ✓ Now stir in the onion, garlic, sesame seeds, caraway seeds, and salt

- ✓ Spread in 1 layer in your parchment-lined baking pan.
- ✓ Bake for 15 minutes until it turns golden brown.
- ✓

Nutrition: Calories 95, Carbs 9g, Fiber 3g, Sugar 0g, Cholesterol 0mg, Total Fat 5g, Protein 4g

170) Tuna Salad Recipe 2

Ingredients:

- 2 (5-ounce) cans water packed tuna, drained
- 2 tablespoons fat-free plain Greek yogurt
- Salt and ground black pepper, as required

- 2 medium carrots, peeled and shredded
- 2 apples, cored and chopped
- 2 cups fresh spinach, torn

Direction: Preparation Time: 15 minutes

Servings: 2

- ✓ In a large bowl, add the tuna, yogurt, salt and black pepper and gently, stir to combine.

- ✓ Add the carrots and apples and stir to combine.
- ✓ Serve immediately.

Nutrition: Calories 306; Total Fat 1.8g ; Saturated Fat 0 g ; Cholesterol 63 mg ; Total Carbs 38 g Sugar 26 g ; Fiber 7.6 g ; Sodium 324 mg ; Potassium 602 mg ; Protein 35.8 g

POULTRY

171) Chicken Soup

Ingredients:

- 1 tablespoon olive oil
- 1 small carrot, peeled and chopped ½ cup onion, chopped
- 1 celery stalk, chopped 2 garlic cloves, minced
- 1 tablespoon fresh thyme, chopped 1 tablespoon fresh rosemary, chopped
- ½ teaspoon ground cumin
- ¼ teaspoon red pepper flakes, crushed lime zest, grated finely
- 5 cups low-sodium chicken broth
- 1¼ cups cooked chicken, chopped
- 2 cups fresh spinach, torn
- 1¼ cups zucchini, chopped
- Ground black pepper, as required
- 2 tablespoons fresh lime juice 1 teaspoon fresh

Direction: Preparation Time: 15 minutes Cooking Time: 23 minutes
Servings: 4

- ✓ In a large soup pan, heat the oil over medium heat and sauté the carrot, onion and celery for about 8-9 minutes.
- ✓ Add the garlic, rosemary and spices and sauté for about 1 minute.
- ✓ Add the broth and bring to a boil over high heat.
- ✓ Now, reduce the heat to medium-low and simmer for about 5 minutes.
- ✓ Add the cooked chicken, spinach and zucchini and simmer for about 6-8 minutes.
- ✓ Stir in the black pepper and lime juice and remove from heat.
- ✓ Serve hot with the garnishing of lime zest. Meal Prep Tip: Transfer the soup into a large bowl and set aside to cool.
- ✓ Divide the soup into 4 containers evenly. Cover the containers and refrigerate for 1-2 days. Reheat in the microwave before serving.

Nutrition: Calories 224 Total Fat 6.8g Saturated Fat 1.4 g Cholesterol 74 mg Total Carbs 7.5 g Sugar 2 g Fiber 2.2 g Sodium 178 mg Potassium 456 mg Protein 31.8 g

172) Chicken Chili

Ingredients:

- 4 cups low-sodium chicken broth, divided
- 3 cups boiled black beans, divided 1 tablespoon extra-virgin olive oil
- 1 large onion, chopped 1 jalapeño pepper, seeded and chopped
- 4 garlic cloves, minced 1 teaspoon dried thyme, crushed
- 1½ tablespoons ground coriander
- 1 tablespoon ground cumin
- ½ tablespoon red chili powder
- 4 cups cooked chicken, shredded
- 1 tablespoon fresh lime juice
- ¼ cup fresh cilantro, chopped

Direction: Preparation Time: 15 minutes Cooking Time: 40 minutes
Servings: 6

- ✓ In a food processor, add 1 cup of broth and 1 can of black beans and pulse until smooth. Transfer the beans puree into a bowl and set aside.
- ✓ In a large pan, heat the oil over medium heat and sauté the onion and jalapeño for about 4-5 minutes.
- ✓ Add the garlic, spices and sea salt and sauté for about 1 minute.
- ✓ Add the beans puree and remaining broth and bring to a boil. Now, reduce the heat to low and simmer for about 20 minutes.
- ✓ Stir in the remaining can of beans, chicken and lime juice and bring to a boil.
- ✓ Now, reduce the heat to low and simmer for about 5-10 minutes.
- ✓ Serve hot with the garnishing of cilantro.
- ✓ Meal Prep Tip: Transfer the chili into a large bowl and set aside to cool.
- ✓ Divide the chili into 6 containers evenly. Cover the containers and refrigerate for 1-2 days.
- ✓ Reheat in the microwave before serving.

Nutrition: Calories 356 Total Fat 7.1 g Saturated Fat 1.2 g Cholesterol 72 mg Total Carbs 33 g Sugar 2.7 g Fiber 11.6 g Sodium 130 mg Potassium 662 mg Protein 39.6 g

173) Chicken with Chickpeas

Ingredients:

- 2 tablespoons olive oil
- 1 pound skinless, boneless chicken breast, cubed
- 2 carrots, peeled and sliced 1 onion, chopped
- 2 celery stalks, chopped 2 garlic cloves, chopped
- 1 tablespoon fresh ginger root, minced
- ½ teaspoon dried oregano, crushed
- ¾ teaspoon ground cumin
- ½ teaspoon paprika
- ¼-13 teaspoon cayenne pepper
- ¼ teaspoon ground turmeric
- 1 cup tomatoes, crushed
- 1½ cups low-sodium chicken broth
- 1 zucchini, sliced
- 1 cup boiled chickpeas, drained
- 1 tablespoon fresh lemon juice

Direction: Preparation Time: 15 minutes Cooking Time: 36 minutes Servings: 4

- ✓ In a large nonstick pan, heat the oil over medium heat and cook the chicken cubes for about 4-5 minutes.
- ✓ With a slotted spoon, transfer the chicken cubes onto a plate.
- ✓ In the same pan, add the carrot, onion, celery and garlic and sauté for about 4-5 minutes.
- ✓ Add the ginger, oregano and spices and sauté for about 1 minute.
- ✓ Add the chicken, tomato and broth and bring to a boil. Now, reduce the heat to low and simmer for about 10 minutes.
- ✓ Add the zucchini and chickpeas and simmer, covered for about 15 minutes. Stir in the lemon juice and serve hot.

Meal Prep Tip:

- ✓ Transfer the chicken mixture into a large bowl and set aside to cool. Divide the mixture into 4 containers evenly. Cover the containers and refrigerate for 1-2 days. Reheat in the microwave before serving.

Nutrition: Calories 308 Total Fat 12.3 g Saturated Fat 2.7 g Cholesterol 66 mg Total Carbs 19 g Sugar 5.3g Fiber 4.7 g Sodium 202 mg Potassium 331 mg Protein 30.7 g

174) Chicken & Broccoli Bake

Ingredients:

- 6 (6-ounce) boneless, skinless chicken breasts
- 3 broccoli heads, cut into florets
- 4 garlic cloves, minced
- ¼ cup olive oil
- 1 teaspoon dried oregano, crushed
- 1 teaspoon dried rosemary, crushed
- Sea Salt and ground black pepper, as required

Direction: Preparation Time: 15 minutes Cooking Time: 45 minutes Servings: 6

- ✓ Preheat the oven to 375 degrees F. Grease a large baking dish. In a large bowl, add all the ingredients and toss to coat well.
- ✓ In the bottom of prepared baking dish, arrange the broccoli florets and top with chicken breasts in a single layer.
- ✓ Bake for about 45 minutes.
- ✓ Remove from the oven and set aside for about 5 minutes before serving.

Meal Prep Tip:

- ✓ Remove the baking dish from the oven and set aside to cool completely. In 6 containers, divide the chicken breasts and broccoli evenly and refrigerate for about 2 days.
- ✓ Reheat in microwave before serving.

Nutrition: Calories 443 Total Fat 21.5 g Saturated Fat 4.7 g Cholesterol 151 mg Total Carbs 9.4 g Sugar 2.2g Fiber 3.6 g Sodium 189 mg Potassium 831 mg Protein 53 g

175) Meatballs Curry

Ingredients:

For Meatballs:

- 1 pound lean ground chicken
- 1 tablespoon onion paste
- 1 teaspoons fresh ginger paste
- 1 teaspoons garlic paste 1 green chili, chopped finely
- 1 tablespoon fresh cilantro leaves, chopped
- 1 teaspoon ground coriander
- ½ teaspoon cumin seeds
- ½ teaspoon red chili powder
- ½ teaspoon ground turmeric
- 1/8 teaspoon salt

For Curry:

- 3 tablespoons olive oil
- ½ teaspoon cumin seeds
- 1 (1-inch) cinnamon stick
- 2 onions, chopped 1 teaspoons fresh ginger, minced
- 1 teaspoons garlic, minced
- 4 tomatoes, chopped finely
- 2 teaspoons ground coriander
- 1 teaspoon garam masala powder
- ½ teaspoon ground nutmeg
- ½ teaspoon red chili powder
- ½ teaspoon ground turmeric
- Salt, as required 1 cup filtered water 3 tablespoons fresh cilantro, chopped

Direction: Preparation Time: 20 minutes Cooking Time: 25 minutes Servings: 6

For meatballs:

- ✓ In a large bowl, add all ingredients and mix until well combined.
- ✓ Make small equal-sized meatballs from mixture. In a large deep skillet, heat the oil over medium heat and cook the meatballs for about 3-5 minutes or until browned from all sides.
- ✓ Transfer the meatballs into a bowl. In the same skillet, add the cumin seeds and cinnamon stick and sauté for about 1 minute.
- ✓ Add the onions and sauté for about 4-5 minutes.
- ✓ Add the ginger and garlic paste and sauté for about 1 minute.
- ✓ Add the tomato and spices and cook, crushing with the back of spoon for about 2-3 minutes.
- ✓ Add the water and meatballs and bring to a boil.
- ✓ Now, reduce the heat to low and simmer for about 10 minutes.
- ✓ Serve hot with the garnishing of cilantro.

Meal Prep Tip:

- ✓ Transfer the curry into a large bowl and set aside to cool. Divide the curry into 5 containers evenly.
- ✓ Cover the containers and refrigerate for 1-2 days. Reheat in the microwave before serving.

Nutrition: Calories 196 Total Fat 11.4 g Saturated Fat 2.4 g Cholesterol 53 mg Total Carbs 7.9 g Sugar 3.9 g Fiber 2.1 g Sodium 143 mg Potassium 279 mg Protein 16.7 g

176) Chicken, Oats & Chickpeas Meatloaf

Ingredients:

- ½ cup cooked chickpeas
- 2 egg whites
- 2½ teaspoons poultry seasoning
- Ground black pepper, as required
- 10 ounce lean ground chicken 1 cup red bell pepper, seeded and minced
- 1 cup celery stalk, minced
- 1/3 cup steel-cut oats 1 cup tomato puree, divided
- 2 tablespoons dried onion flakes, crushed
- 1 tablespoon prepared mustard

Direction: Preparation Time: 20 minutes Cooking Time: 1¼ hours Servings: 4

- ✓ Preheat the oven to 350 degrees F. Grease a 9x5-inch loaf pan. In a food processor, add chickpeas, egg whites, poultry seasoning and black pepper and pulse until smooth.
- ✓ Transfer the mixture into a large bowl. Add the chicken, veggies oats, ½ cup of tomato puree and onion flakes and mix until well combined.
- ✓ Transfer the mixture into prepared loaf pan evenly.
- ✓ With your hands, press, down the mixture slightly. In another bowl mix together mustard and remaining tomato puree. Place the mustard mixture over loaf pan evenly.
- ✓ Bake for about 1-1¼ hours or until desired doneness. Remove from the oven and set aside for about 5 minutes before slicing..
- ✓ Cut into desired sized slices and serve.

Meal Prep Tip:

- ✓ In a resealable plastic bag, place the cooled meatloaf slices and seal the bag. Refrigerate for about 2-4 days. Reheat in the microwave on High for about 1 minute before serving.

Nutrition: Calories 229 Total Fat 5.6 g Saturated Fat 1.4 g Cholesterol 50 mg Total Carbs 23.7 g Sugar 5.2 g Fiber 4.7 g Sodium 227 mg Potassium 509 mg Protein 21.4 g

177) Herbed Turkey Breast

Ingredients:

- ½ cup olive oil
- 2 tablespoons fresh lemon juice
- 1 tablespoon scallion, chopped
- ½ teaspoon dried marjoram, crushed
- ½ teaspoon dried sage, crushed
- ½ teaspoon dried thyme, crushed
- Salt and ground black pepper, as required
- 1 (2-pound) boneless, skinless turkey breast half

Direction: Preparation Time: 15 minutes Cooking Time: 1 hour 50 minutes Servings: 6

- ✓ Preheat the oven to 325 degrees F. Arrange a rack into a greased shallow roasting pan. In a small pan, all the ingredients except turkey breast over medium heat and bring to a boil, stirring frequently.
- ✓ Remove from the heat and set aside to cool. Place turkey breast into the prepared roasting pan. Place some of the herb mixture over the top of turkey breast.
- ✓ Cover the roasting pan and bake for about 1¼-1¾ hours, basting with the remaining herb mixture occasionally.
- ✓ Remove from the oven and set aside for about 10-15 minutes before slicing.
- ✓ With a sharp knife, cut into desired slices and serve.

Meal Prep Tip:

- ✓ Transfer the turkey breast slices onto a wire rack to cool completely.
- ✓ With foil pieces, wrap the turkey breast slices and refrigerate for about 1-2 days. Reheat in the microwave before serving.

Nutrition: Calories 319 Total Fat 17.5 g Saturated Fat 2.4 g Cholesterol 93 mg Total Carbs 0.3 g Sugar 0.1 g Fiber 0.1 g Sodium 75 mg

178) Turkey with Lentils

Ingredients:

- 3 tablespoons olive oil, divided 1 onion, chopped
- 1 tablespoon fresh ginger, minced
- 4 garlic cloves, minced
- 3 plum tomatoes, chopped finely
- 2 cups dried red lentils, soaked for 30 minutes and drained
- 2 cups filtered water
- 2 teaspoons cumin seeds
- ½ teaspoon cayenne pepper
- 1 pound lean ground turkey
- 1 jalapeño pepper, seeded and chopped
- 2 scallions, chopped
- ¼ cup fresh cilantro, chopped

Direction: Preparation Time: 15 minutes Cooking Time: 51 minutes Servings: 7

- ✓ In a Dutch oven, heat 1 tablespoon of oil over medium heat and sauté the onion, ginger and garlic for about 5 minutes.
- ✓ Stir in tomatoes, lentils and water and bring to a boil Now, reduce the heat to medium-low and simmer, covered for about 30 minutes.
- ✓ Meanwhile, in a skillet, heat remaining oil over medium heat and sauté the cumin seeds and cayenne pepper for about 1 minute.
- ✓ Transfer the mixture into a small bowl and set aside. In the same skillet, add turkey and cook for about 4-5 minutes
- ✓ Add the jalapeño and scallion and cook for about 4-5 minutes. Add the spiced oil mixture and stir to combine well.
- ✓ Transfer the turkey mixture in simmering lentils and simmer for about 10-15 minutes or until desired doneness.
- ✓ Serve hot.

Meal Prep Tip:

- ✓ Transfer the turkey mixture into a large bowl and set aside to cool. Divide the mixture into 4 containers evenly. Cover the containers and refrigerate for 1-2 days. Reheat in the microwave before serving.

Nutrition: Calories 361 Total Fat 11.5.4 g Saturated Fat 2.4 g Cholesterol 46 mg Total Carbs 37 g Sugar 3.4 g Fiber 18 g Sodium 937mg Potassium 331 mg Protein 27.9 g

179) Stuffed Chicken Breasts Greek-style

Ingredients:

- 4 oz. chicken breasts, skinless and boneless
- ¼ cup onion, minced
- 4 artichoke hearts, minced
- 1 teaspoon oregano, crushed
- 4 lemon slices

What you will need from the store cupboard:

- 1 cup canned chicken broth, fat-free
- 1-1/2 lemon juice
- 1 tablespoon olive oil
- 2 teaspoons of cornstarch
- Ground pepper Salt, optional

Direction: Servings: 4 Cooking Time: 20 Minutes

- ✓ Take out all the fat from the chicken. Wash and pat dry. Season your chicken with pepper and salt.
- ✓ Pound the chicken to make it flat and thin. Bring together the oregano, onion, and artichoke hearts.
- ✓ Now spoon equal amounts of the mix at the center of your chicken.
- ✓ Roll up the log and secure using a skewer or toothpick. Heat oil in your skillet over medium temperature.
- ✓ Add the chicken. Brown all sides evenly.
- ✓ Pour the lemon juice and broth.
- ✓ Add lemon slices on top of the chicken.
- ✓ Simmer covered for 10 minutes. Transfer to a platter.
- ✓ Remove the skewers or toothpick.
- ✓ Mix cornstarch with a fork. Transfer to skillet and stir over high temperature. Put lemon sauce on the chicken.

Nutrition: Calories 224, Carbohydrates 8g, Fiber 1g, Cholesterol 82mg, Total Fat 5g, Protein 21g, Sodium 339mg

180) Chicken & Tofu

Ingredients:

- 2 tablespoons olive oil, divided 2 tablespoons orange juice
- 1 tablespoon Worcestershire sauce 1 tablespoon low-sodium soy sauce
- 1 teaspoon ground turmeric 1 teaspoon dry mustard
- 8 oz. chicken breast, cooked and sliced into cubes
- 8 oz. extra-firm tofu, drained and sliced into cubed
- 2 carrots, sliced into thin strips 1 cup mushroom, sliced
- 2 cups fresh bean sprouts
- 3 green onions, sliced
- 1 red sweet pepper, sliced into strips

Direction: Preparation Time: 1 hour and 15 minutes Cooking Time: 25 minutes Servings: 6

- ✓ In a bowl, mix half of the oil with the orange juice, Worcestershire sauce, soy sauce, turmeric and mustard.
- ✓ Coat all sides of chicken and tofu with the sauce.
- ✓ Marinate for 1 hour. In a pan over medium heat, add 1 tablespoon oil.
- ✓ Add carrot and cook for 2 minutes.
- ✓ Add mushroom and cook for another 2 minutes.
- ✓ Add bean sprouts, green onion and sweet pepper.
- ✓ Cook for two to three minutes. Stir in the chicken and heat through.

Nutrition: Calories 285 Total Fat 9 g Saturated Fat 1 g Cholesterol 32 mg Sodium 331 mg Total Carbohydrate 30 g Dietary Fiber 4 g Total Sugars 4 g Protein 20 g Potassium 559 mg

181) Chicken & Peanut Stir-Fry

Ingredients:

- 3 tablespoons lime juice
- ½ teaspoon lime zest
- 4 cloves garlic, minced
- 2 teaspoons chili bean sauce
- 1 tablespoon fish sauce
- 1 tablespoon water
- 2 tablespoons peanut butter
- 3 teaspoons oil, divided
- 1 lb. chicken breast, sliced into strips
- 1 red sweet pepper, sliced into strips
- 3 green onions, sliced thinly
- 2 cups broccoli, shredded
- 2 tablespoons peanuts, chopped

Direction: Preparation Time: 15 minutes Cooking Time: 15 minutes Servings: 4

- ✓ In a bowl, mix the lime juice, lime zest, garlic, chili bean sauce, fish sauce, water and peanut butter.
- ✓ Mix well. In a pan over medium high heat, add 2 teaspoons of oil.
- ✓ Cook the chicken until golden on both sides.
- ✓ Pour in the remaining oil. Add the pepper and green onions.
- ✓ Add the chicken, broccoli and sauce. Cook for 2 minutes. Top with peanuts before serving.

Nutrition: Calories 368 Total Fat 11 g Saturated Fat 2 g Cholesterol 66 mg Sodium 556 mg Total Carbohydrate 34 g Dietary Fiber 3 g Total Sugars 4 g Protein 32 g Potassium 482 mg

182) Honey Mustard Chicken

Ingredients:

- 2 tablespoons honey mustard
- 2 teaspoons olive oil
- Salt to taste
- 1 lb. chicken tenders
- 1 lb. baby carrots, steamed
- Chopped parsley

Direction: Preparation Time: 15 minutes Cooking Time: 12 minutes Servings: 4

- ✓ Preheat your oven to 450 degrees F.
- ✓ Mix honey mustard, olive oil and salt.
- ✓ Coat the chicken tenders with the mixture. Place the chicken on a single layer on the baking pan.
- ✓ Bake for 10 to 12 minutes. Serve with steamed carrots and garnish with parsley.

Nutrition: Calories 366 Total Fat 8 g Saturated Fat 2 g Cholesterol 63 mg Sodium 543 mg Total Carbohydrate 46 g Dietary Fiber 8 g Total Sugars 13 g Protein 33 g Potassium 377 mg

183) Lemon Garlic Turkey

Ingredients:

- 4 turkey breasts fillet
- 2 cloves garlic, minced
- 1 tablespoon olive oil
- 3 tablespoons lemon juice
- 1 oz. Parmesan cheese, shredded Pepper to taste
- 1 tablespoon fresh sage, snipped 1 teaspoon lemon zest

Direction: Preparation Time: 1 hour and 10 minutes Cooking Time: 5 minutes Servings: 4

- ✓ Pound the turkey breast until flat. In a bowl, mix the olive oil, garlic and lemon juice.
- ✓ Add the turkey to the bowl. Marinate for 1 hour.
- ✓ Broil for 5 minutes until turkey is fully cooked.
- ✓ Sprinkle cheese on top on the last minute of cooking. In a bowl, mix the pepper, sage and lemon zest.
- ✓ Sprinkle this mixture on top of the turkey before serving.

Nutrition: Calories 188 Total Fat 7 g Saturated Fat 2 g Cholesterol 71 mg Sodium 173 mg Total Carbohydrate 2 g Dietary Fiber 0 g Total Sugars 0 g Protein 29 g Potassium 264 mg

184) Chicken & Spinach

Ingredients:

- 2 tablespoons olive oil
- 1 lb. chicken breast fillet, sliced into small pieces
- Salt and pepper to taste
- 4 cloves garlic, minced
- 1 tablespoon lemon juice
- ½ cup dry white wine
- 1 teaspoon lemon zest
- 10 cups fresh spinach, chopped
- 4 tablespoons Parmesan cheese, grated

Direction: Preparation Time: 15 minutes Cooking Time: 13 minutes Servings: 4

- ✓ Pour oil in a pan over medium heat. Season chicken with salt and pepper.
- ✓ Cook in the pan for 7 minutes until golden on both sides.
- ✓ Add the garlic and cook for 1 minute. Stir in the lemon juice and wine.
- ✓ Sprinkle lemon zest on top. Simmer for 5 minutes.
- ✓ Add the spinach and cook until wilted.
- ✓ Serve with Parmesan cheese.

Nutrition: Calories 334 Total Fat 12 g Saturated Fat 3 g Cholesterol 67 mg Sodium 499 mg Total Carbohydrate 25 g Dietary Fiber 2 g Total Sugars 1 g Protein 29 g Potassium 685 mg

185) Balsamic Chicken 2

Ingredients:

- 6 chicken breast halves, skin removed
- 1 onion, sliced into wedges 1 tablespoon tapioca (quick cooking), crushed
- Salt and pepper to taste
- 1 teaspoon dried thyme, crushed
- 1 teaspoon dried rosemary, crushed
- ¼ cup balsamic vinegar
- 2 tablespoons chicken broth 9 oz. frozen Italian green beans
- 1 red sweet pepper, sliced into strips

Direction: Preparation Time: 15 minutes Cooking Time: 5 hours Servings: 6

- ✓ Put the chicken, onion and tapioca inside a slow cooker. Season with the salt, pepper, thyme and rosemary.
- ✓ Seal the pot and cook on low setting for 4 hours and 30 minutes.
- ✓ Add the sweet pepper and green beans.
- ✓ Cook for 30 more minutes.
- ✓ Pour sauce over the chicken and vegetables before serving.

Nutrition: Calories 234 Total Fat 2 g Saturated Fat 1 g Cholesterol 100 mg Sodium 308 mg Total Carbohydrate 10 g Dietary Fiber 2 g Total Sugars 5 g Protein 41 g Potassium 501 mg

186) Greek Chicken Lettuce Wraps

Ingredients:

- 2 tablespoons freshly squeezed lemon juice
- 1 teaspoon lemon zest
- 5 teaspoons olive oil, divided
- 3 teaspoons garlic, minced and divided
- 1 teaspoon dried oregano
- ¼ teaspoon red pepper, crushed
- 1 lb. chicken tenders
- 1 cucumber, sliced in half and grated
- Salt and pepper to taste
- ¾ cup non-fat Greek yogurt
- 2 teaspoons fresh mint, chopped
- 2 teaspoons fresh dill, chopped
- 4 lettuce leaves
- ½ cup red onion, sliced 1 cup tomatoes, chopped

Direction: Preparation Time: 1 hour and 15 minutes Cooking Time: 8 minutes Servings: 4

- ✓ In a bowl, mix the lemon juice, lemon zest, half of oil, half of garlic, and red pepper. Coat the chicken with the marinade.
- ✓ Marinate it for 1 hour. Toss grated cucumber in salt. Squeeze to release liquid.
- ✓ Add the yogurt, dill, salt, pepper, remaining garlic and remaining oil.
- ✓ Grill the chicken for 4 minutes per side.
- ✓ Shred the chicken and put on top of the lettuce leaves.
- ✓ Top with the yogurt mixture, onion and tomatoes.
- ✓ Wrap the lettuce leaves and secure with a toothpick.

Nutrition: Calories 353 Total Fat 9 g Saturated Fat 1 g Cholesterol 58 mg Sodium 559 mg Total Carbohydrate 33 g Dietary Fiber 6 g Total Sugars 6 g Protein 37 g Potassium 459 mg

187) Lemon Chicken with Kale

Ingredients:

- 1 tablespoon olive oil
- 1 lb. chicken thighs, trimmed
- Salt and pepper to taste
- ½ cup low-sodium chicken stock
- 1 lemon, sliced
- 1 tablespoon fresh tarragon, chopped
- 4 cloves garlic, minced
- 6 cups baby kale

Direction: Preparation Time: 10 minutes Cooking Time: 19 minutes Servings: 4

- ✓ Pour olive oil in a pan over medium heat. Season chicken with salt and pepper.
- ✓ Cook until golden brown on both sides.
- ✓ Pour in the stock. Add the lemon, tarragon and garlic. Simmer for 15 minutes.
- ✓ Add the kale and cook for 4 minutes.

Nutrition: Calories 374 Total Fat 19 g Saturated Fat 4 g Cholesterol 76 mg Sodium 378 mg Total Carbohydrate 26 g Dietary Fiber 3 g Total Sugars 2 g Protein 25 g Potassium 677 mg

MEAT

188) Pork Chops with Grape Sauce

Ingredients:

- Cooking spray
- 4 pork chops
- ¼ cup onion, sliced
- 1 clove garlic, minced
- 1/2 cup low-sodium chicken broth
- ¾ cup apple juice
- 1 tablespoon cornstarch
- 1 tablespoon balsamic vinegar
- 1 teaspoon honey
- 1 cup seedless red grapes, sliced in half

Direction: Preparation Time: 15 minutes
Cooking Time: 25 minutes Servings: 4

- ✓ Spray oil on your pan.
- ✓ Put it over medium heat.
- ✓ Add the pork chops to the pan.
- ✓ Cook for 5 minutes per side.
- ✓ Remove and set aside.
- ✓ Add onion and garlic.
- ✓ Cook for 2 minutes.
- ✓ Pour in the broth and apple juice.
- ✓ Bring to a boil.
- ✓ Reduce heat to simmer.
- ✓ Put the pork chops back to the skillet.
- ✓ Simmer for 4 minutes.
- ✓ In a bowl, mix the cornstarch, vinegar and honey.
- ✓ Add to the pan.
- ✓ Cook until the sauce has thickened.
- ✓ Add the grapes.
- ✓ Pour sauce over the pork chops before serving.

Nutrition: Calories 188; Total Fat 4 g; Saturated Fat 1 g; Cholesterol 47 mg; Sodium 117 mg; Total Carbohydrate 18 g; Dietary Fiber 1 g; Total Sugars 13 g; Protein 19 g; Potassium 759 mg

189) Roasted Pork & Apples

Ingredients:

- Salt and pepper to taste
- 1/2 teaspoon dried, crushed
- 1 lb. pork tenderloin
- 1 tablespoon canola oil
- 1 onion, sliced into wedges
- 3 cooking apples, sliced into wedges
- 2/3 cup apple cider
- Sprigs fresh sage

Direction: Preparation Time: 15 minutes
Cooking Time: 30 minutes Servings: 4

- ✓ In a bowl, mix salt, pepper and sage.
- ✓ Season both sides of pork with this mixture.
- ✓ Place a pan over medium heat.
- ✓ Brown both sides.
- ✓ Transfer to a roasting pan.
- ✓ Add the onion on top and around the pork.
- ✓ Drizzle oil on top of the pork and apples.
- ✓ Roast in the oven at 425 degrees F for 10 minutes.
- ✓ Add the apples, roast for another 15 minutes.
- ✓ In a pan, boil the apple cider and then simmer for 10 minutes.
- ✓ Pour the apple cider sauce over the pork before serving.

Nutrition: Calories 239; Total Fat 6 g; Saturated Fat 1 g; Cholesterol 74 mg; Sodium 209 mg; Total Carbohydrate 22 g; Dietary Fiber 3 g; Total Sugars 16 g; Protein 24 g; Potassium 655 mg

190) Pork with Cranberry Relish

Ingredients:

- 12 oz. pork tenderloin, fat trimmed and sliced crosswise
- Salt and pepper to taste
- ¼ cup all-purpose flour
- 2 tablespoons olive oil
- 1 onion, sliced thinly
- ¼ cup dried cranberries
- ¼ cup low-sodium chicken broth
- 1 tablespoon balsamic vinegar

Direction: Preparation Time: 30 minutes
Cooking Time: 30 minutes Servings: 4

- ✓ Flatten each slice of pork using a mallet.
- ✓ In a dish, mix the salt, pepper and flour.
- ✓ Dip each pork slice into the flour mixture.
- ✓ Add oil to a pan over medium high heat.
- ✓ Cook pork for 3 minutes per side or until golden crispy.
- ✓ Transfer to a serving plate and cover with foil.
- ✓ Cook the onion in the pan for 4 minutes.
- ✓ Stir in the rest of the ingredients.
- ✓ Simmer until the sauce has thickened.

Nutrition: Calories 211; Total Fat 9 g; Saturated Fat 2 g; Cholesterol 53 mg; Sodium 116 mg; Total Carbohydrate 15 g; Dietary Fiber 1 g; Total Sugars 6 g; Protein 18 g; Potassium 378 mg

191) Sesame Pork with Mustard Sauce

Ingredients:

- 2 tablespoons low-sodium teriyaki sauce
- ¼ cup chili sauce
- 2 cloves garlic, minced
- 2 teaspoons ginger, grated
- 2 pork tenderloins
- 2 teaspoons sesame seeds
- ¼ cup low fat sour cream
- 1 teaspoon Dijon mustard
- Salt to taste
- 1 scallion, chopped

Direction: Preparation Time: 25 minutes
Cooking Time: 25 minutes Servings: 4

- ✓ Preheat your oven to 425 degrees F.
- ✓ Mix the teriyaki sauce, chili sauce, garlic and ginger.
- ✓ Put the pork on a roasting pan.
- ✓ Brush the sauce on both sides of the pork.
- ✓ Bake in the oven for 15 minutes.
- ✓ Brush with more sauce.
- ✓ Top with sesame seeds.
- ✓ Roast for 10 more minutes.
- ✓ Mix the rest of the ingredients.
- ✓ Serve the pork with mustard sauce.

Nutrition: Calories 135 ; Total Fat 3 g; Saturated Fat 1 g; Cholesterol 56X mg; Sodium 302 mg; Total Carbohydrate 7 g; Dietary Fiber 1 g; Total Sugars 15 g; Protein 20 g; Potassium 755 mg

192) Steak with Mushroom Sauce

Ingredients:

- 12 oz. sirloin steak, sliced and trimmed
- 2 teaspoons grilling seasoning
- 2 teaspoons oil
- 6 oz. broccoli, trimmed
- 2 cups frozen peas
- 3 cups fresh mushrooms, sliced
- 1 cup beef broth (unsalted)
- 1 tablespoon mustard
- 2 teaspoons cornstarch
- Salt to taste

Direction: Preparation Time: 20 minutes
Cooking Time: 5 minutes Servings: 4

- ✓ Preheat your oven to 350 degrees F.
- ✓ Season meat with grilling seasoning.
- ✓ In a pan over medium high heat, cook the meat and broccoli for 4 minutes.
- ✓ Sprinkle the peas around the steak.
- ✓ Put the pan inside the oven and bake for 8 minutes.
- ✓ Remove both meat and vegetables from the pan.
- ✓ Add the mushrooms to the pan.
- ✓ Cook for 3 minutes.
- ✓ Mix the broth, mustard, salt and cornstarch.
- ✓ Add to the mushrooms.
- ✓ Cook for 1 minute.
- ✓ Pour sauce over meat and vegetables before serving.

Nutrition: Calories 226; Total Fat 6 ; Saturated Fat 2 g; Cholesterol 51 mg ; Sodium 356 mg; Total Carbohydrate 16 g; Dietary Fiber 5 g; Total Sugars 6 g; Protein 26 g; Potassium 780 mg

193) Steak with Tomato & Herbs

Ingredients:

- 8 oz. beef loin steak, sliced in half
- Salt and pepper to taste
- Cooking spray
- 1 teaspoon fresh basil, snipped
- ¼ cup green onion, sliced
- ½ cup tomato, chopped

Direction: Preparation Time: 30 minutes
Cooking Time: 30 minutes Servings: 2

- ✓ Season the steak with salt and pepper.
- ✓ Spray oil on your pan.
- ✓ Put the pan over medium high heat.
- ✓ Once hot, add the steaks.
- ✓ Reduce heat to medium.
- ✓ Cook for 10 to 13 minutes for medium, turning once.
- ✓ Add the basil and green onion.
- ✓ Cook for 2 minutes.
- ✓ Add the tomato.
- ✓ Cook for 1 minute.
- ✓ Let cool a little before slicing.

Nutrition: Calories 170; Total Fat 6 g; Saturated Fat 2 g; Cholesterol 66 mg; Sodium 207 mg; Total Carbohydrate 3 g; Dietary Fiber 1 g; Total Sugars 5 g; Protein 25 g; Potassium 477 mg

194) Barbecue Beef Brisket

Ingredients:

- 4 lb. beef brisket (boneless), trimmed and sliced
- 1 bay leaf
- 2 onions, sliced into rings
- ½ teaspoon dried thyme, crushed
- ¼ cup chili sauce
- 1 clove garlic, minced
- Salt and pepper to taste
- 2 tablespoons light brown sugar
- 2 tablespoons cornstarch
- 2 tablespoons cold water

Direction: Preparation Time: 25 minutes
Cooking Time: 10 hours Servings: 10

- ✓ Put the meat in a slow cooker.
- ✓ Add the bay leaf and onion.
- ✓ In a bowl, mix the thyme, chili sauce, salt, pepper and sugar.
- ✓ Pour the sauce over the meat.
- ✓ Mix well.
- ✓ Seal the pot and cook on low heat for 10 hours.
- ✓ Discard the bay leaf.
- ✓ Pour cooking liquid in a pan.
- ✓ Add the mixed water and cornstarch.
- ✓ Simmer until the sauce has thickened.
- ✓ Pour the sauce over the meat.

Nutrition: Calories 182; Total Fat 6 g; Saturated Fat 2 g; Cholesterol 57 mg; Sodium 217 mg; Total Sugars 4 g; Protein 20 g; Potassium 383 mg

195) Beef & Asparagus

Ingredients:

- 2 teaspoons olive oil
- 1 lb. lean beef sirloin, trimmed and sliced
- 1 carrot, shredded
- Salt and pepper to taste
- 12 oz. asparagus, trimmed and sliced
- 1 teaspoon dried herbs de Provence, crushed
- ½ cup Marsala
- ¼ teaspoon lemon zest

Direction: Preparation Time: 15 minutes
Cooking Time: 10 minutes Servings: 4

- ✓ Pour oil in a pan over medium heat.
- ✓ Add the beef and carrot.
- ✓ Season with salt and pepper.
- ✓ Cook for 3 minutes.
- ✓ Add the asparagus and herbs.
- ✓ Cook for 2 minutes.
- ✓ Add the Marsala and lemon zest.
- ✓ Cook for 5 minutes, stirring frequently.

Nutrition: Calories 327; Total Fat 7 g; Saturated Fat 2 g; Cholesterol 69 mg ; Sodium 209 mg; Total Carbohydrate 29 g; Dietary Fiber 2 g; Total Sugars 3 g; Protein 28 g; Potassium 576 mg

196) Italian Beef

Ingredients:

- Cooking spray
- 1 lb. beef round steak, trimmed and sliced
- 1 cup onion, chopped
- 2 cloves garlic, minced
- 1 cup green bell pepper, chopped
- 1/2 cup celery, chopped
- 2 cups mushrooms, sliced
- 14 1/2 oz. canned diced tomatoes
- 1/2 teaspoon dried basil
- ¼ teaspoon dried oregano
- 1/8 teaspoon crushed red pepper
- 2 tablespoons Parmesan cheese, grated

Direction: Preparation Time: 20 minutes
Cooking Time: 1 hour and 20 minutes Servings: 4

- ✓ Spray oil on the pan over medium heat.
- ✓ Cook the meat until brown on both sides.
- ✓ Transfer meat to a plate.
- ✓ Add the onion, garlic, bell pepper, celery and mushroom to the pan.
- ✓ Cook until tender.
- ✓ Add the tomatoes, herbs, and pepper.
- ✓ Put the meat back to the pan.
- ✓ Simmer while covered for 1 hour and 15 minutes.
- ✓ Stir occasionally.
- ✓ Sprinkle Parmesan cheese on top of the dish before serving.

Nutrition: Calories 212; Total Fat 4 g; Saturated Fat 1 g; Cholesterol 51 mg; Sodium 296 mg; Total Sugars 6 g; Protein 30 g; Potassium 876 mg

197) Lamb with Broccoli & Carrots

Ingredients:

- 2 cloves garlic, minced
- 1 tablespoon fresh ginger, grated
- ¼ teaspoon red pepper, crushed
- 2 tablespoons low-sodium soy sauce
- 1 tablespoon white vinegar
- 1 tablespoon cornstarch
- 12 oz. lamb meat, trimmed and sliced
- 2 teaspoons cooking oil
- 1 lb. broccoli, sliced into florets
- 2 carrots, sliced into strips
- ¾ cup low-sodium beef broth
- 4 green onions, chopped
- 2 cups cooked spaghetti squash pasta

Direction: Preparation Time: 20 minutes
Cooking Time: 10 minutes Servings: 4

- ✓ Combine the garlic, ginger, red pepper, soy sauce, vinegar and cornstarch in a bowl.
- ✓ Add lamb to the marinade.
- ✓ Marinate for 10 minutes.
- ✓ Discard marinade.
- ✓ In a pan over medium heat, add the oil.
- ✓ Add the lamb and cook for 3 minutes.
- ✓ Transfer lamb to a plate.
- ✓ Add the broccoli and carrots.
- ✓ Cook for 1 minute.
- ✓ Pour in the beef broth.
- ✓ Cook for 5 minutes.
- ✓ Put the meat back to the pan.
- ✓ Sprinkle with green onion and serve on top of spaghetti squash.

Nutrition: Calories 205; Total Fat 6 g; Saturated Fat 1 g; Cholesterol 40 mg; Sodium 659 mg; Total Carb. 17 g

198) Rosemary Lamb

Ingredients:

- Salt and pepper to taste
- 2 teaspoons fresh rosemary, snipped
- 5 lb. whole leg of lamb, trimmed and cut with slits on all sides
- 3 cloves garlic, slivered
- 1 cup water

Direction: Preparation Time: 15 minutes
Cooking Time: 2 hours Servings: 14

- ✓ Preheat your oven to 375 degrees F.
- ✓ Mix salt, pepper and rosemary in a bowl.
- ✓ Sprinkle mixture all over the lamb.
- ✓ Insert slivers of garlic into the slits.
- ✓
- ✓ Put the lamb on a roasting pan.
- ✓ Add water to the pan.
- ✓ Roast for 2 hours.
- ✓

Nutrition: Calories 136; Total Fat 4 g; Saturated Fat 1g cholesterol 71 mg; Sodium 218 mg; Protein 23 g; Potassium 248 mg

199) Mediterranean Lamb Meatballs

Ingredients:

- 12 oz. roasted red peppers
- 1 1/2 cups whole wheat breadcrumbs
- 2 eggs, beaten
- 1/3 cup tomato sauce
- 1/2 cup fresh basil
- ¼ cup parsley, snipped
- Salt and pepper to taste
- 2 lb. lean ground lamb

Direction: Preparation Time: 10 minutes
Cooking Time: 20 minutes Servings: 8

- ✓ Preheat your oven to 350 degrees F.
- ✓ In a bowl, mix all the ingredients and then form into meatballs.
- ✓ Put the meatballs on a baking pan.
- ✓ Bake in the oven for 20 minutes.

Nutrition: Calories 94; Total Fat 3 g; Saturated Fat 1 g; Cholesterol 35 mg Sodium 170 mg; Total Carbohydrate 2 g; Dietary Fiber 1 g; Total Sugars 0 g

200) Shredded Beef

Ingredients:

- 1.5lb lean steak 1 cup low sodium gravy
- 2tbsp mixed spices

Direction: Servings: 2 Cooking Time: 35 Minutes

- ✓ Mix all the ingredients in your Instant Pot. Cook on Stew for 35 minutes.
- ✓ Release the pressure naturally. Shred the beef.

Nutrition: Calories: 200 Carbs: 2 Sugar: 0 Fat: 5 Protein: 48 GL: 1

201) Classic Mini Meatloaf

Ingredients:

- 1 pound 80/20 ground beef
- ¼ medium yellow onion, peeled and diced
- ½ medium green bell pepper, seeded and diced 1 large egg
- 3 tablespoons blanched finely ground almond flour
- 1 tablespoon Worcestershire sauce
- ½ teaspoon garlic powder
- 1 teaspoon dried parsley
- 2 tablespoons tomato paste
- ¼ cup water
- 1 tablespoon powdered erythritol

Direction: Servings: 6 Cooking Time: 25 Minutes

- ✓ In a large bowl, combine ground beef, onion, pepper, egg, and almond flour. Pour in the
- ✓ Worcestershire sauce and add the garlic powder and parsley to the bowl.
- ✓ Mix until fully combined. Divide the mixture into two and place into two (4") loaf baking pans.
- ✓ In a small bowl, mix the tomato paste, water, and erythritol. Spoon half the mixture over each loaf.
- ✓ Working in batches if necessary, place loaf pans into the air fryer basket.
- ✓ Adjust the temperature to 350°F and set the timer for 25 minutes or until internal temperature is 180°F. Serve warm.

Nutrition: Calories: 170 Protein: 14.9 G Fiber: 0.9 G Net Carbohydrates: 2.6 G Sugar Alcohol: 1.5 G Fat: 9.4 G Sodium: 85 Mg Carbohydrates: 5.0 G Sugar: 1.5 G

202) Skirt Steak With Asian Peanut Sauce

Ingredients:

- ⅓ cup light coconut milk
- 1 teaspoon curry powder
- 1 teaspoon coriander powder
- 1 teaspoon reduced-sodium soy sauce
- 1¼ pound skirt steak Cooking spray
- ½ cup Asian Peanut Sauce

Direction: Servings: 4 Cooking Time: 15 Minutes

- ✓ In a large bowl, whisk together the coconut milk, curry powder, coriander powder, and soy sauce.
- ✓ Add the steak and turn to coat.
- ✓ Cover the bowl and refrigerate for at least 30 minutes and no longer than 24 hours.
- ✓ Preheat the barbecue or coat a grill pan with cooking spray and place the steak over medium-high heat.
- ✓ Grill the meat until it reaches an internal temperature of 145°F, about 3 minutes per side.
- ✓ Remove the steak from the grill and let it rest for 5 minutes. Slice the steak into 5-ounce pieces and serve each with 2 tablespoons of the Asian Peanut Sauce.
- ✓ REFRIGERATE: Store the cooled steak in a reseal able container for up to 1 week. Reheat each piece in the microwave for 1 minute.

Nutrition: Calories: 361 Fat: 22g Saturated Fat: 7g Protein: 36g Total Carbs: 8g Fiber: 2g Sodium: 349mg

203) Roasted Pork Loin With Grainy Mustard Sauce

Ingredients:

- (2-pound) boneless pork loin roast Sea salt
- Freshly ground black pepper
- 3 tablespoons olive oil
- 1½ cups heavy (whipping) cream
- 3 tablespoons grainy mustard, such as Pommery

Direction: Servings: 8 Cooking Time: 70 Minutes

- ✓ Preheat the oven to 375°F. Season the pork roast all over with sea salt and pepper.
- ✓ Place a large skillet over medium-high heat and add the olive oil.
- ✓ Brown the roast on all sides in the skillet, about 6 minutes in total, and place the roast in a baking dish.
- ✓ Roast until a meat thermometer inserted in the thickest part of the roast reads 155°F, about 1 hour.
- ✓ When there is approximately 15 minutes of roasting time left, place a small saucepan over medium heat and add the heavy cream and mustard. Stir the sauce until it simmers, then reduce the heat to low.
- ✓ Simmer the sauce until it is very rich and thick, about 5 minutes.
- ✓ Remove the pan from the heat and set aside. Let the pork rest for 10 minutes before slicing and serve with the sauce.

Nutrition: Calories 368 Fat: 29g Protein: 25g Carbs: 2g Fiber: 0g Net Carbs: 2g Fat 70%/Protein 25%/Carbs 5%

204) Meatballs In Tomato Gravy

Ingredients:

For Meatballs:

- 1 pound lean ground lamb
- 1 tablespoon homemade tomato paste
- ¼ cup fresh cilantro leaves, chopped 1 small onion, chopped finely
- 2 garlic cloves, minced
- ½ teaspoon ground cumin
- 1/8 teaspoon salt Ground black pepper, as required

For Tomato Gravy:

- 3 tablespoons olive oil, divided 2 medium onions, chopped finely
- 2 garlic cloves, minced
- ½ tablespoon fresh ginger, minced
- 1 teaspoon dried thyme, crushed
- 1 teaspoon dried oregano, crushed
- 3 large tomatoes, chopped finely Ground black pepper, as required
- 1½ cups warm low-sodium chicken broth

Direction: Servings: 6 Cooking Time: 30 Minutes

- ✓ For meatballs: in a large bowl, add all the ingredients and mix until well combined. Make small equal-sized balls from mixture and set aside.
- ✓ For gravy: in a large pan, heat 1 tablespoon of oil over medium heat.
- ✓ Add the meatballs and cook for about 4-5 minutes or until lightly browned from all sides. With a slotted spoon, transfer the meatballs onto a plate.
- ✓ In the same pan, heat the remaining oil over medium heat and sauté the onion for about 8-10 minutes. Add the garlic, ginger and herbs and sauté for about 1 minute.
- ✓ . Add the tomatoes and cook for about 3-4 minutes, crushing with the back of spoon. Add the warm broth and bring to a boil.
- ✓ Carefully, place the meatballs and cook for 5 minutes, without stirring.
- ✓ Now, reduce the heat to low and cook partially covered for about 15-20 minutes, stirring gently 2-3 times. Serve hot.

Meal Prep Tip:

- ✓ Transfer the meatballs mixture into a large bowl and set aside to cool. Divide the mixture into 6 containers evenly. Cover the containers and refrigerate for 1-2 days.
- ✓ Reheat in the microwave before serving.

Nutrition: Calories 248 Total Fat 12.9 g Saturated Fat 3 g Cholesterol 68 mg Total Carbs 10 g Sugar 4.8 g Fiber 2.5 g Sodium 138 mg

205) Garlic-braised Short Rib

Ingredients:

- 4 (4-ounce) beef short ribs
- Sea salt
- Freshly ground black pepper
- 1 tablespoon olive oil
- 2 teaspoons minced garlic
- ½ cup dry red wine
- 3 cups Rich Beef Stock (here)

Direction: Servings: 4 Cooking Time: 2 Hours, 20 Minutes

- ✓ Preheat the oven to 325°F. Season the beef ribs on all sides with salt and pepper.
- ✓ Place a deep ovenproof skillet over medium-high heat and add the olive oil.
- ✓ Sear the ribs on all sides until browned, about 6 minutes in total.
- ✓ Transfer the ribs to a plate. Add the garlic to the skillet and sauté until translucent, about 3 minutes.
- ✓ Whisk in the red wine to deglaze the pan.
- ✓ Be sure to scrape all the browned bits from the meat from the bottom of the pan.
- ✓ Simmer the wine until it is slightly reduced, about 2 minutes.
- ✓ Add the beef stock, ribs, and any accumulated juices on the plate back to the skillet and bring the liquid to a boil.
- ✓ Cover the skillet and place it in the oven to braise the ribs until the meat is fall-off-the-bone tender, about 2 hours.
- ✓ Serve the ribs with a spoonful of the cooking liquid drizzled over each serving.

Nutrition: Calories: 481 Fat: 38g Protein: 29g Carbs: 5g Fiber: 3g Net Carbs: 2g Fat 70%/Protein 25%/Carbs 5%

206) Pulled Pork

Ingredients:

- 2 tablespoons chili powder
- 1 teaspoon garlic powder
- ½ teaspoon onion powder
- ½ teaspoon ground black pepper
- ½ teaspoon cumin

Direction: Servings: 8 Cooking Time: 2½ Hours

- ✓ (4-pound) pork shoulder In a small bowl, mix chili powder, garlic powder, onion powder, pepper, and cumin.
- ✓ Rub the spice mixture over the pork shoulder, patting it into the skin.
- ✓ Place pork shoulder into the air fryer basket.
- ✓ Adjust the temperature to 350°F and set the timer for 150 minutes.
- ✓ Pork skin will be crispy and meat easily shredded with two forks when done.
- ✓ The internal temperature should be at least 145°F.

Nutrition: Calories: 537 Protein: 42.6 G Fiber: 0.8 G Net Carbohydrates: 0.7 G Fat: 35.5 G Sodium: 180 Mg Carbohydrates: 1.5 G Sugar: 0.2 G

207) Rosemary-garlic Lamb Racks

Ingredients:

- 4 tablespoons extra-virgin olive oil
- 2 tablespoons finely chopped fresh rosemary
- 2 teaspoons minced garlic Pinch sea salt
- 2 (1-pound) racks French-cut lamb chops (8 bones each)

Direction: Servings: 4 Cooking Time: 25 Minutes

- ✓ In a small bowl, whisk together the olive oil, rosemary, garlic, and salt. Place the racks in a sealable freezer bag and pour the olive oil mixture into the bag.
- ✓ Massage the meat through the bag so it is coated with the marinade. Press the air out of the bag and seal it.
- ✓ Marinate the lamb racks in the refrigerator for 1 to 2 hours. Preheat the oven to 450°F. Place a large ovenproof skillet over medium-high heat.
- ✓ Take the lamb racks out of the bag and sear them in the skillet on all sides, about 5 minutes in total.
- ✓ Arrange the racks upright in the skillet, with the bones interlaced, and roast them in the oven until they reach your desired doneness, about 20 minutes for medium-rare or until the internal temperature reaches 125°F.
- ✓ Let the lamb rest for 10 minutes and then cut the racks into chops. Serve 4 chops per person.

Nutrition: Calories: 354 Fat: 30g Protein: 21g Carbs: 0g Fiber: 0g Net Carbs: 0g Fat 70%/Protein 30%/Carbs 0%

208) Irish Pork Roast

Ingredients:

- 1 ½ lb. parsnips, peeled and sliced into small pieces
- 1 ½ lb. carrots, sliced into small pieces
- 3 tablespoons olive oil,
- divided 2 teaspoons fresh thyme leaves, divided
- Salt and pepper to taste
- 2 lb. pork loin roast
- 1 teaspoon honey
- 1 cup dry hard cider Applesauce

Direction: Preparation Time: 40 minutes Cooking Time: 1 hour Servings: 8

- ✓ Preheat your oven to 400 degrees F.
- ✓ Drizzle half of the oil over the parsnips and carrots. Season with half of thyme, salt and pepper.
- ✓ Arrange on a roasting pan. Rub the pork with the remaining oil.
- ✓ Season with the remaining thyme.
- ✓ Season with salt and pepper. Put it on the roasting pan on top of the vegetables.
- ✓ Roast for 65 minutes.
- ✓ Let cool before slicing.
- ✓ Transfer the carrots and parsnips in a bowl and mix with honey.
- ✓ Add the cider. Place in a pan and simmer over low heat until the sauce has thickened.
- ✓ Serve the pork with the vegetables and applesauce.

Nutrition: Calories 272 Total Fat 8 g Saturated Fat 2 g Cholesterol 61 mg Sodium 327 mg Total Carbohydrate 23 g Dietary Fiber 6 g Total Sugars 10 g Protein 24 g

209) Lamb & Chickpeas

Ingredients:

- 1 lb. lamb leg (boneless), trimmed and sliced into small pieces
- 2 tablespoons olive oil 1 teaspoon ground coriander
- Salt and pepper to taste
- ½ teaspoon ground cumin
- ¼ teaspoon red pepper, crushed
- ¼ cup fresh mint, chopped
- 2 teaspoons lemon zest
- 2 cloves garlic, minced
- 30 oz. unsalted chickpeas, rinsed and drained
- 1 cup tomatoes, chopped
- 1 cup English cucumber, chopped
- ¼ cup fresh parsley, snipped 1 tablespoon red wine vinegar

Direction: Preparation Time: 30 minutes Cooking Time: 30 minutes Servings: 4

- ✓ Preheat your oven to 375 degrees F.
- ✓ Place the lamb on a baking dish.
- ✓ Toss in half of the following: oil, cumin and coriander.
- ✓ Season with red pepper, salt and pepper.
- ✓ Mix well. Roast for 20 minutes. In a bowl, combine the rest of the ingredients with the remaining seasonings.
- ✓ Add salt and pepper. Serve lamb with chickpea mixture.

Nutrition: Calories 366 Total Fat 15 g Saturated Fat 3 g Cholesterol 74 mg Sodium 369 mg Total Carbohydrate 27 g Dietary Fiber 7 g Total Sugars 3 g Protein 32 g Potassium 579 mg

210) Braised Lamb with Vegetables

Ingredients:

- Salt and pepper to taste
- 2 ½ lb. boneless lamb leg, trimmed and sliced into cubes
- 1 tablespoon olive oil
- 1 onion, chopped
- 1 carrot, chopped
- 14 oz. canned diced tomatoes 1 cup low-sodium beef broth
- 1 tablespoon fresh rosemary
- chopped 4 cloves garlic, minced
- 1 cup pearl onions
- 1 cup baby turnips, peeled and sliced into wedges
- 1 ½ cups baby carrots
- 1 ½ cups peas
- 2 tablespoons fresh parsley, chopped

Direction: Preparation Time: 30 minutes Cooking Time: 2 hours and 15 minutes Servings: 6

- ✓ Sprinkle salt and pepper on both sides of the lamb. Pour oil in a deep skillet.
- ✓ Cook the lamb for 6 minutes. Transfer lamb to a plate.
- ✓ Add onion and carrot. Cook for 3 minutes. Stir in the tomatoes, broth, rosemary and garlic. Simmer for 5 minutes.
- ✓ Add the lamb back to the skillet.
- ✓ Reduce heat to low. Simmer for 1 hour and 15 minutes. Add the pearl onion, baby carrot and baby turnips.
- ✓ Simmer for 30 minutes. Add the peas.
- ✓ Cook for 1 minute. Garnish with parsley before serving.

Nutrition: Calories 420 Total Fat 14 g Saturated Fat 4 g Cholesterol 126 mg Sodium 529 mg Total Carbohydrate 16 g Dietary Fiber 4 g Total Sugars 7 g Protein 43 g Potassium 988 mg

211) Beef Salad

Ingredients:

- For Steak:
- 1½ pounds skirt steak, trimmed and cut into 4 pieces

Salt and ground black pepper, as required

For Salad:

- 2 medium green bell pepper, seeded and sliced thinly
- 2 large tomatoes, sliced
- 1 cup onion, sliced thinly
- 8 cups mixed fresh baby greens

For Dressing:

- 2 teaspoons Dijon mustard
- 4 tablespoons balsamic vinegar
- ½ cup olive oil
- Salt and ground black pepper, as required

Direction: Preparation Time: 20 minutes Cooking Time: 8 minutes Servings: 6

- ✓ Preheat the grill to medium-high heat. Grease the grill grate. Sprinkle the beef steak with a little salt and black pepper. Place the steak onto the grill and cook, covered for about 3-4 minutes per side. Transfer the steak onto a cutting board for about 10 minutes before slicing. With a sharp knife, cut the beef steaks into thin slices.
- ✓ Meanwhile, in a large bowl, mix together all salad ingredients. For dressing: in another bowl, add all the ingredients and beat until well combined.
- ✓ Pour the dressing over salad and gently toss to coat well. Divide the salad onto serving plates evenly. Top each plate with the steak slices and serve.
- ✓ Meanwhile, in a large bowl, mix together all salad ingredients. For dressing: in another bowl, add all the ingredients and beat until well combined. Pour the dressing over salad and gently toss to coat well. Divide the salad onto serving plates evenly. Top each plate with the steak slices and serve.

Nutrition: Calories 313 Total Fat 21.4 g Saturated Fat 5.1 g Cholesterol 50 mg Total Carbs 6.4 g Sugar 3.4 g Fiber 1.7 g Sodium 88 mg Potassium 443mg Protein 24 g

212) Beef Curry

Ingredients:

- 1 cup fat-free plain Greek yogurt
- ½ teaspoon garlic paste
- ½ teaspoon ginger paste
- ½ teaspoon ground cloves
- ½ teaspoon ground cumin
- 2 teaspoons red pepper flakes, crushed
- ¼ teaspoon ground turmeric
- Salt, as required
- 2 pounds round steak, cut into pieces
- ¼ cup olive oil
- 1 medium yellow onion, thinly sliced
- 1½ tablespoons fresh lemon juice
- ¼ cup fresh cilantro, chopped

Direction: Preparation Time: 20 minutes Cooking Time: 40 minutes Servings: 6

- ✓ In a large bowl, add the yogurt, garlic paste, ginger paste and spices and mix well.
- ✓ Add the steak pieces and generously coat with the yogurt mixture. Set aside for at least 15 minutes.
- ✓ In a large skillet, heat the oil over medium-high heat and sauté the onion for about 4-5 minutes.
- ✓ Add the steak pieces with marinade and stir to combine. Immediately, adjust the heat to low and simmer, covered and cook for about 25 minutes, stirring occasionally.
- ✓ Stir in the lemon juice and simmer for about 10 more minutes.
- ✓ Garnish with fresh cilantro and serve hot.

Meal Prep Tip:

- ✓ Transfer the curry into a large bowl and set aside to cool.
- ✓ Divide the curry into 6 containers evenly.
- ✓ Cover the containers and refrigerate for 1-2 days.
- ✓ Reheat in the microwave before serving.

Nutrition: Calories 389 Total Fat 18.2 g Saturated Fat 4.8 g Cholesterol 136 mg Total Carbs 4.3 g Sugar 2.4 g Fiber 0.7 g 149 mg

213) Beef with Barley & Veggies

Ingredients:

- ¾ cup filtered water
- ¼ cup pearl barley
- 2 teaspoons olive oil
- 7 ounces lean ground beef
- 1 cup fresh mushrooms, sliced
- ¾ cup onion, chopped
- 2 cups frozen green beans
- ¼ cup low-sodium beef broth
- 2 tablespoon fresh parsley, chopped

Direction: Preparation Time: 15 minutes Cooking Time: 1 hour 5 minutes Servings: 2

- ✓ In a pan, add water, barley and pinch of salt and bring to a boil over medium heat.
- ✓ Now, reduce the heat to low and simmer, covered for about 30-40 minutes or until all the liquid is absorbed.
- ✓ Remove from heat and set aside.
- ✓ In a skillet, heat oil over medium-high heat and cook beef for about 8-10 minutes.
- ✓ Add the mushroom and onion and cook f or about 6-7 minutes.
- ✓ Add the green beans and cook for about 2-3 minutes. Stir in cooked barley and broth and cook for about 3-5 minutes more.
- ✓ Stir in the parsley and serve hot.

Meal Prep Tip:

- ✓ Transfer the beef mixture into a large bowl and set aside to cool.
- ✓ Divide the mixture into 2 containers evenly. Cover the containers and refrigerate for 1-2 days. Reheat in the microwave before serving.

Nutrition: Calories 374 Total Fat 11.4 g Saturated Fat 3.1 g Cholesterol 89 mg Total Carbs 32.7g Sugar 1.1 g Fiber 4.2 g Sodium 136 mg Potassium 895 mg Protein 36.6 g

214) Beef with Broccoli

Ingredients:

- 2 tablespoons olive oil, divided
- 2 garlic cloves, minced
- 1 pound beef sirloin steak, trimmed and sliced into thin strips
- ¼ cup low-sodium chicken broth
- 2 teaspoons fresh ginger, grated
- 1 tablespoon ground flax seeds
- ½ teaspoon red pepper flakes, crushed
- Salt and ground black pepper, as required
- 1 large carrot, peeled and sliced thinly
- 2 cups broccoli florets
- 1 medium scallion, sliced thinly

Direction: Preparation Time: 10 minutes Cooking Time: 14 minutes Servings: 4

- ✓ In a large skillet, heat 1 tablespoon of oil over medium-high heat and sauté the garlic for about 1 minute.
- ✓ Add the beef and cook for about 4-5 minutes or until browned. With a slotted spoon, transfer the beef into a bowl.
- ✓ Remove the excess liquid from skillet. In a bowl, add the broth, ginger, flax seeds, red pepper flakes, salt and black pepper.
- ✓ In the same skillet, heat remaining oil over medium heat.
- ✓ Add the carrot, broccoli and ginger mixture and cook for about 3-4 minutes or until desired doneness. Stir in beef and scallion and cook for about 3-4 minutes.

Meal Prep Tip:

- ✓ Transfer the beef mixture into a large bowl and set aside to cool.
- ✓ Divide the mixture into 4 containers evenly. Cover the containers and refrigerate for 1-2 days. Reheat in the microwave before serving.

Nutrition: Calories 211 Total Fat 14.9 g Saturated Fat 3.9 g Cholesterol 101 mg Total Carbs 6.9 g Sugar 1.9 g Fiber 2.4 g Sodium 108 mg Potassium 706 mg Protein 36.5 g

215) Pan Grilled Steak

Ingredients:

- 8 medium garlic cloves, crushed
- 1 (2-inch) piece fresh ginger, sliced thinly
- ¼ cup olive oil
- Salt and ground black pepper, as required
- ½ pounds flank steak, trimmed

Direction: Preparation Time: 10 minutes Cooking Time: 16 minutes Servings: 4

- ✓ In a large sealable bag, mix together all ingredients except steak.
- ✓ Add the steak and coat with marinade generously. Seal the bag and refrigerate to marinate for about 24 hours.
- ✓ Remove from refrigerator and keep in room temperature for about 15 minutes.
- ✓ Discard the excess marinade from steak. Heat a lightly greased grill pan over medium-high heat and cook the steak for about 6-8 minutes per side.
- ✓ Remove from grill pan and set aside for about 10 minutes before slicing.
- ✓ With a sharp knife cut into desired slices and serve.

Meal Prep Tip:

- ✓ Transfer the teak slices onto a wire rack to cool completely. With foil pieces, wrap the steak slices and refrigerate for about 1-2 days. Reheat in the microwave before serving.

Nutrition: Calories 447 Total Fat 26.8 g Saturated Fat 7.7 g Cholesterol 94 mg Total Carbs 2.1g Sugar 0.1 g Fiber 0.2 g Sodium 96 mg Potassium 601 mg Protein 47.7 g

216) Lamb Stew Recipe 1

Ingredients:

- 1 teaspoon ground cumin
- 1 teaspoon ground coriander
- ½ teaspoon cayenne pepper
- ½ teaspoon ground cinnamon
- 2 tablespoons olive oil
- 3 pounds lamb stew meat, trimmed and cubed
- Sea Salt and ground black pepper, as required
- 1 onion, chopped
- 2 garlic cloves, minced
- 2¼ cups low-sodium chicken broth
- 2 cups tomatoes, chopped finely
- 1 medium head cauliflower, cut into 1-inch florets

Direction: Preparation Time: 15 minutes Cooking Time: 2¼ hours Servings: 8

- ✓ Preheat the oven to 300 degrees F.
- ✓ In a small bowl, mix together spices and set aside.
- ✓ In a large ovenproof pan, heat oil over medium heat and cook the lamb with a little salt and black pepper for about 10 minutes or until browned from all sides.
- ✓ With a slotted spoon, transfer the lamb into a bowl.
- ✓ In the same pan, add onion and sauté for about 3-4 minutes. Add the garlic and spice mixture and sauté for about 1 minute.
- ✓ Add the cooked lamb, broth and tomatoes and bring to a gentle boil.
- ✓ Immediately, cover the pan and transfer into oven. Bake for about 1½ hours.
- ✓ Remove from oven and stir in cauliflower. Bake for about 30 minutes more or until cauliflower is done completely. Serve hot.

Meal Prep Tip:

- ✓ Transfer the stew into a large bowl and set aside to cool. Divide the stew into 8 containers evenly.
- ✓ Cover the containers and refrigerate for 1-2 days. Reheat in the microwave before serving.

Nutrition: Calories 375 Total Fat 16.2 g Saturated Fat 5 g Cholesterol 153 mg Total Carbs 5.6 g Sugar 2.6 g Fiber 1.8 g Sodium 162 mg Potassium 808 mg Protein 49.7 g

217) Lamb Curry

Ingredients:

For Spice Mixture:
- 2 teaspoons ground coriander
- 2 teaspoons ground cumin
- 1 teaspoon ground cinnamon
- ½ teaspoon ground ginger
- 1 tablespoons sweet paprika
- ½ tablespoon cayenne pepper
- 1 teaspoon red chili powder
- Salt and ground black pepper, as required

For Curry:
- 1 tablespoon olive oil
- 2 pounds boneless lamb, trimmed and cubed into 1-inch size
- 2 cups onions, chopped
- ½ cup fat-free plain Greek yogurt, whipped
- 1½ cups water

Direction: Preparation Time: 15 minutes Cooking Time: 2¼ hours Servings: 8

- ✓ For spice mixture: in a bowl, add all spices and mix well. Set aside. In a large
- ✓ Dutch oven, heat the oil over medium-high heat and stir fry the lamb cubes for about 5 minutes.
- ✓ Add the onion and cook for about 4-5 minutes. Stir in the spice mixture and cook for about 1 minute.
- ✓ Add the yogurt and water and bring to a boil over high heat.
- ✓ Now, reduce the heat to low and simmer, covered for about 1-2 hours or until desired doneness of lamb. Uncover and simmer for about 3-4 minutes. Serve hot.

Meal Prep Tip:
- ✓ Transfer the curry into a large bowl and set aside to cool.
- ✓ Divide the curry into 8 containers evenly.
- ✓ Cover the containers and refrigerate for 1-2 days. Reheat in the microwave before serving.

Nutrition: Calories 254 Total Fat 10.5 g Saturated Fat 3.3 g Cholesterol 102 mg Total Carbs 4.7 g Sugar 1.9 g Fiber 1.4 g Sodium 99 mg Potassium 468 mg Protein 34 g

218) Yummy Meatballs in Tomato Gravy

Ingredients:

For Meatballs:
- 1 pound lean ground lamb
- 1 tablespoon homemade tomato paste
- ¼ cup fresh cilantro leaves, chopped
- 1 small onion, chopped finely
- 2 garlic cloves, minced
- ½ teaspoon ground cumin
- 1/8 teaspoon salt
- Ground black pepper, as required

For Tomato Gravy:
- 3 tablespoons olive oil, divided
- 2 medium onions, chopped finely
- 2 garlic cloves, minced
- ½ tablespoon fresh ginger, minced
- 1 teaspoon dried thyme, crushed
- 1 teaspoon dried oregano, crushed
- 3 large tomatoes, chopped finely
- Ground black pepper, as required
- 1½ cups warm low-sodium chicken broth

Direction: Preparation Time: 20 minutes Cooking Time: 30 minutes Servings: 6

- ✓ For meatballs: in a large bowl, add all the ingredients and mix until well combined.
- ✓ Make small equal-sized balls from mixture and set aside.
- ✓ For gravy: in a large pan, heat 1 tablespoon of oil over medium heat.
- ✓ Add the meatballs and cook for about 4-5 minutes or until lightly browned from all sides.
- ✓ With a slotted spoon, transfer the meatballs onto a plate. In the same pan, heat the remaining oil over medium heat and sauté the onion for about 8-10 minutes.
- ✓ Add the garlic, ginger and herbs and sauté for about 1 minute.
- ✓ Add the tomatoes and cook for about 3-4 minutes, crushing with the back of spoon.
- ✓ Add the warm broth and bring to a boil. Carefully, place the meatballs and cook for 5 minutes, without stirring.
- ✓ Now, reduce the heat to low and cook partially covered for about 15-20 minutes, stirring gently 2-3 times. Serve hot.

Meal Prep Tip:
- ✓ Transfer the meatballs mixture into a large bowl and set aside to cool. Divide the mixture into 6 containers evenly. Cover the containers and refrigerate for 1-2 days. Reheat in the microwave before serving.

Nutrition: Calories 248 Total Fat 12.9 g Saturated Fat 3 g Cholesterol 68 mg Total Carbs 10 g Sugar 4.8 g Fiber 2.5 g Sodium 138 mg Potassium 591 mg Protein 23.4 g

219) Spiced Leg of Lamb

Ingredients:

For Marinade:
- 2/3 cup fat-free plain Greek yogurt
- 1 tablespoon homemade tomato puree
- 1 tablespoon fresh lemon juice
- 3-4 garlic cloves, minced
- 2 tablespoons fresh rosemary, chopped
- 2 teaspoons ground coriander
- 1 teaspoon ground cumin
- 1 teaspoon ground cinnamon 1 teaspoon red pepper flakes, crushed
- ¼ teaspoon sweet paprika
- Sea salt and freshly ground black pepper, as required
- 1 (4½-pound) bone-in leg of lamb

Direction: Preparation Time: 15 minutes Cooking Time: 1 hour 40 minutes Servings: 6

- ✓ In a large bowl, add yogurt, tomato puree, lemon juice, garlic, rosemary, and spices and mix until well combined.
- ✓ Add leg of lamb and coat with marinade generously. Cover and refrigerate to marinate for about 8-10 hours, flipping occasionally.
- ✓ Remove the marinated leg of lamb from refrigerator and keep in room temperature for about 25-30 minutes before roasting.
- ✓ Preheat the oven to 425 degree F. Line a large roasting pan with a greased foil piece.
- ✓ Arrange the leg of lamb into prepared roasting pan. Roast for 20 minutes.
- ✓ Remove the roasting pan from oven and change the side of leg of lamb.
- ✓ Now, Now, reduce the temperature of oven to 325 degree F.
- ✓ Roast for 40 minutes. Now loosely cover the roasting pan with a large piece of foil. Roast for 40 minutes more. Remove from oven and place onto a cutting board for about 10-15 minutes before slicing.
- ✓ With a sharp knife cut the leg of lamb in desired sized slices and serve.

Meal Prep Tip:
- ✓ Transfer the leg slices onto a wire rack to cool completely. With foil pieces, wrap the leg slices and refrigerate for about 1-2 days. Reheat in the microwave before serving.

Nutrition: Calories 478 Total Fat 15.5 g Saturated Fat 6.1 g Cholesterol 226 mg Total Carbs 3.3 g Sugar 1.3 g Fiber 0.9 g Sodium 226 mg Potassium 48 mg Protein 72.3 g

220) Baked Lamb & Spinach

Ingredients:

- 2 tablespoons olive oil
- 2 pounds lamb necks, trimmed and cut into
- 2-inch pieces crosswise
- Salt, as required
- 2 medium onions, chopped
- 3 tablespoons fresh ginger, minced
- 4 garlic cloves, minced
- 2 tablespoons ground coriander
- 1 tablespoon ground cumin
- 1 teaspoon ground turmeric
- ¼ cup fat-free plain Greek yogurt
- ½ cup tomatoes, chopped 2 cups boiling water
- 30 ounces frozen spinach, thawed and squeezed
- 1½ tablespoons garam masala
- 1 tablespoon fresh lemon juice Ground black pepper, as required

Direction: Preparation Time: 15 minutes Cooking Time: 2 hours 55 minutes Servings: 6

- ✓ Preheat the oven to 300 degrees F. In a large
- ✓ Dutch oven, heat the oil over medium-high heat and stir fry the lamb necks with a little salt for about 4-5 minutes or until browned completely.
- ✓ With a slotted spoon, transfer the lamb onto a plate and Now, reduce the heat to medium.
- ✓ In the same pan, add the onion and sauté for about 10 minutes.
- ✓ Add the ginger, garlic and spices and sauté for about 1 minute.
- ✓ Add the yogurt and tomatoes and cook for about 3-4 minutes.
- ✓ With an immersion blender, blend the mixture until smooth. Add the lamb, boiling water and salt and bring to a boil. Cover the pan and transfer into the oven.
- ✓ Bake for about 2½ hours. Now, remove the pan from oven and place over medium heat. Stir in spinach and garam masala and cook for about 3-5 minutes. Stir in lemon juice, salt and black pepper and remove from heat.
- ✓ Serve hot.

Meal Prep Tip:
- ✓ Transfer the lamb mixture into a large bowl and set aside to cool. Divide the mixture into 6 containers evenly. Cover the containers and refrigerate for 1-2 days. Reheat in the microwave before serving.

Nutrition: Calories 469 Total Fat 32.4 g Saturated Fat 13.4 g Cholesterol 0 mg Total Carbs 12.9 g Sugar 3.1 g Fiber 4.7 g Sodium 304 mg Potassium 957 mg Protein 34.1 g

221) Pork Salad

Ingredients:

- 1½ pounds pork tenderloin, trimmed and sliced thinly
- Salt and ground black pepper, as required
- 3 tablespoon olive oil
- 2 carrots, peeled and grated
- 3 cups Napa cabbage, shredded
- 2 scallions, chopped
- 2 tablespoon fresh lime juice
- ¼ cup fresh mint leaves, chopped

Direction: Preparation Time: 15 minutes Cooking Time: 6 minutes Servings: 5

- ✓ Season the pork with salt and black pepper lightly.
- ✓ In a large skillet, heat the oil over medium heat and cook the pork slices for about 2-3 minutes per sides or until cooked through.
- ✓ Remove from the heat and set aside to cool slightly.
- ✓ In a large bowl, add the pork and remaining ingredients except mint leaves and toss to coat well. Serve with the garnishing of mint leaves.

Meal Prep Tip:
- ✓ In 5 containers, divide salad. Refrigerate the containers for about 1 day. Just before serving, stir the salad well

Nutrition: Calories 292 Total Fat 13.3 g Saturated Fat 2.9 g Cholesterol 99 mg Total Carbs 5.7 g Sugar 2.7 g Fiber 2.1 g Sodium 104 mg Potassium 760 mg Protein 36.6 g

222) Pork with Bell Peppers

Ingredients:

- 1 tablespoon fresh ginger, chopped finely
- 4 garlic cloves, chopped finely
- 1 cup fresh cilantro, chopped and divided
- ¼ cup plus
- 1 tablespoon olive oil, divided
- 1 pound tender pork, trimmed, sliced thinly
- 2 onions, sliced thinly
- 1 green bell pepper, seeded and sliced thinly
- 1 red bell pepper, seeded and sliced thinly
- 1 tablespoon fresh lime juice

Direction: Preparation Time: 15 minutes Cooking Time: 13 minutes Servings: 4

- ✓ In a large bowl, mix together ginger, garlic, ½ cup of cilantro and ¼ cup of oil.
- ✓ Add the pork and coat with mixture generously.
- ✓ Refrigerate to marinate for about 2 hours.
- ✓ Heat a large skillet over medium-high heat and stir fry the pork mixture for about 4-5 minutes.
- ✓ Transfer the pork into a bowl. In the same skillet, heat remaining oil over medium heat and sauté the onion for about 3 minutes. Stir in the bell pepper and stir fry for about 3 minutes.
- ✓ Stir in the pork, lime juice and remaining cilantro and cook for about 2 minutes.
- ✓ Serve hot.

Meal Prep Tip:

- ✓ Transfer the pork mixture into a large bowl and set aside to cool.
- ✓ Divide the mixture into 4 containers evenly.
- ✓ Cover the containers and refrigerate for 1-2 days. Reheat in the microwave before serving.

Nutrition: Calories 360 Total Fat 21.8 g Saturated Fat 3.9 g Cholesterol 83 mg Total Carbs 11 g Sugar 5.4 g Fiber 2.2 g Sodium 71 mg Potassium 706 mg Protein 31.2 g

223) Roasted Pork Shoulder

Ingredients:

- 1 head garlic, peeled and crushed
- ¼ cup fresh rosemary, minced
- 2 tablespoons fresh lemon juice
- 2 tablespoons balsamic vinegar
- 1 (4-pound) pork shoulder, trimmed

Direction: Preparation Time: 10 minutes Cooking Time: 6 hours Servings: 12

- ✓ In a bowl, add all the ingredients except pork shoulder and mix well.
- ✓ In a large roasting pan place pork shoulder and coat with marinade generously. With a large plastic wrap, cover the roasting pan and refrigerate to marinate for at least 1-2 hours.
- ✓ Remove the roasting pan from refrigerator.
- ✓ Remove the plastic wrap from roasting pan and keep in room temperature for 1 hour. Preheat the oven to 275 degrees F.
- ✓ Arrange the roasting pan in oven and roast for about 6 hours.
- ✓ Remove from the oven and set aside for about 15-20 minutes. With a sharp knife, cut the pork shoulder into desired slices and serve.

Meal Prep Tip:

- ✓ Transfer the pork slices onto a wire rack to cool completely. With foil pieces, wrap the pork slices and refrigerate for about 1-2 days. Reheat in the microwave before serving.

Nutrition: Calories 450 Total Fat 32.6g Saturated Fat 12 g Cholesterol 136 mg Total Carbs 1.5 g Sugar 0.1 g Fiber 0.6 g Sodium 104 mg Potassium 522 mg Protein 35.4 g

224) Pork Chops in Peach Glaze

Ingredients:

- 2 (6-ounce) boneless pork chops, trimmed
- Sea Salt and ground black pepper, as required
- ½ of ripe yellow peach, peeled, pitted and chopped
- 1 tablespoon olive oil
- 2 tablespoons shallot, minced
- 2 tablespoons garlic, minced
- 2 tablespoons fresh ginger, minced
- 4-6 drops liquid stevia
- 1 tablespoon balsamic vinegar
- ¼ teaspoon red pepper flakes, crushed
- ¼ cup filtered water

Direction: Preparation Time: 15 minutes Cooking Time: 16 minutes Servings: 2

- ✓ Season the pork chops with sea salt and black pepper generously. In a blender, add the peach pieces and pulse until a puree forms.
- ✓ Reserve the remaining peach pieces. In a skillet, heat the oil over medium heat and sauté the shallots for about 1-2 minutes.
- ✓ Add the garlic and ginger and sauté for about 1 minute. Stir in the remaining ingredients and bring to a boil.
- ✓ Now, reduce the heat to medium-low and simmer for about 4-5 minutes or until a sticky glaze forms.
- ✓ Remove from the heat and reserve 1/3 of the glaze and set aside. Coat the chops with remaining glaze.
- ✓ Heat a nonstick skillet over medium-high heat and sear the chops for about 4 minutes per side.
- ✓ Transfer the chops onto a plate and coat with the remaining glaze evenly. Serve immediately.

Meal Prep Tip:

- ✓ Transfer the pork chops into a large bowl and set aside to cool.
- ✓ Divide the chops into 2 containers evenly.
- ✓ Cover the containers and refrigerate for 1-2 days. Reheat in the microwave before serving.

Nutrition: Calories 359 Total Fat 13.5 g Saturated Fat 3.2 g Cholesterol 124 mg Total Carbs 12 g Sugar 3.8 g Fiber 1.5 g Sodium 102 mg Potassium 938 mg Protein 46.2 g

225) Ground Pork with Spinach

Ingredients:

- 1 tablespoon olive oil
- ½ of white onion, chopped
- 2 garlic cloves, chopped finely
- 1 jalapeño pepper, chopped finely
- 1 pound lean ground pork
- 1 teaspoon ground coriander
- 1 teaspoon ground cumin
- ½ teaspoon ground turmeric
- ½ teaspoon ground cinnamon
- ½ teaspoon ground fennel seeds
- Salt and ground black pepper, as required
- ½ cup fresh cherry tomatoes, quartered
- 1¼ pounds collard greens leaves, stemmed and chopped
- 1 teaspoon fresh lemon juice

Direction: Preparation Time: 15 minutes Cooking Time: 15 minutes Servings: 4

- ✓ In a large skillet, heat the oil over medium heat and sauté the onion for about 4 minutes.
- ✓ Add the garlic and jalapeño pepper and sauté for about 1 minute.
- ✓ Add the pork and spices and cook for about 6 minutes breaking into pieces with the spoon.
- ✓ Stir in the tomatoes and greens and cook, stirring gently for about 4 minutes. Stir in the lemon juice and remove from heat. Serve hot.

Meal Prep Tip:

- ✓ Transfer the pork mixture into a large bowl and set aside to cool. Divide the mixture into 4 containers evenly. Cover the containers and refrigerate for 1-2 days. Reheat in the microwave before serving.

Nutrition: Calories 316 Total Fat 21.8 g Saturated Fat 0.5 g Cholesterol 0 mg Total Carbs 11.4 g Sugar 1.4 g Fiber 5.7 g Sodium 27 mg Potassium 107 mg Protein 23 g

FISH AND SEAFOOD

226) Baked Salmon with Garlic Parmesan Topping

Ingredients:

- 1 lb. wild caught salmon filets
- 2 tbsp. margarine
- What you'll need from store cupboard:
- ¼ cup reduced fat parmesan cheese, grated
- ¼ cup light mayonnaise
- 2-3 cloves garlic, diced
- 2 tbsp. parsley
- Salt and pepper

Direction: Preparation time: 5 minutes,
Cooking time: 20 minutes, Servings: 4

- ✓ Heat oven to 350 and line a baking pan with parchment paper.
- ✓ Place salmon on pan and season with salt and pepper.
- ✓ In a medium skillet, over medium heat, melt butter. Add garlic and cook, stirring 1 minute.
- ✓ Reduce heat to low and add remaining Ingredients. Stir until everything is melted and combined.
- ✓ Spread evenly over salmon and bake 15 minutes for thawed fish or 20 for frozen. Salmon is done when it flakes easily with a fork. Serve.

Nutrition: Calories 408; Total Carbs 4g; Protein 41g; Fat 24g; Sugar 1g; Fiber 0g

227) Blackened Shrimp

Ingredients:

- 1 1/2 lbs. shrimp, peel & devein
- 4 lime wedges
- 4 tbsp. cilantro, chopped
- What you'll need from store cupboard:
- 4 cloves garlic, diced
- 1 tbsp. chili powder
- 1 tbsp. paprika
- 1 tbsp. olive oil
- 2 tsp. Splenda brown sugar
- 1 tsp. cumin
- 1 tsp. oregano
- 1 tsp. garlic powder
- 1 tsp. salt
- 1/2tsp. pepper

Direction: Preparation time: 5 minutes
Cooking time: 5 minutes Servings: 4

- ✓ In a small bowl combine seasonings and Splenda brown sugar.
- ✓ Heat oil in a skillet over med-high heat. Add shrimp, in a single layer, and cook 1-2 minutes per side.
- ✓ Add seasonings, and cook, stirring, 30 seconds.
- ✓ Serve garnished with cilantro and a lime wedge.

Nutrition: Calories 252; Total Carbs 7g; Net Carbs 6g; Protein 39g; Fat 7g; Sugar 2g; Fiber 1g

228) Cajun Catfish

Ingredients:

- 4 (8 oz.) catfish fillets
- What you'll need from store cupboard:
- 2 tbsp. olive oil
- 2 tsp. garlic salt
- 2 tsp. thyme
- 2 tsp. paprika
- 1/2tsp. cayenne pepper
- 1/2tsp. red hot sauce
- ¼ tsp. black pepper
- Nonstick cooking spray

Direction: Preparation time: 5 minutes
Cooking time: 15 minutes Servings: 4

- ✓ Heat oven to 450 degrees. Spray a 9x13-inch baking dish with cooking spray.
- ✓ In a small bowl whisk together everything but catfish. Brush both sides of fillets, using all the spice mix.
- ✓ 3. Bake 10-13 minutes or until fish flakes easily with a fork. Serve.

Nutrition: Calories 366; Total Carbs 0g; Protein 35g; Fat 24g; Sugar 0g; Fiber 0g

229) Cajun Flounder & Tomatoes

Ingredients:

- 4 flounder fillets
- 2 1/2 cups tomatoes, diced
- ¾ cup onion, diced
- ¾ cup green bell pepper, diced
- What you'll need from store cupboard:
- 2 cloves garlic, diced fine
- 1 tbsp. Cajun seasoning
- 1 tsp. olive oil

Direction: Preparation time: 10 minutes
Cooking time: 15 minutes Servings: 4

- ✓ Heat oil in a large skillet over med-high heat. Add onion and garlic and cook 2 minutes, or until soft. Add tomatoes, peppers and spices, and cook 2-3 minutes until tomatoes soften.
- ✓ Lay fish over top. Cover, reduce heat to medium and cook, 5-8 minutes, or until fish flakes easily with a fork. Transfer fish to serving plates and top with sauce.

Nutrition: Calories 194; Total Carbs 8g; Net Carbs 6g; Protein 32g; Fat 3g; Sugar 5g; Fiber 2g

230) Cajun Shrimp & Roasted Vegetables

Ingredients:

- 1 lb. large shrimp, peeled and deveined
- 2 zucchinis, sliced
- 2 yellow squash, sliced
- 1/2 bunch asparagus, cut into thirds
- 2 red bell pepper, cut into chunks
- What you'll need from store cupboard:
- 2 tbsp. olive oil
- 2 tbsp. Cajun Seasoning
- Salt & pepper, to taste

Direction: Preparation time: 5 minutes
Cooking time: 15 minutes Servings: 4

- ✓ Heat oven to 400 degrees.
- ✓ Combine shrimp and vegetables in a large bowl. Add oil and seasoning and toss to coat.
- ✓ Spread evenly in a large baking sheet and bake 15-20 minutes, or until vegetables are tender. Serve.

Nutrition: Calories 251; Total Carbs 13g; Net Carbs 9g; Protein 30g; Fat 9g; Sugar 6g; Fiber 4g

231) Cilantro Lime Grilled Shrimp

Ingredients:

- 1 1/2 lbs. large shrimp raw, peeled, deveined with tails on
- Juice and zest of 1 lime
- 2 tbsp. fresh cilantro chopped
- What you'll need from store cupboard:
- ¼ cup olive oil
- 2 cloves garlic, diced fine
- 1 tsp. smoked paprika
- ¼ tsp. cumin
- 1/2 teaspoon salt
- ¼ tsp. cayenne pepper

Direction: Preparation time: 5 minutes, Cooking time: 5 minutes, Servings: 6

- ✓ Place the shrimp in a large Ziploc bag.
- ✓ Mix remaining Ingredients in a small bowl and pour over shrimp. Let marinate 20-30 minutes.
- ✓ Heat up the grill. Skewer the shrimp and cook 2-3 minutes, per side, just until they turn pick. Be careful not to overcook them. Serve garnished with cilantro.

Nutrition: Calories 317; Total Carbs 4g; Protein 39g; Fat 15g; Sugar 0g; Fiber 0g

232) Crab Frittata

Ingredients:

- 4 eggs
- 2 cups lump crabmeat
- 1 cup half-n-half
- 1 cup green onions, diced
- What you'll need from store cupboard:
- 1 cup reduced fat parmesan cheese, grated
- 1 tsp. salt
- 1 tsp. pepper
- 1 tsp. smoked paprika
- 1 tsp. Italian seasoning
- Nonstick cooking spray

Direction: Preparation time: 10 minutes Cooking time: 50 minutes Servings: 4

- ✓ Heat oven to 350 degrees. Spray an 8-inch springform pan, or pie plate with cooking spray.
- ✓ In a large bowl, whisk together the eggs and half-n-half. Add seasonings and parmesan cheese, stir to mix.
- ✓ Stir in the onions and crab meat. Pour into prepared pan and bake 35-40 minutes, or eggs are set and top is lightly browned.
- ✓ Let cool 10 minutes, then slice and serve warm or at room temperature.

Nutrition: Calories 276; Total Carbs 5g; Net Carbs 4g; Protein 25g; Fat 17g Sugar 1g, Fiber 1g

233) Crunchy Lemon Shrimp

Ingredients:

- 1 lb. raw shrimp, peeled and deveined
- 2 tbsp. Italian parsley, roughly chopped
- 2 tbsp. lemon juice, divided
- What you'll need from store cupboard:
- 2/3 cup panko bread crumbs
- 2 1/2 tbsp. olive oil, divided
- Salt and pepper, to taste

Direction: Preparation time: 5 minutes Cooking time: 10 minutes, Servings: 4

- ✓ Heat oven to 400 degrees.
- ✓ Place the shrimp evenly in a baking dish and sprinkle with salt and pepper.
- ✓ Drizzle on 1 tablespoon lemon juice and 1 tablespoon of olive oil. Set aside.
- ✓ In a medium bowl, combine parsley, remaining lemon juice, bread crumbs, remaining olive oil, and ¼ tsp. each of salt and pepper. Layer the panko mixture evenly on top of the shrimp.
- ✓ Bake 8-10 minutes or until shrimp are cooked through and the panko is golden brown.

Nutrition: Calories 283; Total Carbs 15g; Net Carbs 14g; Protein 28g; Fat 12g; Sugar 1g; Fiber 1g

234) Grilled Tuna Steaks

Ingredients:

- 6 6 oz. tuna steaks
- 3 tbsp. fresh basil, diced
- What you'll need from store cupboard:
- 4 1/2 tsp. olive oil
- ¾ tsp. salt
- ¼ tsp. pepper
- Nonstick cooking spray

Direction: Preparation time: 5 minutes Cooking time: 10 minutes, Servings: 6

- ✓ Heat grill to medium heat. Spray rack with cooking spray.
- ✓ Drizzle both sides of the tuna with oil. Sprinkle with basil, salt and pepper.
- ✓ Place on grill and cook 5 minutes per side, tuna should be slightly pink in the center. Serve.

Nutrition: Calories 343; Total Carbs 0g; Protein 51g; Fat 14g; Sugar 0g; Fiber 0g

235) Red Clam Sauce & Pasta

Ingredients:

- 1 onion, diced
- ¼ cup fresh parsley, diced
- What you'll need from store cupboard:
- 2 6 1/2 oz. cans clams, chopped, undrained
- 14 1/2 oz. tomatoes, diced, undrained
- 6 oz. tomato paste
- 2 cloves garlic, diced
- 1 bay leaf
- 1 tbsp. sunflower oil
- 1 tsp. Splenda
- 1 tsp. basil
- 1/2 tsp. thyme
- 1/2 Homemade Pasta, cook & drain

Direction: Preparation time: 10 minutes, Cooking time: 3 hours, Servings: 4

- ✓ Heat oil in a small skillet over med-high heat. Add onion and cook until tender,
- ✓ Add garlic and cook 1 minute more. Transfer to crock pot.
- ✓ Add remaining Ingredients, except pasta, cover and cook on low 3-4 hours.
- ✓ Discard bay leaf and serve over cooked pasta.

Nutrition: Calories 223; Total Carbs 32g; Net Carbs 27g; Protein 12g; Fat 6g; Sugar 15g Fiber 5g

236) Salmon Milano

Ingredients:
- 2 1/2 lb. salmon filet
- 2 tomatoes, sliced
- 1/2 cup margarine
- What you'll need from store cupboard:
- 1/2 cup basil pesto

Direction: Preparation time: 10 minutes,
Cooking time: 20 minutes, Servings: 6

- ✓ Heat the oven to 400 degrees. Line a 9x15-inch baking sheet with foil, making sure it covers the sides. Place another large piece of foil onto the baking sheet and place the salmon filet on top of it.
- ✓ Place the pesto and margarine in blender or food processor and pulse until smooth. Spread evenly over salmon.
- ✓ Place tomato slices on top.
- ✓ Wrap the foil around the salmon, tenting around the top to prevent foil from touching the salmon as much as possible.
- ✓ Bake 15-25 minutes, or salmon flakes easily with a fork. Serve.

Nutrition: Calories 444; Total Carbs 2g; Protein 55g; Fat 24g; Sugar 1g; Fiber 0g

237) Shrimp & Artichoke Skillet

Ingredients:
- 1 1/2 cups shrimp, peel & devein
- 2 shallots, diced
- 1 tbsp. margarine
- What you'll need from store cupboard
- 2 12 oz. jars artichoke hearts, drain & rinse
- 2 cups white wine
- 2 cloves garlic, diced fine

Direction: Preparation time: 5 minutes
Cooking time: 10 minutes Servings: 4

- ✓ Melt margarine in a large skillet over med-high heat. Add shallot and garlic and cook until they start to brown, stirring frequently.
- ✓ Add artichokes and cook 5 minutes. Reduce heat and add wine. Cook 3 minutes, stirring occasionally.
- ✓ Add the shrimp and cook just until they turn pink. Serve.

Nutrition: Calories 487; Total Carbs 26g; Net Carbs 17g; Protein 64g; Fat 5; Sugar 3g; Fiber 9g

238) Tuna Carbonara

Ingredients:
- 1/2 lb. tuna fillet, cut in pieces
- 2 eggs
- 4 tbsp. fresh parsley, diced
- What you'll need from store cupboard:
- 1/2 Homemade Pasta, cook & drain,
- 1/2 cup reduced fat parmesan cheese
- 2 cloves garlic, peeled
- 2 tbsp. extra virgin olive oil
- Salt & pepper, to taste

Direction: Preparation time: 5 minutes
Cooking time: 25 minutes Servings: 4

- ✓ In a small bowl, beat the eggs, parmesan and a dash of pepper.
- ✓ Heat the oil in a large skillet over med-high heat.
- ✓ Add garlic and cook until browned. Add the tuna and cook 2-3 minutes, or until tuna is almost cooked through. Discard the garlic.
- ✓ Add the pasta and reduce heat. Stir in egg mixture and cook, stirring constantly, 2 minutes. If the sauce is too thick, thin with water, a little bit at a time, until it has a creamy texture.
- ✓ Salt and pepper to taste and serve garnished with parsley.

Nutrition: Calories 409; Total Carbs 7g; Net Carbs 6g; Protein 25g

239) Mediterranean Fish Fillets

Ingredients:
- 4 cod fillets
- 1 lb. grape tomatoes, halved
- 1 cup olives, pitted and sliced
- 2 tbsp. capers
- 1 tsp. dried thyme
- 2 tbsp. olive oil
- 1 tsp. garlic, minced
- Pepper
- Salt

Direction: Preparation Time: 10 minutes
Cooking Time: 3 minutes Servings: 4

- ✓ Pour 1 cup water into the instant pot then place steamer rack in the pot.
- ✓ Spray heat-safe baking dish with cooking spray.
- ✓ Add half grape tomatoes into the dish and season with pepper and salt.
- ✓ Arrange fish fillets on top of cherry tomatoes. Drizzle with oil and season with garlic, thyme, capers, pepper, and salt.
- ✓ Spread olives and remaining grape tomatoes on top of fish fillets.
- ✓ Place dish on top of steamer rack in the pot.
- ✓ Seal pot with a lid and select manual and cook on high for 3 minutes.
- ✓ Once done, release pressure using quick release. Remove lid.
- ✓ Serve and enjoy.

Nutrition: Calories 212; Fat 11.9 g; Carbs 7.1 g; Sugar 3 g; Protein 21.4 g; Cholesterol 55 mg

240) Lemony Salmon

Ingredients:
- 1 pound salmon fillet, cut into 3 pieces
- 3 teaspoons fresh dill, chopped
- 5 tablespoons fresh lemon juice, divided
- Salt and ground black pepper, as required

Direction: Preparation Time: 10 minutes
Cooking Time: 3 Minutes Servings: 3

- ✓ Arrange a steamer trivet in Instant Pot and pour ¼ cup of lemon juice.
- ✓ Season the salmon with salt and black pepper evenly.
- ✓ Place the salmon pieces on top of trivet, skin side down and drizzle with remaining lemon juice.
- ✓ Now, sprinkle the salmon pieces with dill evenly.
- ✓ Close the lid and place the pressure valve to "Seal" position.
- ✓ Press "Steam" and use the default time of 3 minutes.
- ✓ Press "Cancel" and allow a "Natural" release.
- ✓ Open the lid and serve hot.

Nutrition: Calories 20 Fats 9.6g, Carbs 1.1g, Sugar 0.5g, Proteins 29.7g, Sodium 74mg

241) Shrimp with Green Beans

Ingredients:

- ¾ pound fresh green beans, trimmed
- 1 pound medium frozen shrimp, peeled and deveined
- 2 tablespoons fresh lemon juice
- 2 tablespoons olive oil
- Salt and ground black pepper, as required

Direction: Preparation Time: 10 minutes
Cooking Time: 2 Minutes Servings: 4

- ✓ Arrange a steamer trivet in the Instant Pot and pour cup of water.
- ✓ Arrange the green beans on top of trivet in a single layer and top with shrimp.
- ✓ Drizzle with oil and lemon juice.
- ✓ Sprinkle with salt and black pepper.
- ✓ Close the lid and place the pressure valve to "Seal" position.
- ✓ Press "Steam" and just use the default time of 2 minutes.
- ✓ Press "Cancel" and allow a "Natural" release.
- ✓ Open the lid and serve.

Nutrition: Calories 223, Fats 1g, Carbs 7.9g, Sugar 1.4g, Proteins 27.4g, Sodium 322mg

242) Crab Curry

Ingredients:

- 0.5lb chopped crab
- 1 thinly sliced red onion
- 0.5 cup chopped tomato
- 3tbsp curry paste
- 1tbsp oil or ghee

Direction: Preparation Time: 10 minutes
Cooking Time: 20 Minutes Servings: 2

- ✓ Set the Instant Pot to sauté and add the onion, oil, and curry paste.
- ✓ When the onion is soft, add the remaining ingredients and seal.
- ✓ Cook on Stew for 20 minutes.
- ✓ Release the pressure naturally.

Nutrition: Calories 2; Carbs 11; Sugar 4; Fat 10; Protein 24; GL 9

243) Mixed Chowder

Ingredients:

- 1lb fish stew mix
- 2 cups white sauce
- 3tbsp old bay seasoning

Direction: Preparation Time: 10 minutes
Cooking Time: 35 Minutes Servings: 2

- ✓ Mix all the ingredients in your Instant Pot.
- ✓ Cook on Stew for 35 minutes.
- ✓ Release the pressure naturally.

Nutrition: : Calories 320; Carbs 9; Sugar 2; Fat 16; Protein GL 4

244) Mussels in Tomato Sauce

Ingredients:

- 2 tomatoes, seeded and chopped finely
- 2 pounds mussels, scrubbed and de-bearded
- 1 cup low-sodium chicken broth
- 1 tablespoon fresh lemon juice
- 2 garlic cloves, minced

Direction: Preparation Time: 10 minutes
Cooking Time: 3 Minutes Servings: 4

- ✓ In the pot of Instant Pot, place tomatoes, garlic, wine and bay leaf and stir to combine.
- ✓ Arrange the mussels on top.
- ✓ Close the lid and place the pressure valve to "Seal" position.
- ✓ Press "Manual" and cook under "High Pressure" for about 3 minutes.
- ✓ Press "Cancel" and carefully allow a "Quick" release.
- ✓ Open the lid and serve hot.

Nutrition: Calories 213, Fats 25.2g, Carbs 11g, Sugar 1. Proteins 28.2g, Sodium 670mg

245) Citrus Salmon

Ingredients:

- 4 (4-ounce) salmon fillets
- 1 cup low-sodium chicken broth
- 1 teaspoon fresh ginger, minced
- 2 teaspoons fresh orange zest, grated finely
- 3 tablespoons fresh orange juice
- 1 tablespoon olive oil
- Ground black pepper, as required

Direction: Preparation Time: 10 minutes
Cooking Time: 7 Minutes Servings: 4

- ✓ In Instant Pot, add all ingredients and mix.
- ✓ Close the lid and place the pressure valve to "Seal" position.
- ✓ Press "Manual" and cook under "High Pressure" for about 7 minutes.
- ✓ Press "Cancel" and allow a "Natural" release.
- ✓ Open the lid and serve the salmon fillets with the topping of cooking sauce.

Nutrition: Calories 190, Fats 10.5g, Carbs 1.8g, Sugar 1g, Proteins 22. Sodium 68mg

246) Herbed Salmon

Ingredients:

- 4 (4-ounce) salmon fillets
- ¼ cup olive oil
- 2 tablespoons fresh lemon juice
- 1 garlic clove, minced
- ¼ teaspoon dried oregano
- Salt and ground black pepper, as required
- 4 fresh rosemary sprigs
- 4 lemon slices

Direction: Preparation Time: 10 minutes
Cooking Time: 3 Minutes Servings: 4

- ✓ For dressing: in a large bowl, add oil, lemon juice, garlic, oregano, salt and black pepper and beat until well co combined.
- ✓ Arrange a steamer trivet in the Instant Pot and pour 11/2 cups of water in Instant Pot.
- ✓ Place the salmon fillets on top of trivet in a single layer and top with dressing.
- ✓ Arrange 1 rosemary sprig and 1 lemon slice over each fillet.
- ✓ Close the lid and place the pressure valve to "Seal" position.
- ✓ Press "Steam" and just use the default time of 3 minutes.
- ✓ Press "Cancel" and carefully allow a "Quick" release.
- ✓ Open the lid and serve hot.

Nutrition: Calories 262, Fats 17g, Carbs 0.7g, Sugar 0.2g, Proteins 22.1g, Sodium 91mg

247) Salmon in Green Sauce

Ingredients:

- 4 (6-ounce) salmon fillets
- 1 avocado, peeled, pitted and chopped
- 1/2 cup fresh basil, chopped
- 3 garlic cloves, chopped
- 1 tablespoon fresh lemon zest, grated finely

Direction: Preparation Time: 10 minutes
Cooking Time: 12 Minutes Servings: 4

- ✓ Grease a large piece of foil.
- ✓ In a large bowl, add all ingredients except salmon and water and with a fork, mash completely.
- ✓ Place fillets in the center of foil and top with avocado mixture evenly.
- ✓ Fold the foil around fillets to seal them.
- ✓ Arrange a steamer trivet in the Instant Pot and pour 1/2 cup of water.
- ✓ Place the foil packet on top of trivet.
- ✓ Close the lid and place the pressure valve to "Seal" position.
- ✓ Press "Manual" and cook under "High Pressure" for about minutes.
- ✓ Meanwhile, preheat the oven to broiler.
- ✓ Press "Cancel" and allow a "Natural" release.
- ✓ Open the lid and transfer the salmon fillets onto a broiler pan.
- ✓ Broil for about 3-4 minutes.
- ✓ Serve warm.

Nutrition: Calories 333, Fats 20.3g, Carbs 5.5g, Sugar 0.4g, Proteins 34.2g, Sodium 79mg

248) Braised Shrimp

Ingredients:

- 1 pound frozen large shrimp, peeled and deveined
- 2 shallots, chopped
- ¾ cup low-sodium chicken broth
- 2 tablespoons fresh lemon juice
- 2 tablespoons olive oil
- 1 tablespoon garlic, crushed
- Ground black pepper, as required

Direction: Preparation Time: 10 minutes
Cooking Time: 4 Minutes Servings: 4

- ✓ In the Instant Pot, place oil and press "Sauté". Now add the shallots and cook for about 2 minutes.
- ✓ Add the garlic and cook for about 1 minute.
- ✓ Press "Cancel" and stir in the shrimp, broth, lemon juice and black pepper.
- ✓ Close the lid and place the pressure valve to "Seal" position.
- ✓ Press "Manual" and cook under "High Pressure" for about 1 minute.
- ✓ Press "Cancel" and carefully allow a "Quick" release.
- ✓ Open the lid and serve hot.

Nutrition: Calories 209, Fats 9g, Carbs 4.3g, Sugar 0.2g, Proteins 26.6g, Sodium 293mg

249) Shrimp Coconut Curry

Ingredients:

- 0.5lb cooked shrimp
- 1 thinly sliced onion
- 1 cup coconut yogurt
- 3tbsp curry paste
- 1tbsp oil or ghee

Direction: Preparation Time: 10 minutes
Cooking Time: 20 Minutes Servings: 2

- ✓ Set the Instant Pot to sauté and add the onion, oil, and curry paste.
- ✓ When the onion is soft, add the remaining ingredients and seal.
- ✓ Cook on Stew for 20 minutes.
- ✓ Release the pressure naturally.

Nutrition: Calories: 380 Carbs 13; Sugar 4; Fat 22; Protein 40; GL 14

250) Trout Bake

Ingredients:

- 1lb trout fillets, boneless
- 1lb chopped winter vegetables
- 1 cup low sodium fish broth
- 1tbsp mixed herbs
- sea salt as desired

Direction: Preparation Time: 10 minutes
Cooking Time: 35 Minutes Servings: 2

- ✓ Mix all the ingredients except the broth in a foil pouch.
- ✓ Place the pouch in the steamer basket your Instant Pot.
- ✓ Pour the broth into the Instant Pot.
- ✓ Cook on Steam for 35 minutes.
- ✓ Release the pressure naturally.

Nutrition: : Calories 310; Carbs 14; Sugar 2; Fat 12; Protein 40; GL 5

251) Sardine Curry

Ingredients:
- 5 tins of sardines in tomato
- 1lb chopped vegetables
- 1 cup low sodium fish broth
- 3tbsp curry paste

Direction: Preparation Time: 10 minutes
Cooking Time: 35 Minutes **Servings:** 2

- ✓ Mix all the ingredients in your Instant Pot.
- ✓ Cook on Stew for 35 minutes.
- ✓ Release the pressure naturally.

Nutrition: Calories 320; Carbs 8; Sugar 2; Fat 16; Protein GL 3

252) Swordfish Steak

Ingredients:
- 1lb swordfish steak, whole
- 1lb chopped Mediterranean vegetables
- 1 cup low sodium fish broth
- 2tbsp soy sauce

Direction: Preparation Time: 10 minutes
Cooking Time: 35 Minutes **Servings:** 2

- ✓ Mix all the ingredients except the broth in a foil pouch.
- ✓ Place the pouch in the steamer basket for your Instant Pot.
- ✓ Pour the broth into the Instant Pot. Lower the steamer basket into the Instant Pot.
- ✓ Cook on Steam for 35 minutes.
- ✓ Release the pressure naturally.

Nutrition: Calories 270; Carbs 5; Sugar 1; Fat 10; Protein 48; GL 1

253) Lemon Sole

Ingredients:
- 1lb sole fillets, boned and skinned
- 1 cup low sodium fish broth
- 2 shredded sweet onions
- juice of half a lemon
- 2tbsp dried cilantro

Direction: Preparation Time: 10 minutes
Cooking Time: 5 Minutes **Servings:** 2

- ✓ Mix all the ingredients in your Instant Pot.
- ✓ Cook on Stew for 5 minutes.
- ✓ Release the pressure naturally.

Nutrition: Calories 230; Carbs Sugar 1; Fat 6; Protein 46; GL 1

254) Tuna Sweet corn Casserole

Ingredients:
- 3 small tins of tuna
- 0.5lb sweet corn kernels
- 1lb chopped vegetables
- 1 cup low sodium vegetable broth
- 2tbsp spicy seasoning

Direction: Preparation Time: 10 minutes
Cooking Time: 35 Minutes **Servings:** 2

- ✓ Mix all the ingredients in your Instant Pot.
- ✓ Cook on Stew for 35 minutes.
- ✓ Release the pressure naturally.

Nutrition: Calories: 300; Carbs: 6 ; Sugar: 1 ; Fat: 9 ; Protein: ; GL: 2

255) Lemon Pepper Salmon

Ingredients:
- 3 tbsps. ghee or avocado oil
- 1 lb. skin-on salmon filet
- 1 julienned red bell pepper
- 1 julienned green zucchini
- 1 julienned carrot
- ¾ cup water
- A few sprigs of parsley, tarragon, dill, basil or a combination
- 1/2 sliced lemon
- 1/2 tsp. black pepper
- ¼ tsp. sea salt

Direction: Preparation Time: 10 minutes
Cooking Time: 10 Minutes **Servings:** 4

- ✓ Add the water and the herbs into the bottom of the Instant Pot and put in a wire steamer rack making sure the handles extend upwards.
- ✓ Place the salmon filet onto the wire rack, with the skin side facing down.
- ✓ Drizzle the salmon with ghee, season with black pepper and salt, and top with the lemon slices.
- ✓ Close and seal the Instant Pot, making sure the vent is turned to "Sealing".
- ✓ Select the "Steam" setting and cook for 3 minutes.
- ✓ While the salmon cooks, julienne the vegetables, and set aside.
- ✓ Once done, quick release the pressure, and then press the "Keep Warm/Cancel" button.
- ✓ Uncover and wearing oven mitts, carefully remove the steamer rack with the salmon.
- ✓ Remove the herbs and discard them.
- ✓ Add the vegetables to the pot and put the lid back on.
- ✓ Select the "Sauté" function and cook for 1-2 minutes.
- ✓ Serve the vegetables with salmon and add the remaining fat to the pot.
- ✓ Pour a little of the sauce over the fish and vegetables if desired.

Nutrition: Calories 296, Carbs 8g, Fat 15 g, Protein 31 g, Potassium (K) 1084 mg, Sodium (Na) 284 mg

256) Almond Crusted Baked Chili Mahi Mahi

Ingredients:
- 4 mahi mahi fillets 1 lime
- 2 teaspoons olive oil Salt and pepper to taste
- ½ cup almonds
- ¼ teaspoon paprika
- ¼ teaspoon onion powder
- ¾ teaspoon chili powder
- ½ cup red bell pepper, chopped
- ¼ cup onion, chopped
- ¼ cup fresh cilantro, chopped

Direction: Preparation Time: 20 minutes Cooking Time: 15 minutes **Servings:** 4

- ✓ Preheat your oven to 325 degrees F. Line your baking pan with parchment paper. Squeeze juice from the lime.
- ✓ Grate zest from the peel. Put juice and zest in a bowl. Add the oil, salt and pepper. In another bowl, add the almonds, paprika, onion powder and chili powder.
- ✓ Put the almond mixture in a food processor. Pulse until powdery.
- ✓ Dip each fillet in the oil mixture.
- ✓ Dredge with the almond and chili mixture.
- ✓ Arrange on a single layer in the oven. Bake for 12 to 15 minutes or until fully cooked.
- ✓ Serve with red bell pepper, onion and cilantro.

Nutrition: Calories 322 Total Fat 12 g Saturated Fat 2 g Cholesterol 83 mg Sodium 328 mg Total Carbohydrate 28 g Dietary Fiber 4 g Total Sugars 10 g Protein 28 g Potassium 829 mg

257) Salmon & Asparagus

Ingredients:

- 2 salmon fillets
- 8 spears asparagus, trimmed
- 2 tablespoons balsamic vinegar
- 1 teaspoon olive oil
- 1 teaspoon dried dill
- Salt and pepper to taste

Direction: Preparation Time: 15 minutes Cooking Time: 10 minutes Servings: 2

- ✓ Preheat your oven to 325 degrees F.
- ✓ Dry salmon with paper towels.
- ✓ Arrange the asparagus around the salmon fillets on a baking pan. In a bowl, mix the rest of the ingredients.
- ✓ Pour mixture over the salmon and vegetables.
- ✓ Bake in the oven for 10 minutes or until the fish is fully cooked.

Nutrition: Calories 328 Total Fat 15 g Saturated Fat 3 g Cholesterol 67 mg Sodium 365 mg Total Carbohydrate 6 g Dietary Fiber 4 g Total Sugars 5 g Protein 28 g Potassium 258 mg

258) Halibut with Spicy Apricot Sauce

Ingredients:

- 4 fresh apricots, pitted
- ⅓ cup apricot preserves
- ½ cup apricot nectar
- ½ teaspoon dried oregano
- 3 tablespoons scallion, sliced
- 1 teaspoon hot pepper sauce Salt to taste
- 4 halibut steaks
- 1 tablespoon olive oil

Direction: Preparation Time: 15 minutes Cooking Time: 17 minutes Servings: 4

- ✓ Put the apricots, preserves, nectar, oregano, scallion, hot pepper sauce and salt in a saucepan.
- ✓ Bring to a boil and then simmer for 8 minutes. Set aside.
- ✓ Brush the halibut steaks with olive oil.
- ✓ Grill for 7 to 9 minutes or until fish is flaky.
- ✓ Brush one tablespoon of the sauce on both sides of the fish. Serve with the reserved sauce.

Nutrition:: Calories 304 Total Fat 8 g Saturated Fat 1 g Cholesterol 73 mg Sodium 260 mg Total Carbohydrate 27 g Dietary Fiber 2 g Total Sugars 16 g Protein 29 g Potassium 637 mg

259) Popcorn Shrimp

Ingredients:

- Cooking spray
- ½ cup all-purpose flour
- 2 eggs, beaten
- 2 tablespoons water
- 1 ½ cups panko breadcrumbs
- 1 tablespoon garlic powder
- 1 tablespoon ground cumin
- 1 lb. shrimp, peeled and deveined
- ½ cup ketchup
- 2 tablespoons fresh cilantro, chopped
- 2 tablespoons lime juice Salt to taste

Direction: Preparation Time: 15 minutes Cooking Time: 8 minutes Servings: 4

- ✓ Coat the air fryer basket with cooking spray
- ✓ Put the flour in a dish. In the second dish, beat the eggs and water.
- ✓ In the third dish, mix the breadcrumbs, garlic powder and cumin.
- ✓ Dip each shrimp in each of the three dishes, first in the dish with flour, then the egg and then breadcrumb mixture.
- ✓ Place the shrimp in the air fryer basket.
- ✓ Cook at 360 degrees F for 8 minutes, flipping once halfway through.
- ✓ Combine the rest of the ingredients as dipping sauce for the shrimp.

Nutrition: Calories 297 Total Fat 4 g Saturated Fat 1 g Cholesterol 276 mg Sodium 291 mg Total Carbohydrate 35 g Dietary Fiber 1 g Total Sugars 9 g Protein 29 g Potassium 390 mg

260) Shrimp Lemon Kebab

Ingredients:

- 1 ½ lb. shrimp, peeled and deveined but with tails intact
- ⅓ cup olive oil
- ¼ cup lemon juice
- 2 teaspoons lemon zest
- 1 tablespoon fresh parsley, chopped
- 8 cherry tomatoes, quartered
- 2 scallions, sliced

Direction: Preparation Time: 10 minutes Cooking Time: 5 minutes Servings: 4

- ✓ Mix the olive oil, lemon juice, lemon zest and parsley in a bowl.
- ✓ Marinate the shrimp in this mixture for 15 minutes.
- ✓ Thread each shrimp into the skewers.
- ✓ Grill for 4 to 5 minutes, turning once halfway through.
- ✓ Serve with tomatoes and scallions.

Nutrition: Calories 271 Total Fat 12 g Saturated Fat 2 g Cholesterol 259 mg Sodium 255 mg Total Carbohydrate 4 g Dietary Fiber 1 g Total Sugars 1 g Protein 25 g Potassium 429 mg

261) Grilled Herbed Salmon with Raspberry Sauce & Cucumber Dill Dip

Ingredients:

- 3 salmon fillets
- 1 tablespoon olive oil
- Salt and pepper to taste
- 1 teaspoon fresh sage, chopped
- 1 tablespoon fresh parsley, chopped
- 2 tablespoons Apple juice
- 1 cup raspberries
- 1 teaspoon Worcestershire sauce
- 1 cup cucumber, chopped
- 2 tablespoons light mayonnaise
- ½ teaspoon dried dill

Direction: Preparation Time: 15 minutes Cooking Time: 30 minutes Servings: 4

- ✓ Coat the salmon fillets with oil. Season with salt, pepper, sage and parsley.
- ✓ Cover the salmon with foil.
- ✓ Grill for 20 minutes or until fish is flaky.
- ✓ While waiting, mix the apple juice, raspberries and Worcestershire sauce.
- ✓ Pour the mixture into a saucepan over medium heat. Bring to a boil and then simmer for 8 minutes.
- ✓ In another bowl, mix the rest of the ingredients.
- ✓ Serve salmon with raspberry sauce and cucumber dip.

Nutrition: Calories 256 Total Fat 15 g Saturated Fat 3 g Cholesterol 68 mg Sodium 176 mg Total Carbohydrate 6 g Dietary Fiber 1 g Total Sugars 5 g Protein 23 g Potassium 359 mg

262) Tarragon Scallops

Ingredients:

- 1 cup water
- 1 lb. asparagus spears, trimmed
- 2 lemons 1
- ¼ lb. scallops
- Salt and pepper to taste
- 1 tablespoon olive oil
- 1 tablespoon fresh tarragon, chopped

Direction: Preparation Time: 10 minutes Cooking Time: 15 minutes Servings: 4

- ✓ Pour water into a pot. Bring to a boil. Add asparagus spears. Cover and cook for 5 minutes.
- ✓ Drain and transfer to a plate. Slice one lemon into wedges.
- ✓ Squeeze juice and shred zest from the remaining lemon.
- ✓ Season the scallops with salt and pepper.
- ✓ Put a pan over medium heat.
- ✓ Add oil to the pan.
- ✓ Cook the scallops until golden brown.
- ✓ Transfer to the same plate, putting scallops beside the asparagus.
- ✓ Add lemon zest, juice and tarragon to the pan. Cook for 1 minute.
- ✓ Drizzle tarragon sauce over the scallops and asparagus.

Nutrition: Calories 253 Total Fat 12 g Saturated Fat 2 g Cholesterol 47 mg Sodium 436 mg Total Carbohydrate 14 g Dietary Fiber 5 g Total Sugars 3 g Protein 27 g Potassium 773 mg

263) Garlic Shrimp & Spinach

Ingredients:

- 3 tablespoons olive oil, divided
- 6 clove garlic, sliced and divided
- 1 lb. spinach Salt to taste
- 1 tablespoons lemon juice
- 1 lb. shrimp, peeled and deveined
- ¼ teaspoon red pepper, crushed
- 1 tablespoon parsley, chopped
- 1 teaspoon lemon zest

Direction: Preparation Time: 10 minutes Cooking Time: 10 minutes Servings: 4

- ✓ Pour 1 tablespoon olive oil in a pot over medium heat.
- ✓ Cook the garlic for 1 minute.
- ✓ Add the spinach and season with salt.
- ✓ Cook for 3 minutes. Stir in lemon juice.
- ✓ Transfer to a bowl. Pour the remaining oil.
- ✓ Add the shrimp. Season with salt and add red pepper.
- ✓ Cook for 5 minutes.
- ✓ Sprinkle parsley and lemon zest over the shrimp before serving

Nutrition: Calories 226 Total Fat 12 g Saturated Fat 2 g Cholesterol 183 mg Sodium 444 mg Total Carbohydrate 6 g Dietary Fiber 3 g Total Sugars 1 g Protein 26 g Potassium 963 mg

264) Herring & Veggies Soup

Ingredients:

- 2 tablespoons olive oil
- 1 shallot, chopped
- 2 small garlic cloves, minced
- 1 jalapeño pepper, chopped
- 1 head cabbage, chopped 1 small red bell pepper, seeded and chopped finely
- 1 small yellow bell pepper, seeded and chopped finely
- 5 cups low-sodium chicken broth 2 (4-ounce) boneless herring fillets, cubed
- ¼ cup fresh cilantro, minced
- 2 tablespoons fresh lemon juice
- Ground black pepper, as required
- 2 scallions, chopped

Direction: Preparation Time: 15 minutes Cooking Time: 25 minutes Servings: 5

- ✓ In a large soup pan, heat the oil over medium heat and sauté shallot and garlic for 2-3 minutes.
- ✓ Add the cabbage and bell peppers and sauté for about 3-4 minutes.
- ✓ Add the broth and bring to a boil over high heat.
- ✓ Now, reduce the heat to medium-low and simmer for about 10 minutes.
- ✓ Add the herring cubes and cook for about 5-6 minutes.
- ✓ Stir in the cilantro, lemon juice, salt and black pepper and cook for about 1-2 minutes.
- ✓ Serve hot with the topping of scallion.

Meal Prep Tip:

- ✓ Transfer the soup into a large bowl and set aside to cool. Divide the soup into 5 containers evenly. Cover the containers and refrigerate for 1-2 days. Reheat in the microwave before serving.

Nutrition: Calories 215 Total Fat 11.2g Saturated Fat 2.1 g Cholesterol 35 mg Total Carbs 14.7 g Sugar 7 g Fiber 4.5 g Sodium 152 mg Potassium 574 mg Protein 15.1 g

265) Salmon Soup

Ingredients:

- 1 tablespoon olive oil
- 1 yellow onion, chopped
- 1 garlic clove, minced
- 4 cups low-sodium chicken broth
- 1 pound boneless salmon, cubed
- 2 tablespoon fresh cilantro, chopped
- Ground black pepper, as required
- 1 tablespoon fresh lime juice

Direction: Preparation Time: 15 minutes Cooking Time: 20 minutes Servings: 4

- ✓ In a large pan heat the oil over medium heat and sauté the onion for about 5 minutes.
- ✓ Add the garlic and sauté for about 1 minute.
- ✓ Stir in the broth and bring to a boil over high heat. Now, reduce the heat to low and simmer for about 10 minutes.
- ✓ Add the salmon, and soy sauce and cook for about 3-4 minutes. Stir in black pepper, lime juice, and cilantro and serve hot.

Meal Prep Tip:

- ✓ Transfer the soup into a large bowl and set aside to cool.
- ✓ Divide the soup into 4 containers evenly.
- ✓ Cover the containers and refrigerate for 1-2 days. Reheat in the microwave before serving.

Nutrition: Calories 208 Total Fat 10.5 g Saturated Fat 1.5 g Cholesterol 50 mg Total Carbs 3.9 g Sugar 1.2 g Fiber 0.6 g Sodium 121 mg Potassium 331 mg Protein 24.4 g

266) Salmon Curry

Ingredients:

- 6 (4-ounce) salmon fillets
- 1 teaspoon ground turmeric, divided Salt, as required
- 3 tablespoon olive oil, divided
- 1 yellow onion, chopped finely
- 1 teaspoon garlic paste
- 1 teaspoon fresh ginger paste
- 3-4 green chilies, halved
- 1 teaspoon red chili powder
- ½ teaspoon ground cumin
- ½ teaspoon ground cinnamon
- ¾ cup fat-free plain Greek yogurt, whipped
- ¾ cup filtered water 3 tablespoon fresh cilantro, chopped

Direction: Preparation Time: 15 minutes Cooking Time: 30 minutes Servings: 6

- ✓ Season each salmon fillet with ½ teaspoon of the turmeric and salt.
- ✓ In a large skillet, melt 1 tablespoon of the butter over medium heat and cook the salmon fillets for about 2 minutes per side.
- ✓ Transfer the salmon onto a plate. In the same skillet, melt the remaining butter over medium heat and sauté the onion for about 4-5 minutes.
- ✓ Add the garlic paste, ginger paste, green chilies, remaining turmeric and spices and sauté for about 1 minute.
- ✓ Now, reduce the heat to medium-low. Slowly, add the yogurt and water, stirring continuously until smooth.
- ✓ Cover the skillet and simmer for about 10-15 minutes or until desired doneness of the sauce.
- ✓ Carefully, add the salmon fillets and simmer for about 5 minutes. Serve hot with the garnishing of cilantro.

Meal Prep Tip:

- ✓ Transfer the curry into a large bowl and set aside to cool. Divide the curry into 6 containers evenly.
- ✓ Cover the containers and refrigerate for 1-2 days. Reheat in the microwave before serving.

Nutrition: Calories 242 Total Fat 14.3 g Saturated Fat 2 g Cholesterol 51 mg Total Carbs 4.1 g Sugar 2 g Fiber 0.8 g Sodium 98 mg Potassium 493 mg Protein 25.4 g

267) Salmon with Bell Peppers

Ingredients:

- 6 (3-ounce) salmon fillets Pinch of salt
- Ground black pepper, as required
- 1 yellow bell pepper, seeded and cubed
- 1 red bell pepper, seeded and cubed, 4 plum tomatoes, cubed
- 1 small onion, sliced thinly
- ½ cup fresh parsley, chopped
- ¼ cup olive oil
- 2 tablespoons fresh lemon juice

Direction: Preparation Time: 15 minutes Cooking Time: 20 minutes Servings: 6

- ✓ Preheat the oven to 400 degrees F. Season each salmon fillet with salt and black pepper lightly. In a bowl, mix together the bell peppers, tomato and onion.
- ✓ Arrange 6 foil pieces onto a smooth surface. Place 1 salmon fillet over each foil paper and sprinkle with salt and black pepper.
- ✓ Place veggie mixture over each fillet evenly and top with parsley and capers evenly.
- ✓ Drizzle with oil and lemon juice. Fold each foil around salmon mixture to seal it. Arrange the foil packets onto a large baking sheet in a single layer.
- ✓ Bake for about 20 minutes. Serve hot.

Meal Prep Tip:

- ✓ Transfer the salmon mixture into a large bowl and set aside to cool. Divide the salmon mixture into 6 containers evenly.
- ✓ Cover the containers and refrigerate for 1 day. Reheat in the microwave before serving.

Nutrition: Calories 220 Total Fat 14 g Saturated Fat 2 g Cholesterol 38 mg Total Carbs 7.7 g Sugar 4.8 g Fiber 2 g Sodium 74 mg Potassium 647 mg Protein 17.9 g

268) Shrimp Salad

Ingredients:

- For Salad: 1 pound shrimp, peeled and deveined
- Salt and ground black pepper, as required
- 1 teaspoon olive oil
- 1½ cups carrots, peeled and julienned
- 1½ cups red cabbage, shredded1
- ½ cup cucumber, julienned
- 5 cups fresh baby arugula
- ¼ cup fresh basil, chopped
- ¼ cup fresh cilantro, chopped
- 4 cups lettuce, torn
- ¼ cup almonds, chopped
- For Dressing:
- 2 tablespoons natural almond butter
- 1 garlic clove, crushed
- 1 tablespoon fresh cilantro, chopped
- 1 tablespoon fresh lime juice 1 tablespoon unsweetened applesauce
- 2 teaspoons balsamic vinegar
- ½ teaspoon cayenne pepper Salt, as required
- 1 tablespoon water 1/3 cup olive oil

Direction: Preparation Time: 20 minutes Cooking Time: 4 minutes
Servings: 6

- ✓ Slowly, add the oil, beating continuously until smooth. For salad: in a bowl, add shrimp, salt, black pepper and oil and toss to coat well. Heat a skillet over medium-high heat and cook the shrimp for about 2 minutes per side.
- ✓ Remove from the heat and set aside to cool. In a large bowl, add the shrimp, vegetables and mix well. For dressing: in a bowl, add all ingredients except oil and beat until well combined.
- ✓ Place the dressing over shrimp mixture and gently, toss to coat well. Serve immediately.

Meal Prep Tip:

- ✓ Divide dressing in 6 large mason jars evenly. Place the remaining ingredients in the layers of carrots, followed by cabbage, cucumber, arugula, basil, cilantro, shrimp, lettuce and almonds.
- ✓ Cover each jar with the lid tightly and refrigerate for about 1 day. Shake the jars well just before serving.

Nutrition: Calories 274 Total Fat 17.7 g Saturated Fat 2.4 g Cholesterol 159 mg Total Carbs 10 g Sugar 3.8 g Fiber 2.9 g Sodium 242 mg Potassium 481 mg Protein 20.5 g

269) Shrimp & Veggies Curry

Ingredients:

- 2 teaspoons olive oil
- 1½ medium white onions, sliced
- 2 medium green bell peppers, seeded and sliced
- 3 medium carrots, peeled and sliced thinly
- 3 garlic cloves, chopped finely
- 1 tablespoon fresh ginger, chopped finely
- 2½ teaspoons curry powder
- 1½ pounds shrimp, peeled and deveined
- 1 cup filtered water
- 2 tablespoons fresh lime juice
- Salt and ground black pepper, as required
- 2 tablespoons fresh cilantro, chopped

Direction: Preparation Time: 20 minutes Cooking Time: 20 minutes
Servings: 6

- ✓ In a large skillet, heat oil over medium-high heat and sauté the onion for about 4-5 minutes.
- ✓ Add the bell peppers and carrot and sauté for about 3-4 minutes. Add the garlic, ginger and curry powder and sauté for about 1 minute.
- ✓ Add the shrimp and sauté for about 1 minute. Stir in the water and cook for about 4-6 minutes, stirring occasionally.
- ✓ Stir in lime juice and remove from heat. Serve hot with the garnishing of cilantro.

Meal Prep Tip:

- ✓ Transfer the curry into a large bowl and set aside to cool. Divide the curry into 6 containers evenly.
- ✓ Cover the containers and refrigerate for 1-2 days. Reheat in the microwave before serving.

Nutrition: Calories 193 Total Fat 3.8 g Saturated Fat 0.9 g Cholesterol 239 mg Total Carbs 12 g Sugar 4.7 g Fiber 2.3 g Sodium 328 mg

270) Shrimp with Zucchini

Ingredients:

- 3 tablespoons olive oil
- 1 pound medium shrimp, peeled and deveined
- 1 shallot, minced 4 garlic cloves, minced
- ¼ teaspoon red pepper flakes, crushed
- Salt and ground black pepper, as required
- ¼ cup low-sodium chicken broth
- 2 tablespoons fresh lemon juice
- 1 teaspoon fresh lemon zest, grated finely
- ½ pound zucchini, spiralized with Blade C

Direction: Preparation Time: 20 minutes Cooking Time: 8 minutes
Servings: 4

- ✓ In a large skillet, heat the oil and butter over medium-high heat and cook the shrimp, shallot, garlic, red pepper flakes, salt and black pepper for about 2 minutes, stirring occasionally.
- ✓ Stir in the broth, lemon juice and lemon zest and bring to a gentle boil.
- ✓ Stir in zucchini noodles and cook for about 1-2 minutes.
- ✓ Serve hot.

Meal Prep Tip:

- ✓ Transfer the shrimp mixture into a large bowl and set aside to cool.
- ✓ Divide the shrimp mixture into 4 containers. Cover the containers and refrigerate for about 1-2 days.
- ✓ Reheat in microwave before serving.

Nutrition: Calories 245 Total Fat 12.6 g Saturated Fat 2.2 g Cholesterol 239 mg Total Carbs 5.8 g Sugar 1.2 g Fiber 08 g Sodium 289 mg Potassium 381 mg Protein 27 g

271) Shrimp with Broccoli

Ingredients:

- 2 tablespoons olive oil, divided
- 4 cups broccoli, chopped
- 2-3 tablespoons filtered water
- 1½ pounds large shrimp, peeled and deveined
- 2 garlic cloves, minced
- 1 (1-inch) piece fresh ginger, minced
- Salt and ground black pepper, as required

Direction: Preparation Time: 15 minutes Cooking Time: 12 minutes Servings: 6

- : In a large skillet, heat 1 tablespoon of oil over medium-high heat and cook the broccoli for about 1-2 minutes stirring continuously.
- Stir in the water and cook, covered for about 3-4 minutes, stirring occasionally.
- With a spoon, push the broccoli to side of the pan. Add the remaining oil and let it heat.
- Add the shrimp and cook for about 1-2 minutes, tossing occasionally.
- Add the remaining ingredients and sauté for about 2-3 minutes. Serve hot.

Meal Prep Tip:

- Transfer the shrimp mixture into a large bowl and set aside to cool.
- Divide the shrimp mixture into 6 containers evenly.
- Cover the containers and refrigerate for 1 day. Reheat in the microwave before serving.

Nutrition: Calories 197 Total Fat 6.8 g Saturated Fat 1.3 g Cholesterol 239 mg Total Carbs 6.1 g Sugar 1.1 g Fiber 1.6 g Sodium 324 mg Potassium 389 mg Protein 27.6 g

272) Grilled Salmon with Ginger Sauce

Ingredients:

- 1 tablespoon toasted sesame oil
- 1 tablespoon fresh cilantro, chopped
- 1 tablespoon lime juice
- 1 teaspoon fish sauce
- 1 clove garlic, mashed
- 1 teaspoon fresh ginger, grated
- 1 teaspoon jalapeño pepper, minced
- 4 salmon fillets
- 1 tablespoon olive oil
- Salt and pepper to taste

Direction: Preparation Time: 15 minutes Cooking Time: 8 minutes Servings: 4

- In a bowl, mix the sesame oil, cilantro, lime juice, fish sauce, garlic, ginger and jalapeño pepper.
- Preheat your grill.
- Brush oil on salmon. Season both sides with salt and pepper.
- Grill salmon for 6 to 8 minutes, turning once or twice.
- Take 1 tablespoon from the oil mixture.
- Brush this on the salmon while grilling.
- Serve grilled salmon with the remaining sauce.

Nutrition: Calories 204 Total Fat 11 g Saturated Fat 2 g Cholesterol 53 mg Sodium 320 mg Total Carbohydrate 2 g Dietary Fiber 0 g Total Sugars 2 g Protein 23 g Potassium 437 mg

273) Swordfish with Tomato Salsa

Ingredients:

- 1 cup tomato, chopped
- ¼ cup tomatillo, chopped
- 2 tablespoons fresh cilantro, chopped
- ¼ cup avocado, chopped
- 1 clove garlic, minced
- 1 jalapeño pepper, chopped
- 1 tablespoon lime juice
- Salt and pepper to taste
- 4 swordfish steaks
- 1 clove garlic, sliced in half
- 2 tablespoons lemon juice
- ½ teaspoon ground cumin

Direction: Preparation Time: 20 minutes Cooking Time: 12 minutes Servings: 4

- Preheat your grill. In a bowl, mix the tomato, tomatillo, cilantro, avocado, garlic, jalapeño, lime juice, salt and pepper.
- Cover the bowl with foil and put in the refrigerator.
- Rub each swordfish steak with sliced garlic. Drizzle lemon juice on both sides.
- Season with salt, pepper and cumin.
- Grill for 12 minutes or until the fish is fully cooked. Serve with salsa.

Nutrition: Calories 190 Total Fat 8 g Saturated Fat 2 g Cholesterol 43 mg Sodium 254 mg Total Carbohydrate 6 g Dietary Fiber 3 g Total Sugars 1 g Protein 24 g Potassium 453 mg

274) Salmon & Shrimp Stew

Ingredients:

- 2 tablespoons olive oil
- 1/2 cup onion, chopped finely
- 2 garlic cloves, minced
- 1 Serrano pepper, chopped
- 1 teaspoon smoked paprika
- 4 cups fresh tomatoes, chopped
- 4 cups low-sodium chicken broth
- 1 pound salmon fillets, cubed
- 1 pound shrimp, peeled and deveined
- 2 tablespoons fresh lime juice
- ¼ cup fresh basil, chopped
- ¼ cup fresh parsley, chopped
- Ground black pepper, as required
- 2 scallions, chopped

Direction: Preparation Time: 20 minutes Cooking Time: 21 minutes Servings: 6

- In a large soup pan, melt coconut oil over medium-high heat and sauté the onion for about 5-6 minutes.
- Add the garlic, Serrano pepper and smoked paprika and sauté for about 1 minute.
- Add the tomatoes and broth and bring to a gentle simmer over medium heat.
- Simmer for about 5 minutes.
- Add the salmon and simmer for about 3-4 minutes.
- Stir in the remaining seafood and cook for about 4-5 minutes.
- Stir in the lemon juice, basil, parsley, sea salt and black pepper and remove from heat.
- Serve hot with the garnishing of scallion.

Nutrition: Calories 271; Total Fat 11 g; Saturated Fat 1.8 g; Cholesterol 193 mg; Total Carbs 8.6 g; Sugar 3.8 g; Fiber 2.1 g; Sodium 273 mg; Potassium 763 mg; Protein 34.7 g

275) Salmon Baked

Ingredients:

- 6 (3-ounce) salmon fillets
- Pinch of salt
- Ground black pepper, as required
- 1 yellow bell pepper, seeded and cubed
- 1 red bell pepper, seeded and cubed
- 4 plum tomatoes, cubed
- 1 small onion, sliced thinly
- 1/2 cup fresh parsley, chopped
- ¼ cup olive oil
- 2 tablespoons fresh lemon juice

Direction: Preparation Time: 15 minutes
Cooking Time: 20 minutes Servings: 6

- ✓ Preheat the oven to 400 degrees F.
- ✓ Season each salmon fillet with salt and black pepper lightly.
- ✓ In a bowl, mix together the bell peppers, tomato and onion.
- ✓ Arrange 6 foil pieces onto a smooth surface.
- ✓ Place 1 salmon fillet over each foil paper and sprinkle with salt and black pepper.
- ✓ Place veggie mixture over each fillet evenly and top with parsley and capers evenly.
- ✓ Drizzle with oil and lemon juice.
- ✓ Fold each foil around salmon mixture to seal it.
- ✓ Arrange the foil packets onto a large baking sheet in a single layer.
- ✓ Bake for about 20 minutes.
- ✓ Serve hot.

Nutrition: Calories 220; Total Fat 14 g; Saturated Fat 2 g ; Cholesterol 38 mg; Total Carbs 7.7 g; Sugar 4.8 g; Fiber 2 g; Sodium 74 mg; Potassium 647 mg; Protein 17.9 g

SIDE DISH

276) Lemon Garlic Green Beans

Ingredients:

- 1 1/2 pounds green beans, trimmed
- 2 tablespoons olive oil
- 1 tablespoon fresh lemon juice
- 2 cloves minced garlic
- Salt and pepper

Direction: Preparation time: 5 minutes
Cooking Time: 10 minutes **Servings:** 6

- ✓ Fill a large bowl with ice water and set aside.
- ✓ Bring a pot of salted water to boil then add the green beans.
- ✓ Cook for 3 minutes then drain and immediately place in the ice water.
- ✓ Cool the beans completely then drain them well.
- ✓ Heat the oil in a large skillet over medium-high heat.
- ✓ Add the green beans, tossing to coat, then add the lemon juice, garlic, salt, and pepper.
- ✓ Sauté for 3 minutes until the beans are tender-crisp then serve hot.

Nutrition: Calories 75, Total Fat 4.8g, Saturated Fat 0.7g, Total Carbs 8.5g, Net Carbs 4.6g, Protein 2.1g, Sugar 1.7g, Fiber 3.9g, Sodium 7mg

277) Brown Rice & Lentil Salad

Ingredients:

- 1 cup water
- 1/2 cup instant brown rice
- 2 tablespoons olive oil
- 2 tablespoons red wine vinegar
- 1 tablespoon Dijon mustard
- 1 tablespoon minced onion
- 1/2 teaspoon paprika
- Salt and pepper
- 1 (15-ounce) can brown lentils, rinsed and drained
- 1 medium carrot, shredded
- 2 tablespoons fresh chopped parsley

Direction: Preparation time: 10 minutes
Cooking Time: 10 minutes **Servings:** 4

- ✓ Stir together the water and instant brown rice in a medium saucepan.
- ✓ Bring to a boil then simmer for 10 minutes, covered.
- ✓ Remove from heat and set aside while you prepare the salad.
- ✓ Whisk together the olive oil, vinegar, Dijon mustard, onion, paprika, salt, and pepper in a medium bowl.
- ✓ Toss in the cooked rice, lentils, carrots, and parsley.
- ✓ Adjust seasoning to taste then stir well and serve warm.

Nutrition: Calories 145, Total Fat 7.7g, Saturated Fat 1g, Total Carbs 13.1g, Net Carbs 10.9g, Protein 6g, Sugar 1g, Fiber 2.2g, Sodium 57mg

278) Mashed Butternut Squash

Ingredients:

- 3 pounds whole butternut squash (about 2 medium)
- 2 tablespoons olive oil
- Salt and pepper

Direction: Preparation time: 5 minutes
Cooking Time: 25 minutes **Servings:** 6

- ✓ Preheat the oven to 400F and line a baking sheet with parchment.
- ✓ Cut the squash in half and remove the seeds.
- ✓ Cut the squash into cubes and toss with oil then spread on the baking sheet.
- ✓ Roast for 25 minutes until tender then place in a food processor.
- ✓ Blend smooth then season with salt and pepper to taste.

Nutrition: Calories 90, Total Fat 4.8g, Saturated Fat 0.7g, Total Carbs 12.3g, Net Carbs 10.2g, Protein 1.1g, Sugar 2.3g, Fiber 2.1g, Sodium 4mg

279) Cilantro Lime Quinoa

Ingredients:

- 1 cup uncooked quinoa
- 1 tablespoon olive oil
- 1 medium yellow onion, diced
- 2 cloves minced garlic
- 1 (4-ounce) can diced green chiles, drained
- 1 1/2 cups fat-free chicken broth
- ¾ cup fresh chopped cilantro
- 1/2 cup sliced green onion
- 2 tablespoons lime juice
- Salt and pepper

Direction: Preparation time: 5 minutes
Cooking Time: 25 minutes **Servings:** 6

- ✓ Rinse the quinoa thoroughly in cool water using a fine mesh sieve.
- ✓ Heat the oil in a large saucepan over medium heat.
- ✓ Add the onion and sauté for 2 minutes then stir in the chile and garlic.
- ✓ Cook for 1 minute then stir in the quinoa and chicken broth.
- ✓ Bring to a boil then reduce heat and simmer, covered, until the quinoa absorbs the liquid – about 20 to 25 minutes.
- ✓ Remove from heat then stir in the cilantro, green onions, and lime juice.
- ✓ Season with salt and pepper to taste and serve hot.

Nutrition: Calories 150, Total Fat 4.1g, Saturated Fat 0.5g, Total Carbs 22.5g, Net Carbs 19.8g, Protein 6g, Sugar 1.7g, Fiber 2.7g, Sodium 179mg

280) Oven-Roasted Veggies

Ingredients:

- 1 pound cauliflower florets
- 1/2 pound broccoli florets
- 1 large yellow onion, cut into chunks
- 1 large red pepper, cored and chopped
- 2 medium carrots, peeled and sliced
- 2 tablespoons olive oil
- 2 tablespoons apple cider vinegar
- Salt and pepper

Direction: Preparation time: 5 minutes
Cooking Time: 25 minutes **Servings:** 6

- ✓ Preheat the oven to 425F and line a large rimmed baking sheet with parchment.
- ✓ Spread the veggies on the baking sheet and drizzle with oil and vinegar.
- ✓ Toss well and season with salt and pepper.
- ✓ Spread the veggies in a single layer then roast for 20 to 25 minutes, stirring every 10 minutes, until tender.
- ✓ Adjust seasoning to taste and serve hot.

Nutrition: Calories 100, Total Fat 5g, Saturated Fat 0.7g, Total Carbs 12.4g, Net Carbs 8.2g, Protein 3.2g, Sugar 5.5g, Fiber 4.2g, Sodium 51mg

281) Vegetable Rice Pilaf

Ingredients:

- 1 tablespoon olive oil
- 1/2 medium yellow onion, diced
- 1 cup uncooked long-grain brown rice
- 2 cloves minced garlic
- 1/2 teaspoon dried basil
- Salt and pepper
- 2 cups fat-free chicken broth
- 1 cup frozen mixed veggies

Direction: Preparation time: 5 minutes
Cooking Time: 25 minutes Servings: 6

- ✓ Heat the oil in a large skillet over medium heat.
- ✓ Add the onion and sauté for 3 minutes until translucent.
- ✓ Stir in the rice and cook until lightly toasted.
- ✓ Add the garlic, basil, salt, and pepper then stir to combined.
- ✓ Stir in the chicken broth then bring to a boil.
- ✓ Reduce heat and simmer, covered, for 10 minutes.
- ✓ Stir in the frozen veggies then cover and cook for another 10 minutes until heated through. Serve hot.

Nutrition: Calories 90, Total Fat 2.7g, Saturated Fat 0.4g, Total Carbs 12.6g, Net Carbs 10.4g, Protein 3.9g, Sugar 1.5g, Fiber 2.2g, Sodium 143mg

282) Curry Roasted Cauliflower Florets

Ingredients:

- 8 cups cauliflower florets
- 2 tablespoons olive oil
- 1 teaspoon curry powder
- 1/2 teaspoon garlic powder
- Salt and pepper

Direction: Preparation time: 5 minutes
Cooking Time: 25 minutes Servings: 6

- ✓ Preheat the oven to 425F and line a baking sheet with foil.
- ✓ Toss the cauliflower with the olive oil and spread on the baking sheet.
- ✓ Sprinkle with curry powder, garlic powder, salt, and pepper.
- ✓ Roast for 25 minutes or until just tender. Serve hot.

Nutrition: Calories 75, Total Fat 4.9g, Saturated Fat 0.7g, Total Carbs 7.4g, Net Carbs 3.9g, Protein 2.7g, Sugar 3.3g, Fiber 3.5g, Sodium 40mg

283) Mushroom Barley Risotto

Ingredients:

- 4 cups fat-free beef broth
- 2 tablespoons olive oil
- 1 small onion, diced well
- 2 cloves minced garlic
- 8 ounces thinly sliced mushrooms
- 1/4 tsp. dried thyme
- Salt and pepper
- 1 cup pearled barley
- 1/2 cup dry white wine

Direction: Preparation time: 5 minutes
Cooking Time: 25 minutes Servings: 8

- ✓ Heat the beef broth in a medium saucepan and keep it warm.
- ✓ Heat the oil in a large, deep skillet over medium heat.
- ✓ Add the onions and garlic and sauté for 2 minutes then stir in the mushrooms and thyme.
- ✓ Season with salt and pepper and sauté for 2 minutes more.
- ✓ Add the barley and sauté for 1 minute then pour in the wine.
- ✓ Ladle about 1/2 cup of beef broth into the skillet and stir well to combine.
- ✓ Cook until most of the broth has been absorbed then add another ladle.
- ✓ Repeat until you have used all of the broth and the barley is cooked to al dente.
- ✓ Adjust seasoning to taste with salt and pepper and serve hot.

Nutrition: Calories 155, Total Fat 4.4g, Saturated Fat 0.6g, Total Carbs 21.9g, Net Carbs 17.5g, Protein 5.5g, Sugar 1.2g, Fiber 4.4g, Sodium 455mg

284) Braised Summer Squash

Ingredients:

- 3 tablespoons olive oil
- 3 cloves minced garlic
- 1/4 teaspoon crushed red pepper flakes
- 1 pound summer squash, sliced
- 1 pound zucchini, sliced
- 1 teaspoon dried oregano
- Salt and pepper

Direction: Preparation time: 10 minutes
Cooking Time: 20 minutes Servings: 6

- ✓ Heat the oil in a large skillet over medium heat.
- ✓ Add the garlic and crushed red pepper and cook for 2 minutes.
- ✓ Add the summer squash and zucchini and cook for 15 minutes, stirring often, until just tender.
- ✓ Stir in the oregano then season with salt and pepper to taste. serve hot.

Nutrition: Calories 90, Total Fat 7.4g, Saturated Fat 1.1g, Total Carbs 6.2g, Net Carbs 4.4g, Protein 1.8g, Sugar 4g, Fiber 1.8g, Sodium 10mg

285) Parsley Tabbouleh

Ingredients:

- 1 cup water
- 1/2 cup bulgur
- 1/4 cup fresh lemon juice
- 2 tablespoons olive oil
- 2 cloves minced garlic
- Salt and pepper
- 2 cups fresh chopped parsley
- 2 medium tomatoes, died
- 1 small cucumber, diced
- 1/4 cup fresh chopped mint

Direction: Preparation time: 5 minutes
Cooking Time: 25 minutes Servings: 6

- ✓ Bring the water and bulgur to a boil in a small saucepan then remove from heat.
- ✓ Cover and let stand until the water is fully absorbed, about 25 minutes.
- ✓ Meanwhile, whisk together the lemon juice, olive oil, garlic, salt, and pepper in a medium bowl.
- ✓ Toss in the cooked bulgur along with the parsley, tomatoes, cucumber, and mint.
- ✓ Season with salt and pepper to taste and serve.

Nutrition: Calories 110, Total Fat 5.3g, Saturated Fat 0.9g, Total Carbs 14.4g, Net Carbs 10.5g, Protein 3g, Sugar 2.4g, Fiber 3.9g, Sodium 21mg

286) Garlic Sautéed Spinach

Ingredients:

- 1 1/2 tablespoons olive oil
- 4 cloves minced garlic
- 6 cups fresh baby spinach
- Salt and pepper

Direction: Preparation time: 5 minutes
Cooking Time: 10 minutes Servings: 4

- ✓ Heat the oil in a large skillet over medium-high heat.
- ✓ Add the garlic and cook for 1 minute.
- ✓ Stir in the spinach and season with salt and pepper.
- ✓ Sauté for 1 to 2 minutes until just wilted. Serve hot.

Nutrition: Calories 60, Total Fat 5.5g, Saturated Fat 0.8g, Total Carbs 2.6g, Net Carbs 1.5g, Protein 1.5g, Sugar 0.2g, Fiber 1.1g, Sodium 36mg

287) French Lentils

Ingredients:

- 2 tablespoons olive oil
- 1 medium onion, diced
- 1 medium carrot, peeled and diced
- 2 cloves minced garlic
- 5 1/2 cups water
- 2 ¼ cups French lentils, rinsed and drained
- 1 teaspoon dried thyme
- 2 small bay leaves
- Salt and pepper

Direction: Preparation time: 5 minutes
Cooking Time: 25 minutes **Servings:** 10

- ✓ Heat the oil in a large saucepan over medium heat.
- ✓ Add the onions, carrot, and garlic and sauté for 3 minutes.
- ✓ Stir in the water, lentils, thyme, and bay leaves – season with salt.
- ✓ Bring to a boil then reduce to a simmer and cook until tender, about 20 minutes.
- ✓ Drain any excess water and adjust seasoning to taste. Serve hot.

Nutrition: Calories 185, Total Fat 3.3g, Saturated Fat 0.5g, Total Carbs 27.9g, Net Carbs 14.2g, Protein 11.4g, Sugar 1.7g, Fiber 13.7g, Sodium 11mg

288) Grain-Free Berry Cobbler

Ingredients:

- 4 cups fresh mixed berries
- 1/2 cup ground flaxseed
- ¼ cup almond meal
- ¼ cup unsweetened shredded coconut
- 1/2 tablespoon baking powder
- 1 teaspoon ground cinnamon
- ¼ teaspoon salt
- Powdered stevia, to taste
- 6 tablespoons coconut oil

Direction: Preparation time: 5 minutes
Cooking Time: 25 minutes **Servings:** 10

- ✓ Preheat the oven to 375F and lightly grease a 10-inch cast-iron skillet.
- ✓ Spread the berries on the bottom of the skillet.
- ✓ Whisk together the dry ingredients in a mixing bowl.
- ✓ Cut in the coconut oil using a fork to create a crumbled mixture.
- ✓ Spread the crumble over the berries and bake for 25 minutes until hot and bubbling.
- ✓ Cool the cobbler for 5 to 10 minutes before serving.

Nutrition: Calories 215 Total Fat 16.8g, Saturated Fat 10.4g, Total Carbs 13.1g, Net Carbs 6.7g, Protein 3.7g, Sugar 5.3g, Fiber 6.4g, Sodium 61mg

289) Spicy Spinach

Ingredients:

- 1 tablespoon olive oil
- 1 red onion, chopped finely
- 6 garlic cloves, minced
- 1 (1-inch) piece fresh ginger, minced
- 1 teaspoon garam masala
- 1 teaspoon ground coriander
- ½ teaspoon ground cumin
- ¼ teaspoon ground turmeric
- 6 cups fresh spinach, chopped
- Salt and ground black pepper, as required
- 1-2 tablespoons water

Direction: Preparation Time: 10 minutes Cooking Time: 20 minutes Servings: 3

- ✓ Heat the olive oil in a large nonstick skillet over medium heat and sauté the onion for about 6-7 minutes.
- ✓ Add the garlic, ginger and spices and sauté for about 1 minute.
- ✓ Add the spinach, salt and black pepper and water and cook, covered for about 10 minutes.
- ✓ Uncover and stir fry for about 2 minutes. Serve hot.

Meal Prep Tip:

- ✓ Transfer the spinach mixture into a large bowl and set aside to cool completely. Divide the mixture into 3 containers evenly.
- ✓ Cover the containers and refrigerate for about 1-2 days. Reheat in the microwave before serving.

Nutrition: Calories 80 Total Fat 5.1 g Saturated Fat 0.7 g Cholesterol 0 mg Total Carbs 8 g Sugar 1.9 g Fiber 2.3 g Sodium 52 mg Potassium 331 mg Protein 2.6 g

290) Herbed Asparagus

Ingredients:

- 2 tablespoons olive oil
- 2 tablespoons fresh lemon juice
- 1 tablespoon balsamic vinegar
- 1 teaspoon garlic, minced
- 1 tablespoon fresh parsley, chopped
- 1 teaspoon dried oregano
- Salt and ground black pepper, as required
- 1 pound fresh asparagus, ends removed

Direction: Preparation Time: 10 minutes Cooking Time: 10 minutes Servings: 4

- ✓ Preheat oven to 400 degrees F and lightly grease a rimmed baking sheet.
- ✓ Place the oil, lemon juice, vinegar, garlic, herbs, salt and black pepper in a bowl and beat until well combined.
- ✓ Arrange the asparagus onto the prepared baking sheet in a single layer. Top with half of the herb mixture and toss to coat.
- ✓ Roast for about 8-10 minutes. Remove from the oven and transfer the asparagus onto a platter. Drizzle with the remaining herb mixture and serve.

Meal Prep Tip:

- ✓ Transfer the asparagus into a large bowl and set aside to cool completely.
- ✓ Divide the asparagus into 4 containers evenly. Cover the containers and refrigerate for about 1-2 days. Reheat in the microwave before serving.

Nutrition: Calories 88 Total Fat 7.3 g Saturated Fat 1.1 g Cholesterol 0 mg Total Carbs 5.1 g Sugar 2.4 g Fiber 2.6 g Sodium 5 mg Potassium 256 mg Protein 2.7 g

291) Lemony Brussels Sprout

Ingredients:

- ½ pound Brussels sprouts, halved
- 1 tablespoon olive oil
- 1 garlic clove, minced
- ½ teaspoon red pepper flakes, crushed
- Salt and ground black pepper, as required
- 1 tablespoon fresh lemon juice

Direction: Preparation Time: 10 minutes Cooking Time: 7 minutes Servings: 2

- ✓ : Heat the olive oil in a large skillet over medium heat and cook the garlic and red pepper flakes for about 1 minute, stirring continuously.
- ✓ Stir in the Brussels sprouts, salt and black pepper and sauté for about 4-5 minutes.
- ✓ Stir in lemon juice and sauté for about 1 minute more. Serve hot.

Meal Prep Tip:
- ✓ Transfer the Brussels sprouts into a large bowl and set aside to cool completely.
- ✓ Divide the Brussels sprouts into 2 containers evenly. Cover the containers and refrigerate for about 1-2 days.
- ✓ Reheat in the microwave before serving.

Nutrition: Calories 114 Total Fat 7.5 g Saturated Fat 1.2 g Cholesterol 0 mg Total Carbs 11.2 g Sugar 2.7 g Fiber 4.4 g Sodium 108 mg Potassium 465 mg Protein 4.1 g

292) Gingered Cauliflower

Ingredients:

- 2 cups cauliflower, cut into
- 1-inch florets Salt, as required
- 2 tablespoons olive oil
- 1 teaspoon fresh ginger root, sliced thinly
- 2 fresh thyme sprigs

Direction: Preparation Time: 0 minutes Cooking Time: 0 minutes Servings: 2

- ✓ In a pan of the water, add the cauliflower and salt over medium heat and bring to a boil.
- ✓ Cover and cook for about 10-12 minutes.
- ✓ Drain the cauliflower well and transfer onto a serving platter.
- ✓ Meanwhile, in a small skillet, melt the coconut oil over medium-low heat.
- ✓ Add the ginger and thyme sprigs and swirl the pan occasionally for about 2-3 minutes.
- ✓ Discard the ginger and thyme sprigs.
- ✓ Pour the oil over cauliflower and serve immediately.

Meal Prep Tip:
- ✓ Transfer the cauliflower into a large bowl and set aside to cool completely.
- ✓ Divide the cauliflower into 2 containers evenly.
- ✓ Cover the containers and refrigerate for about 1-2 days. Reheat in the microwave before serving.

Nutrition: Calories 147 Total Fat 14.2 g Saturated Fat 2 g Cholesterol 0 mg Total Carbs 5.7 g Sugar 2.4 g Fiber 2.7 g Sodium 108 mg Potassium 310 mg Protein 2 g

293) Roasted Broccoli

Ingredients:

- 2 cups fresh broccoli florets
- 1 small yellow onion, cut into wedges
- ¼ teaspoon garlic powder
- 1/8 teaspoon paprika
- 1/8 teaspoon freshly ground black pepper
- 2 tablespoons olive oil

Direction: Preparation Time: 10 minutes Cooking Time: 15 minutes Servings: 2

- ✓ Preheat the grill to medium heat. In a large bowl, add all the ingredients and toss to coat well.
- ✓ Transfer the broccoli mixture over a double thickness of a foil paper.
- ✓ Fold the foil paper around broccoli mixture to seal it.
- ✓ Grill for about 10-15 minutes. Serve hot. Meal Prep Tip:
- ✓ Transfer the broccoli mixture into a large bowl and set aside to cool completely.
- ✓ Divide the broccoli mixture into 2 containers evenly.
- ✓ Cover the containers and refrigerate for about 1-2 days. Reheat in the microwave before serving.

Nutrition: Calories 167 Total Fat 14.4 g Saturated Fat 2 g Cholesterol 0 mg Total Carbs 9.7 g Sugar 3.1 g Fiber 3.2 g Sodium 32 mg Potassium 348 mg Protein 3 g

294) Garlicky Cabbage

Ingredients:

- 1 tablespoon olive oil
- 2 garlic cloves, minced
- 1 pound cabbage, shredded
- 2-3 tablespoons filtered water
- 1½ tablespoons fresh lemon juice
- Salt and ground black pepper, as required

Direction: Preparation Time: 10 minutes Cooking Time: 10 minutes Servings: 4

- ✓ In a large skillet, heat the oil over medium heat and sauté the garlic for about 1 minute.
- ✓ Stir in the cabbage and cook, covered for about 2-3 minute.
- ✓ Stir in the water and cook for about 2-3 minutes, stirring continuously.
- ✓ Increase the heat to high and stir in the lemon juice, salt and black pepper.
- ✓ Cook for about 2-3 minutes, stirring continuously. Serve hot.

Meal Prep Tip:
- ✓ Transfer the cabbage mixture into a large bowl and set aside to cool completely. Divide the cabbage mixture into 2 containers evenly. Cover the containers and refrigerate for about 1-2 days. Reheat in the microwave before serving.

Nutrition: Calories 62 Total Fat 3.7 g Saturated Fat 0.6 g Cholesterol 0 mg Total Carbs 7.2 g Sugar 3.8 g Fiber 2.9 g Sodium 168 mg Potassium 206 mg Protein 1.6 g

295) Stir Fried Zucchini

Ingredients:

- 1 tablespoon olive oil
- ½ cup yellow onion, sliced
- 4 cups zucchini, sliced
- 1½ teaspoons garlic, minced
- ¼ cup water
- Salt and ground black pepper, as required

Direction: Preparation Time: 10 minutes Cooking Time: 10 minutes
Servings: 4

- ✓ In a large skillet, heat the oil over medium-high heat and sauté the onion and zucchini for about 4-5 minutes.
- ✓ Add the garlic and sauté for about 1 minute.
- ✓ Add the remaining ingredients and stir to combine.
- ✓ Now, reduce the heat to medium and cook for about 3-4 minutes, stirring occasionally.
- ✓ Serve hot. Meal Prep Tip: Transfer the zucchini mixture into a large bowl and set aside to cool completely.
- ✓ Divide the zucchini mixture into 4 containers evenly.
- ✓ Cover the containers and refrigerate for about 1-2 days. Reheat in the microwave before serving.

Nutrition: Calories 55 Total Fat 3.7 g Saturated Fat 0.5 g Cholesterol 0 mg Total Carbs 5.5 g Sugar 2.6 g Fiber 1.6 g Sodium 51 mg Potassium 321 mg Protein 1.6 g

296) Green Beans with Tomatoes

Ingredients:

- ¼ teaspoon fresh lemon peel, grated finely
- 2 teaspoons olive oil
- Salt and freshly ground white pepper, as required
- 4 cups grape tomatoes
- 1½ pounds fresh green beans, trimmed

Direction: Preparation Time: 15 minutes Cooking Time: 40 minutes
Servings: 8

- ✓ Preheat the oven to 350 degrees F. In a large bowl, mix together lemon peel, oil, salt and white pepper.
- ✓ Add the cherry tomatoes and toss to coat well.
- ✓ Transfer the tomato mixture into a roasting pan.
- ✓ Roast for about 35-40 minutes, stirring once in the middle way.
- ✓ Meanwhile, in a pan of boiling water, arrange a steamer basket.
- ✓ Place the green beans in steamer basket and steam, covered for about 7-8 minutes.
- ✓ Drain the green beans well.
- ✓ Divide the green beans and tomatoes onto serving plates and serve. Meal Prep Tip:
- ✓ Transfer the green beans and tomatoes into a large bowl and set aside to cool completely.
- ✓ Divide the green beans and tomatoes into 8 containers evenly.
- ✓ Cover the containers and refrigerate for about 1-2 days. Reheat in the microwave before serving.

Nutrition: Calories 53 Total Fat 1.5 g Saturated Fat 0.2 g Cholesterol 0 mg Total Carbs 9.6 g Sugar 3.6 g Fiber 4 g Sodium 29 mg Potassium 391 mg Protein 2.3 g

SOUPS AND STEWS

297) Kidney Bean Stew

Ingredients:
- 1lb cooked kidney beans
- 1 cup tomato passata
- 1 cup low sodium beef broth
- 3tbsp Italian herbs

Direction: Preparation time: 15 minutes
Cooking time: 15 minutes Servings: 2

- ✓ Mix all the ingredients in your Instant Pot.
- ✓ Cook on Stew for 15 minutes.
- ✓ Release the pressure naturally.

Nutrition: Calories: 270; Carbs: 16; Sugar: 3; Fat: 10; Protein: 23; GL: 8

298) Cabbage Soup

Ingredients:
- 1lb shredded cabbage
- 1 cup low sodium vegetable broth
- 1 shredded onion
- 2tbsp mixed herbs
- 1tbsp black pepper

Direction: Preparation time: 15 minutes
Cooking time: 35 minutes Servings: 2

- ✓ Mix all the ingredients in your Instant Pot.
- ✓ Cook on Stew for 35 minutes.
- ✓ Release the pressure naturally.

Nutrition: Calories: 60; Carbs: 2; Sugar: 0; Fat: 2; Protein: 4; GL: 1

299) Pumpkin Spice Soup

Ingredients:
- 1lb cubed pumpkin
- 1 cup low sodium vegetable broth
- 2tbsp mixed spice

Direction: Preparation time: 10 minutes
Cooking time: 35 minutes Servings: 2

- ✓ Mix all the ingredients in your Instant Pot.
- ✓ Cook on Stew for 35 minutes.
- ✓ Release the pressure naturally.
- ✓ Blend the soup.

Nutrition: Calories: 100; Carbs: 7; Sugar: 1; Fat: 2; Protein: 3; GL: 1

300) Cream of Tomato Soup

Ingredients:
- 1lb fresh tomatoes, chopped
- 1.5 cups low sodium tomato puree
- 1tbsp black pepper

Direction: Preparation time: 15 minutes
Cooking time: 15 minutes Servings: 2

- ✓ Mix all the ingredients in your Instant Pot.
- ✓ Cook on Stew for 15 minutes.
- ✓ Release the pressure naturally.
- ✓ Blend.

Nutrition: Calories: 20; Carbs: 2; Sugar: 1; Fat: 0; Protein: 3; GL: 1

301) Shiitake Soup

Ingredients:
- 1 cup shiitake mushrooms
- 1 cup diced vegetables
- 1 cup low sodium vegetable broth
- 2tbsp 5 spice seasoning

Direction: Preparation time: 15 minutes
Cooking time: 35 minutes Servings: 2

- ✓ Mix all the ingredients in your Instant Pot.
- ✓ Cook on Stew for 35 minutes.
- ✓ Release the pressure naturally.

Nutrition: Calories: 70; Carbs: 5; Sugar: 1; Fat: 2; Protein: 2; GL: 1

302) Spicy Pepper Soup

Ingredients:
- 1lb chopped mixed sweet peppers
- 1 cup low sodium vegetable broth
- 3tbsp chopped chili peppers
- 1tbsp black pepper

Direction: Preparation time: 15 minutes
Cooking time: 15 minutes Servings: 2

- ✓ Mix all the ingredients in your Instant Pot.
- ✓ Cook on Stew for 15 minutes.
- ✓ Release the pressure naturally. Blend.

Nutrition: Calories: 100; Carbs: 11; Sugar: 4; Fat: 2; Protein: 3; GL: 6

303) Zoodle Won-Ton Soup

Ingredients:
- 1lb spiralized zucchini
- 1 pack unfried won-tons
- 1 cup low sodium beef broth
- 2tbsp soy sauce

Direction: Preparation time: 15 minutes
Cooking time: 5 minutes Servings: 2

- ✓ Mix all the ingredients in your Instant Pot.
- ✓ Cook on Stew for 5 minutes.
- ✓ Release the pressure naturally.

Nutrition: Calories: 300; Carbs: 6; Sugar: 1; Fat: 9; Protein: 43; GL: 2

304) Broccoli Stilton Soup

Ingredients:
- 1lb chopped broccoli
- 0.5lb chopped vegetables
- 1 cup low sodium vegetable broth
- 1 cup Stilton

Direction: Preparation time: 15 minutes
Cooking time: 35 minutes Servings: 2

- ✓ Mix all the ingredients in your Instant Pot.
- ✓ Cook on Stew for 35 minutes.
- ✓ Release the pressure naturally.
- ✓ Blend the soup.

Nutrition: Calories: 280; **Carbs:** 9; **Sugar:** 2; **Fat:** 22; **Protein:** 13; GL: 4

305) Lamb Stew Recipe 2

Ingredients:

- 1lb diced lamb shoulder
- 1lb chopped winter vegetables
- 1 cup low sodium vegetable broth
- 1tbsp yeast extract
- 1tbsp star anise spice mix

Direction: Preparation time: 15 minutes
Cooking time: 35 minutes Servings: 2

- ✓ Mix all the ingredients in your Instant Pot.
- ✓ Cook on Stew for 35 minutes.
- ✓ Release the pressure naturally.

Nutrition: Calories: 320; Carbs: 10; Sugar: 2; Fat: 8; Protein: 42; GL: 3

306) Irish Stew

Ingredients:

- 1.5lb diced lamb shoulder
- 1lb chopped vegetables
- 1 cup low sodium beef broth
- 3 minced onions
- 1tbsp ghee

Direction: Preparation time: 15 minutes
Cooking time: 35 minutes Servings: 2

- ✓ Mix all the ingredients in your Instant Pot.
- ✓ Cook on Stew for 35 minutes.
- ✓ Release the pressure naturally.

Nutrition: Calories: 330; Carbs: 9; Sugar: 2; Fat: 12; Protein: 49; GL: 3

307) Sweet And Sour Soup

Ingredients:

- 1lb cubed chicken breast
- 1lb chopped vegetables
- 1 cup low carb sweet and sour sauce
- 0.5 cup diabetic marmalade

Direction: Preparation time: 15 minutes
Cooking time: 35 minutes Servings: 2

- ✓ Mix all the ingredients in your Instant Pot.
- ✓ Cook on Stew for 35 minutes.
- ✓ Release the pressure naturally.

308) Meatball Stew

Ingredients:

- 1lb sausage meat
- 2 cups chopped tomato
- 1 cup chopped vegetables
- 2tbsp Italian seasonings
- 1tbsp vegetable oil

Direction: Preparation time: 15 minutes
Cooking time: 25 minutes Servings: 2

- ✓ Roll the sausage into meatballs.
- ✓ Put the Instant Pot on Sauté and fry the meatballs in the oil until brown.
- ✓ Mix all the ingredients in your Instant Pot.
- ✓ Cook on Stew for 25 minutes.
- ✓ Release the pressure naturally.

Nutrition: Calories: 300; Carbs: 4; Sugar: 1; Fat: 12; Protein: 40; GL: 2

309) Kebab Stew

Ingredients:

- 1lb cubed, seasoned kebab meat
- 1lb cooked chickpeas
- 1 cup low sodium vegetable broth
- 1tbsp black pepper

Direction: Preparation time: 15 minutes
Cooking time: 35 minutes Servings: 2

- ✓ Mix all the ingredients in your Instant Pot.
- ✓ Cook on Stew for 35 minutes.
- ✓ Release the pressure naturally.

Nutrition: Calories: 290; Carbs: 22; Sugar: 4; Fat: 10; Protein: 34; GL: 6

310) French Onion Soup

Ingredients:

- 6 onions, chopped finely
- 2 cups vegetable broth
- 2tbsp oil
- 2tbsp Gruyere

Direction: Preparation time: 35 minutes
Cooking time: 35 minutes Servings: 2

- ✓ Place the oil in your Instant Pot and cook the onions on Sauté until soft and brown.
- ✓ Mix all the ingredients in your Instant Pot.
- ✓ Cook on Stew for 35 minutes.
- ✓ Release the pressure naturally.

Nutrition: Calories: 110; Carbs: 8; Sugar: 3; Fat: 10; Protein: 3; GL: 4

311) Meatless Ball Soup

Ingredients:

- 1lb minced tofu
- 0.5lb chopped vegetables
- 2 cups low sodium vegetable broth
- 1tbsp almond flour
- salt and pepper

Direction: Preparation time: 15 minutes
Cooking time: 15 minutes Servings: 2

- ✓ Mix the tofu, flour, salt and pepper.
- ✓ Form the meatballs.
- ✓ Place all the ingredients in your Instant Pot.
- ✓ Cook on Stew for 15 minutes.
- ✓ Release the pressure naturally.

Nutrition: Calories: 240; Carbs: 9; Sugar: 3; Fat: 10; Protein: 35; GL: 5

312) Fake-On Stew

Ingredients:

- 0.5lb soy bacon
- 1lb chopped vegetables
- 1 cup low sodium vegetable broth
- 1tbsp nutritional yeast

Direction: Preparation time: 15 minutes
Cooking time: 25 minutes Servings: 2

- ✓ Mix all the ingredients in your Instant Pot.
- ✓ Cook on Stew for 25 minutes.
- ✓ Release the pressure naturally.

Nutrition: Calories: 200; Carbs: 12; Sugar: 3; Fat: 7; Protein: 41; GL: 5

313) Chickpea Soup

Ingredients:
- 1lb cooked chickpeas
- 1lb chopped vegetables
- 1 cup low sodium vegetable broth
- 2tbsp mixed herbs

Direction: Preparation time: 15 minutes
Cooking time: 35 minutes **Servings:** 2

- ✓ Mix all the ingredients in your Instant Pot.
- ✓ Cook on Stew for 35 minutes.
- ✓ Release the pressure naturally.

Nutrition: Calories: 310; **Carbs:** 20; **Sugar:** 3; **Fat:** 5; **Protein:** 27; **GL:** 5

314) Chicken Zoodle Soup

Ingredients:
- 1lb chopped cooked chicken
- 1lb spiralized zucchini
- 1 cup low sodium chicken soup
- 1 cup diced vegetables

Direction: Preparation time: 15 minutes
Cooking time: 35 minutes **Servings:** 2

- ✓ Mix all the ingredients except the zucchini in your Instant Pot.
- ✓ Cook on Stew for 35 minutes.
- ✓ Release the pressure naturally.
- ✓ Stir in the zucchini and allow to heat thoroughly.

Nutrition: Calories: 250; **Carbs:** 5; **Sugar:** 0; **Fat:** 10; **Protein:** 40; **GL:** 1

SMOOTHIES & JUICES

315) Strawberry Smoothie

Ingredients:

- 5 Strawberries, medium
- 6 Ice Cubes
- 1 cup Soy Milk, unsweetened
- 1/2 cup Greek Yoghurt, low-fat

Direction: Preparation Time: 5 Minutes
Cooking Time: 5 Minutes Servings: 1

- ✓ Place strawberries, yogurt, milk, and ice cubes in a high-speed blender.
- ✓ Blend them for 2 to 3 minutes or until you get a smooth and luscious smoothie.
- ✓ Transfer to a serving glass and enjoy it.

Nutrition: Calories 167Kcal; Carbohydrates 11g; Proteins 16g; Fat 6g; Sodium 161mg

316) Berry Mint Smoothie

Ingredients:

- 1 tbsp. Low-carb Sweetener of your choice
- 1 cup Kefir or Low Fat-Yoghurt
- 2 tbsp. Mint
- ¼ cup Orange
- 1 cup Mixed Berries

Direction: Preparation Time: 5 Minutes
Cooking Time: 5 Minutes Servings: 2

- ✓ Place all of the ingredients in a high-speed blender and then blend it until smooth.
- ✓ Transfer the smoothie to a serving glass and enjoy it.

Nutrition: Calories: 137Kcal; Carbohydrates: 11g; Proteins: 6g; Fat: 1g; Sodium: 64mg

317) Greenie Smoothie

Ingredients:

- 1 1/2 cup Water
- 1 tsp. Stevia
- 1 Green Apple, ripe
- 1 tsp. Stevia
- 1 Green Pear, chopped into chunks
- 1 Lime
- 2 cups Kale, fresh
- ¾ tsp. Cinnamon
- 12 Ice Cubes
- 20 Green Grapes
- 1/2 cup Mint, fresh

Direction: Preparation Time: 5 Minutes
Cooking Time: 5 Minutes Servings: 2

- ✓ Pour water, kale, and pear in a high-speed blender and blend them for 2 to 3 minutes until mixed.
- ✓ Stir in all the remaining ingredients into it and blend until it becomes smooth.
- ✓ Transfer the smoothie to serving glass.

Nutrition: Calories: 123Kcal; Carbohydrates: 27g; Proteins: 2g; Fat: 2g; Sodium: 30mg

318) Coconut Spinach Smoothie

Ingredients:

- 1 ¼ cup Coconut Milk
- 2 Ice Cubes
- 2 tbsp. Chia Seeds
- 1 scoop of Protein Powder, preferably vanilla
- 1 cup Spin

Direction: Preparation Time: 5 Minutes
Cooking Time: 5 Minutes Servings: 2

- ✓ Pour coconut milk along with spinach, chia seeds, protein powder, and ice cubes in a high-speed blender.
- ✓ Blend for 2 minutes to get a smooth and luscious smoothie.
- ✓ Serve in a glass and enjoy it.

Nutrition: Calories 251Kcal; Carbs 10.9g; Proteins 20.3g; Fat 15.1g; Sodium: 102mg

319) Oats Coffee Smoothie

Ingredients:

- 1 cup Oats, uncooked & grounded
- 2 tbsp. Instant Coffee
- 3 cup Milk, skimmed
- 2 Banana, frozen & sliced into chunks
- 2 tbsp. Flax Seeds, grounded

Direction: Preparation Time: 5 Minutes
Cooking Time: 5 Minutes Servings: 2

- ✓ Place all of the ingredients in a high-speed blender and blend for 2 minutes or until smooth and luscious.
- ✓ Serve and enjoy.

Nutrition: Calories: 251Kcal; Carbs 10.9g; Proteins: 20.3g; Fat: 15.1g; Sodium: 102mg

320) Veggie Smoothie

Ingredients:

- ¼ of 1 Red Bell Pepper, sliced
- 1/2 tbsp. Coconut Oil
- 1 cup Almond Milk, unsweetened
- ¼ tsp. Turmeric
- 4 Strawberries, chopped
- Pinch of Cinnamon
- 1/2 of 1 Banana, preferably frozen

Direction: Preparation Time: 5 Minutes
Cooking Time: 5 Minutes Servings: 1

- ✓ Combine all the ingredients required to make the smoothie in a high-speed blender.
- ✓ Blend for 3 minutes to get a smooth and silky mixture.
- ✓ Serve and enjoy.

Nutrition: Calories: 169cal; Carbs: 17g; Proteins: 2.3g; Fat: 9.8g; Sodium: 162mg

321) Avocado Smoothie

Ingredients:

- 1 Avocado, ripe & pit removed
- 2 cups Baby Spinach
- 2 cups Water
- 1 cup Baby Kale
- 1 tbsp. Lemon Juice
- 2 sprigs of Mint
- 1/2 cup Ice Cubes

Direction: Preparation Time: 10 Minutes
Cooking Time: 0 Minutes Servings: 2

- ✓ Place all the ingredients needed to make the smoothie in a high-speed blender then blend until smooth.
- ✓ Transfer to a serving glass and enjoy it.

Nutrition: Calories: 214cal; Carbohydrates: 15g; Proteins: 2g; Fat: 17g; Sodium: 25mg

322) Orange Carrot Smoothie

Ingredients:

- 1 1/2 cups Almond Milk
- ¼ cup Cauliflower, blanched & frozen
- 1 Orange
- 1 tbsp. Flax Seed
- 1/3 cup Carrot, grated
- 1 tsp. Vanilla Extract

Direction: Preparation Time: 5 Minutes
Cooking Time: 0 Minutes Servings: 1

- ✓ Mix all the ingredients in a high-speed blender and blend for 2 minutes or until you get the desired consistency.
- ✓ Transfer to a serving glass and enjoy it.

Nutrition: Calories: 216cal; Carbohydrates: 10g; Proteins: 15g; Fat: 7g; Sodium: 25mg

323) Blackberry Smoothie

Ingredients:

- 1 1/2 cups Almond Milk
- 1/2 tsp. Vanilla Extract
- 3 oz. Blackberries, frozen
- 1 tbsp. Lemon Juice
- 1 tsp. Vanilla Extract

Direction: Preparation Time: 5 Minutes
Cooking Time: 0 Minutes Servings: 1

- ✓ Place all the ingredients needed to make the blackberry smoothie in a high-speed blender and blend for 2 minutes until you get a smooth mixture.
- ✓ Transfer to a serving glass and enjoy it.

Nutrition: Calories: 275cal; Carbohydrates: 9g; Proteins: 11g; Fat: 17g; Sodium: 73mg

324) Key Lime Pie Smoothie

Ingredients:

- 1/2 cup Cottage Cheese
- 1 tbsp. Sweetener of your choice
- 1/2 cup Water
- 1/2 cup Spinach
- 1 tbsp. Lime Juice
- 1 cup Ice Cubes

Direction: Preparation Time: 5 Minutes Cooking Time: 2 Minutes
Servings: 2

- ✓ Spoon in the ingredients to a high-speed blender and blend until silky smooth.
- ✓ Transfer to a serving glass and enjoy it.

Nutrition: Calories: 180 cal; Carbohydrates: 7g; Proteins: 36g; Fat: 1 g; Sodium: 35mg

325) Cinnamon Roll Smoothie

Ingredients:

- 1 tsp. Flax Meal or oats, if preferred
- 1 cup Almond Milk
- 1/2 tsp. Cinnamon
- 2 tbsp. Protein Powder
- 1 cup Ice
- ¼ tsp. Vanilla Extract
- 4 tsp. Sweetener of your choice

Direction: Preparation Time: 5 Minutes
Cooking Time: 0 Minutes Servings: 1

- ✓ Pour the milk into the blender, followed by the protein powder, sweetener, flax meal, cinnamon, vanilla extract, and ice.
- ✓ Blend for 40 seconds or until smooth.
- ✓ Serve and enjoy.

Nutrition: : Calories: 145cal; Carbs: 1.6g; Proteins: 26.5g; Fat: 3.25g; Sodium: 30mg

326) Strawberry Cheesecake Smoothie

Ingredients:

- ¼ cup Soy Milk, unsweetened
- 1/2 cup Cottage Cheese, low-fat
- 1/2 tsp. Vanilla Extract
- 2 oz. Cream Cheese
- 1 cup Ice Cubes
- 1/2 cup Strawberries
- 4 tbsp. Low-carb Sweetener of your choice

Direction: Preparation Time: 5 Minutes
Cooking Time: 0 Minutes Servings: 1

- ✓ Add all the ingredients for making the strawberry cheesecake smoothie to a high-speed blender until you get the desired smooth consistency.
- ✓ Serve and enjoy.

Nutrition: Calories: 347cal; Carbs: 10.05g; Proteins: 17.5g; Fat: 24g; Sodium: 45mg

327) Peanut Butter Banana Smoothie

Ingredients:

- ¼ cup Greek Yoghurt, plain
- 1/2 tbsp. Chia Seeds
- 1/2 cup Ice Cubes
- 1/2 of 1 Banana
- 1/2 cup Water
- 1 tbsp. Peanut Butter

Direction: Preparation Time: 5 Minutes
Cooking Time: 2 Minutes
Servings: 1

- ✓ Place all the ingredients needed to make the smoothie in a high-speed blender and blend to get a smooth and luscious mixture.
- ✓ Transfer the smoothie to a serving glass and enjoy it.

Nutrition: Calories: 202cal; Carbohydrates: 14g; Proteins: 10g; Fat: 9g; Sodium: 30mg

328) Avocado Turmeric Smoothie

Ingredients:

- 1/2 of 1 Avocado
- 1 cup Ice, crushed
- ¾ cup Coconut Milk, full-fat
- 1 tsp. Lemon Juice
- ¼ cup Almond Milk
- 1/2 tsp. Turmeric
- 1 tsp. Ginger, freshly grated

Direction: Preparation Time: 5 Minutes
Cooking Time: 2 Minutes Servings: 1

- ✓ Place all the ingredients excluding the crushed ice in a high-speed blender and blend for 2 to 3 minutes or until smooth.
- ✓ Transfer to a serving glass and enjoy it.

Nutrition: Calories: 232cal; Carbs: 4.1g; Proteins: 1.7g; Fat: 22.4g; Sodium: 25mg

329) Blueberry Smoothie

Ingredients:

- 1 tbsp. Lemon Juice
- 1 ¾ cup Coconut Milk, full-fat
- 1/2 tsp. Vanilla Extract
- 3 oz. Blueberries, frozen

Direction: Preparation Time: 5 Minutes
Cooking Time: 2 Minutes Servings: 2

- ✓ Combine coconut milk, blueberries, lemon juice, and vanilla extract in a high-speed blender.
- ✓ Blend for 2 minutes for a smooth and luscious smoothie.
- ✓ Serve and enjoy.

330) Matcha Green Smoothie

Ingredients:

- ¼ cup Heavy Whipping Cream
- 1/2 tsp. Vanilla Extract
- 1 tsp. Matcha Green Tea Powder
- 2 tbsp. Protein Powder
- 1 tbsp. Hot Water
- 1 ¼ cup Almond Milk, unsweetened
- 1/2 of 1 Avocado, medium

Direction: Preparation Time: 5 Minutes
Cooking Time: 2 Minutes Servings: 2

- ✓ Place all the ingredients in the high-blender for one to two minutes.
- ✓ Serve and enjoy.

Nutrition: Calories: 229cal; **Carbs:** 1.5g; **Proteins:** 14.1g; **Fat:** 43g; **Sodium:** 35mg

DESSERTS

331) Slow Cooker Peaches

Ingredients:

- 4 cups peaches, sliced
- 2/3 cup rolled oats
- 1/3 cup Bisques
- 1/4 teaspoon cinnamon
- 1/2 cup brown sugar
- 1/2 cup granulated sugar

Direction: Preparation Time: 10 minutes
Cooking time: 4 hours 20 minutes Servings: 4-6

- ✓ Spray the slow cooker pot with a cooking spray.
- ✓ Mix oats, Bisques, cinnamon and all the sugars in the pot.
- ✓ Add peaches and stir well to combine. Cook on low for 4-6 hours.

Nutrition: 617 calories; 3.6 g fat; 13 g total carbs; 9 g protein

332) Pumpkin Custard 1

Ingredients:

- 1/2 cup almond flour
- 4 eggs
- 1 cup pumpkin puree
- 1/2 cup stevia/erythritol blend, granulated
- 1/8 teaspoon sea salt
- 1 teaspoon vanilla extract or maple flavoring
- 4 tablespoons butter, ghee, or coconut oil melted
- 1 teaspoon pumpkin pie spice

Direction: Preparation Time: 10 minutes
Cooking time: 2 hours 30 minutes Servings: 6

- ✓ Grease or spray a slow cooker with butter or coconut oil spray.
- ✓ In a medium mixing bowl, beat the eggs until smooth. Then add in the sweetener.
- ✓ To the egg mixture, add in the pumpkin puree along with vanilla or maple extract.
- ✓ Then add almond flour to the mixture along with the pumpkin pie spice and salt. Add melted butter, coconut oil or ghee.
- ✓ Transfer the mixture into a slow cooker. Close the lid. Cook for 2-2 ¾ hours on low.
- ✓ When through, serve with whipped cream, and then sprinkle with little nutmeg if need be. Enjoy!
- ✓ Set slow-cooker to the low setting. Cook for 2-2.45 hours, and begin checking at the two hour mark. Serve warm with stevia sweetened whipped cream and a sprinkle of nutmeg.

Nutrition: 147 calories; 12 g fat; 4 g total carbs; 5 g protein

333) Blueberry Lemon Custard Cake

Ingredients:

- 6 eggs, separated
- 2 cups light cream
- 1/2 cup coconut flour
- 1/2 teaspoon salt
- 2 teaspoon lemon zest
- 1/2 cup granulated sugar substitute
- 1/3 cup lemon juice
- 1/2 cup blueberries fresh
- 1 teaspoon lemon liquid stevia

Direction: Preparation Time: 10 minutes
Cooking time: 3 hours Servings: 12

- ✓ Into a stand mixer, add the egg whites and whip them well until stiff peaks have formed; set aside.
- ✓ Whisk the yolks together with the remaining ingredients except blueberries, to form batter.
- ✓ When done, fold egg whites into the formed batter a little at a time until slightly combined.
- ✓ Grease the crock pot and then pour in the mixture. Then sprinkle batter with the blueberries.
- ✓ Close the lid then cook for 3 hours on low. When the cooking time is over, open the lid and let cool for an hour, and then let chill in the refrigerator for at least 2 hours or overnight.
- ✓ Serve cold with little sugar free whipped cream and enjoy!

Nutrition: 165 calories; 10 g fat; 14 g total carbs; 4 g protein

334) Sugar Free Carrot Cake

Ingredients:

- 2 eggs
- 1 1/2 almond flour
- 1/2 cup butter, melted
- ¼ cup heavy cream
- 1 teaspoon baking powder
- 1 teaspoon vanilla extract or almond extract, optional
- 1 cup sugar substitute
- 1 cup carrots, finely shredded
- 1 teaspoon cinnamon
- ¼ teaspoon nutmeg
- 1/8 teaspoon allspice
- 1 teaspoon ginger
- 1/2 teaspoon baking soda
- For cream cheese frosting:
- 1 cup confectioner's sugar substitute
- ¼ cup butter, softened
- 1 teaspoon almond extract
- 4 oz. cream cheese, softened

Direction: Cooking time: 4 hours
Servings: 8 Ingredients

- ✓ Grease a loaf pan well and then set it aside.
- ✓ Using a mixer, combine butter together with eggs, vanilla, sugar substitute and heavy cream in a mixing bowl, until well blended.
- ✓ Combine almond flour together with baking powder, spices and the baking soda in a another bowl until well blended.
- ✓ When done, combine the wet ingredients together with the dry ingredients until well blended, and then stir in carrots.
- ✓ Pour the mixer into the prepared loaf pan, and then place the pan into a slow cooker on a trivet. Add 1 cup water inside.
- ✓ Cook for about 4-5 hours on low. Be aware that the cake will be very moist.
- ✓ When the cooking time is over, let the cake cool completely.
- ✓ To prepare the cream cheese frosting: blend the cream cheese together with extract, butter and powdered sugar substitute until frosting is formed.
- ✓ Top the cake with the frosting.

Nutrition: 299 calories; 25.4 g fat; 15 g total carbs; 4 g protein

335) Sugar Free Chocolate Molten Lava Cake

Ingredients:

- 3 egg yolks
- 1 1/2 cups Swerve sweetener, divided
- 1 teaspoon baking powder
- 1/2 cup flour, gluten free
- 3 whole eggs
- 5 tablespoons cocoa powder, unsweetened, divided
- 4 oz. chocolate chips, sugar free
- 1/2 teaspoon salt
- 1/2 teaspoon vanilla liquid stevia
- 1/2 cup butter, melted, cooled
- 2 cups hot water
- 1 teaspoon vanilla extract

Direction: Preparation Time: 10 minutes
Cooking time: 3 hours Servings: 12

- ✓ Grease the crockpot well with cooking spray.
- ✓ Whisk 1 ¼ cups of swerve together with flour, salt, baking powder and 3 tablespoons cocoa powder in a bowl.
- ✓ Stir the cooled melted butter together with eggs, yolks, liquid stevia and the vanilla extract in a separate bowl.
- ✓ When done, add the wet ingredients to the dry ingredient until nicely combined, and then pour the mixture into the prepared crock pot.
- ✓ Then top the mixture in the crockpot with chocolate chips.
- ✓ Whisk the rest of the swerve sweetener and the remaining cocoa powder with the hot water, and then pour this mixture over the chocolate chips top.
- ✓ Close the lid and cook for 3 hours on low. When the cooking time is over, let cool a bit and then serve. Enjoy!

Nutrition: 157 calories; 13 g fat; 10.5 g total carbs; 3.9 g protein

336) Chocolate Quinoa Brownies

Ingredients:

- 2 eggs
- 3 cups quinoa, cooked
- 1 teaspoon vanilla liquid stevia
- 1 ¼ chocolate chips, sugar free
- 1 teaspoon vanilla extract
- 1/3 cup flaxseed ground
- ¼ teaspoon salt
- 1/3 cup cocoa powder, unsweetened
- 1/2 teaspoon baking powder
- 1 teaspoon pure stevia extract
- 1/2 cup applesauce, unsweetened
- Sugar- frees frosting:
- ¼ cup heavy cream
- 1 teaspoon chocolate liquid stevia
- ¼ cup cocoa powder, unsweetened
- 1/2 teaspoon vanilla extract

Direction: Preparation Time: 10 minutes
Cooking time: 2 hours Servings: 16

- ✓ Add all the ingredients to a food processor. Then process until well incorporated.
- ✓ Line a crock pot with a parchment paper, and then spread the batter into the lined pot.
- ✓ Close the lid and cook for 4 hours on LOW or 2 hours on HIGH. Let cool.
- ✓ Prepare the frosting. Whisk all the ingredients together and then microwave for 20 seconds. Taste and adjust on sweetener if desired.
- ✓ When the frosting is ready, stir it well again and then pour it over the sliced brownies.
- ✓ Serve and enjoy!

Nutrition: 133 calories; 7.9 g fat; 18.4 g total carbs; 4.3 g protein

337) Blueberry Crisp

Ingredients:

- 1/4 cup butter, melted
- 24 oz. blueberries, frozen
- 3/4 teaspoon salt
- 1 1/2 cups rolled oats, coarsely ground
- 3/4 cup almond flour, blanched
- 1/4 cup coconut oil, melted
- 6 tablespoons sweetener
- 1 cup pecans or walnuts, coarsely chopped

Direction: Preparation Time: 10 minutes
Cooking time: 3-4 hours Servings: 10

- ✓ Using a non-stick cooking spray, spray the slow cooker pot well.
- ✓ Into a bowl, add ground oats and chopped nuts along with salt, blanched almond flour, brown sugar, stevia granulated sweetener, and then stir in the coconut/butter mixture. Stir well to combine.
- ✓ When done, spread crisp topping over blueberries. Cook for 3-4 hours, until the mixture has become bubbling hot and you can smell the blueberries.
- ✓ Serve while still hot with the whipped cream or the ice cream if desired. Enjoy!

Nutrition: 261 calories; 16.6 g fat; 32 g total carbs; 4 g protein

338) Maple Custard

Ingredients:

- 1 teaspoon maple extract
- 2 egg yolks
- 1 cup heavy cream
- 2 eggs
- 1/2 cup whole milk
- 1/4 teaspoon salt
- 1/4 cup Sukrin Gold or any sugar-free brown sugar substitute
- 1/2 teaspoon cinnamon

Direction: Preparation Time: 10 minutes
Cooking time: 2 hours Servings: 6

- ✓ Combine all ingredients together in a blender, process well.
- ✓ Grease 6 ramekins and then pour the batter evenly into each ramekin.
- ✓ To the bottom of the slow cooker, add 4 ramekins and then arrange the remaining 2 against the side of a slow cooker, and not at the top of bottom ramekins.
- ✓ Close the lid and cook on high for 2 hours, until the center is cooked through but the middle is still jiggly.
- ✓ Let cool at a room temperature for an hour after removing from the slow cooker, and then chill in the fridge for at least 2 hours.
- ✓ Serve and enjoy with a sprinkle of cinnamon and little sugar free whipped cream.

Nutrition: 190 calories; 18 g fat; 2 g total carbs; 4 g protein

339) Raspberry Cream Cheese Coffee Cake

Ingredients:

- 1 1/4 almond flour
- 2/3 cup water
- 1/2 cup Swerve
- 3 eggs
- 1/4 cup coconut flour
- 1/4 cup protein powder
- 1/4 teaspoon salt
- 1/2 teaspoon vanilla extract
- 1 1/2 teaspoon baking powder
- 6 tablespoons butter, melted

For the Filling:

- 1 1/2 cup fresh raspberries
- 8 oz. cream cheese
- 1 large egg
- 1/3 cup powdered Swerve
- 2 tablespoon whipping cream

Direction: Preparation Time: 10 minutes
Cooking time: 4 hours **Servings:** 12

- Grease the slow cooker pot. Prepare the cake batter. In a bowl, combine almond flour together with coconut flour, sweetener, baking powder, protein powder and salt, and then stir in the melted butter along with eggs and water until well combined. Set aside.
- Prepare the filling.
- Beat cream cheese thoroughly with the sweetener until have smoothened, and then beat in whipping cream along with the egg and vanilla extract until well combined.
- Assemble the cake. Spread around 2/3 of batter in the slow cooker as you smoothen the top using a spatula or knife.
- Pour cream cheese mixture over the batter in the pan, evenly spread it, and then sprinkle with raspberries. Add the rest of batter over filling.
- Cook for 3-4 hours on low. Let cool completely.
- Serve and enjoy!

Nutrition: 239 calories; 19.18 g fat; 6.9 g total carbs; 7.5 g protein

340) Pumpkin Pie Bars

Ingredients:

- For the Crust:
- 3/4 cup coconut, shredded
- 4 tablespoons butter, unsalted, softened
- 1/4 cup cocoa powder, unsweetened
- 1/4 teaspoon salt
- 1/2 cup raw sunflower seeds or sunflower seed flour
- 1/4 cup confectioners Swerve
- Filling:
- 2 teaspoons cinnamon liquid stevia
- 1 cup heavy cream
- 1 can pumpkin puree
- 6 eggs
- 1 tablespoon pumpkin pie spice
- 1/2 teaspoon salt
- 1 tablespoon vanilla extract
- 1/2 cup sugar-free chocolate chips, optional

Direction: Preparation Time: 10 minutes
Cooking time: 3 hours **Servings:** 16

- Add all the crust ingredients to a food processor. Then process until fine crumbs are formed.
- Grease the slow cooker pan well. When done, press crust mixture onto the greased bottom.
- In a stand mixer, combine all the ingredients for the filling, and then blend well until combined.
- Top the filling with chocolate chips if using, and then pour the mixture onto the prepared crust.
- Close the lid and cook for 3 hours on low. Open the lid and let cool for at least 30 minutes, and then place the slow cooker into the refrigerator for at least 3 hours.
- Slice the pumpkin pie bar and serve it with sugar free whipped cream. Enjoy!

Nutrition: 169 calories; 15 g fat; 6 g total carbs; 4 g protein

341) Dark Chocolate Cake

Ingredients:

- 1 cup almond flour
- 3 eggs
- 2 tablespoons almond flour
- 1/4 teaspoon salt
- 1/2 cup Swerve Granular
- 3/4 teaspoon vanilla extract
- 2/3 cup almond milk, unsweetened
- 1/2 cup cocoa powder
- 6 tablespoons butter, melted
- 1 1/2 teaspoon baking powder
- 3 tablespoon unflavored whey protein powder or egg white protein powder
- 1/3 cup sugar-free chocolate chips, optional

Direction: Preparation Time: 10 minutes
Cooking time: 3 hours **Servings:** 10

- Grease the slow cooker well.
- Whisk the almond flour together with cocoa powder, sweetener, whey protein powder, salt and baking powder in a bowl. Then stir in butter along with almond milk, eggs and the vanilla extract until well combined, and then stir in the chocolate chips if desired.
- When done, pour into the slow cooker. Allow to cook for 2-2 1/2 hours on low.
- When through, turn off the slow cooker and let the cake cool for about 20-30 minutes.
- When cooled, cut the cake into pieces and serve warm with lightly sweetened whipped cream. Enjoy!

Nutrition: 205 calories; 17 g fat; 8.4 g total carbs; 12 g protein

342) Lemon Custard

Ingredients:

- 2 cups whipping cream or coconut cream
- 5 egg yolks
- 1 tablespoon lemon zest
- 1 teaspoon vanilla extract
- 1/4 cup fresh lemon juice, squeezed
- 1/2 teaspoon liquid stevia
- Lightly sweetened whipped cream

Direction: Preparation Time: 10 minutes
Cooking time: 3 hours
Servings: 4

- Whisk egg yolks together with lemon zest, liquid stevia, lemon zest and vanilla in a bowl, and then whisk in heavy cream.
- Divide the mixture among 4 small jars or ramekins.
- To the bottom of a slow cooker add a rack, and then add ramekins on top of the rack and add enough water to cover half of ramekins.
- Close the lid and cook for 3 hours on low. Remove ramekins.
- Let cool to room temperature, and then place into the refrigerator to cool completely for about 3 hours.
- When through, top with the whipped cream and serve. Enjoy!

Nutrition: 319 calories; 30 g fat; 3 g total carbs; 7 g protein

343) Coffee & Chocolate Ice Cream

Ingredients:

- 3 cups brewed coffee
- ½ cup low calorie chocolate flavored syrup
- ¾ cup low fat half and half

Direction: Preparation Time: 4 minutes Cooking Time: 0 minutes Servings: 15

- ✓ Mix the ingredients in a bowl.
- ✓ Pour into popsicle molds. Freeze for 4 hours.

Nutrition: Calories 21 Total Fat 0 g Saturated Fat 0 g Cholesterol 1 mg Sodium 28 mg Total Carbohydrate 4 g Dietary Fiber 0 g Total Sugars 3 g Protein 0 g Potassium 450 mg

344) Choco Banana Bites

Ingredients:

- : 2 bananas, sliced into rounds
- ¼ cup dark chocolate cubes

Direction: Preparation Time: 2 hours and 5 minutes Cooking Time: 5 minutes Servings: 4

- ✓ Melt chocolate in the microwave or in a saucepan over medium heat.
- ✓ Coat each banana slice with melted chocolate.
- ✓ Place on a metal pan. Freeze for 2 hours.

Nutrition: Calories 102 Total Fat 3 g Saturated Fat 2 g Cholesterol 0 mg Sodium 4 mg Total Carbohydrate 20 g Dietary Fiber 2 g Total Sugars 13 g Protein 1 g Potassium 211 mg

345) Blueberries with Yogurt

Ingredients:

- 1 cup nonfat Greek yogurt
- ¼ cup blueberries
- ¼ cup almonds

Direction: Preparation Time: 5 minutes Cooking Time: 0 minute Serving: 1

- ✓ Add yogurt and blueberries in a food processor.
- ✓ Pulse until smooth. Top with almonds before serving.

Nutrition: Calories 154 Total Fat 1 g Saturated Fat 0 g Cholesterol 11 mg Sodium 81 mg Total Carbohydrate 13 g Dietary Fiber 1 g Total Sugars 11 g Protein 23 g Potassium 346 mg

346) Roasted Mangoes

Ingredients:

- 2 mangoes, peeled and sliced into cubes
- 2 tablespoons coconut flakes
- 2 teaspoons crystallized ginger, chopped
- 2 teaspoons orange zest

Direction: Preparation Time: 5 minutes Cooking Time: 10 minutesServings: 4

- ✓ Preheat your oven to 350 degrees F. Put the mango cubes in custard cups.
- ✓ Top with the ginger and orange zest. Bake in the oven for 10 minutes.

Nutrition: Calories 89 Total Fat 2 g Saturated Fat 1 g Cholesterol 0 mg Sodium 14 mg Total Carbohydrate 20 g Dietary Fiber 2 g Total Sugars 17 g Protein 1 g Potassium 177 mg

347) Figs with Yogurt

Ingredients:

- 8 oz. low fat yogurt
- ½ teaspoon vanilla
- 2 figs, sliced
- 1 tablespoon walnuts, toasted and chopped
- Lemon zest

Direction: Preparation Time: 8 hours and 5 minutes Cooking Time: 0 minutes Servings: 2

- ✓ Refrigerate yogurt in a bowl for 8 hours.
- ✓ After 8 hours, take it out of the refrigerator and stir in yogurt and vanilla.
- ✓ Stir in the figs. Sprinkle walnuts and lemon zest on top before serving.

Nutrition: Calories 157 Total Fat 4 g Saturated Fat 1 g Cholesterol 7 mg Sodium 80 mg Total Carbohydrate 24 g Dietary Fiber 2 g Total Sugars 1 g Protein 7 g Potassium 557mg

348) Grilled Peaches

Ingredients:

- 1 cup balsamic vinegar
- ⅛ teaspoon ground cinnamon
- 1 tablespoon honey
- 3 peaches, pitted and sliced in half
- 2 teaspoons olive oil
- 6 gingersnaps, crushed

Direction: Preparation Time: 5 minutes Cooking Time: 3 minutes Servings: 6

- ✓ Pour the vinegar into a saucepan. Bring it to a boil. Lower heat and simmer for 10 minutes.
- ✓ Remove from the stove. Stir in cinnamon and honey.
- ✓ Coat the peaches with oil. Grill peaches for 2 to 3 minutes.
- ✓ Drizzle each one with syrup. Top with the gingersnaps.

Nutrition: : Calories 135 Total Fat 3 g Saturated Fat 1 g Cholesterol 0 mg Sodium 42 mg Total Carbohydrate 25 g Dietary Fiber 2 g Total Sugars 18 g Protein 1 g Potassium 251 mg

349) Fruit Salad

Ingredients:

- 8 oz. light cream cheese
- 6 oz. Greek yogurt
- 1 tablespoon honey
- 1 teaspoon orange zest
- 1 teaspoon lemon zest
- 1 orange, sliced into sections
- 3 kiwi fruit, peeled and sliced 1 mango, cubed
- 1 cup blueberries

Direction: Preparation Time: 5 minutes Cooking Time: 0 minute Servings: 6

- ✓ Beat cream cheese using an electric mixer.
- ✓ Add yogurt and honey. Beat until smooth.
- ✓ Stir in the orange and lemon zest.
- ✓ Toss the fruits to mix.
- ✓ Divide in glass jars. Top with the cream cheese mixture.

Nutrition: Calories 131 Total Fat 3 g Saturated Fat 2 g Cholesterol 9 mg Sodium 102 mg Total Carbohydrate 23 g Dietary Fiber 3 g Total Sugars 18 g Protein 5 g Potassium 234 mg

350) Strawberry & Watermelon Pops

Ingredients:

- ¾ cup strawberries, sliced
- 2 cups watermelon, cubed
- ¼ cup lime juice
- 2 tablespoons brown sugar
- ⅛ teaspoon salt

Direction: Preparation Time: 6 hours and 10 minutes Cooking Time: 0 minutes Servings: 6

- ✓ Put the strawberries inside popsicle molds. In a blender, pulse the rest of the ingredients until well mixed.
- ✓ Pour the puree into a sieve before pouring into the molds. Freeze for 6 hours.

Nutrition: Calories 57 Total Fat 0 g Saturated Fat 0 g Cholesterol 0 mg Sodium 180 mg Total Carbohydrate 14 g Dietary Fiber 2 g Total Sugars 11 g Protein 1 g Potassium 180 mg

351) Frozen Vanilla Yogurt

Ingredients:

- 3 cups fat-free plain Greek yogurt
- 4-6 drops liquid stevia
- 1 teaspoon organic vanilla extract
- ¼ cup fresh strawberries, hulled and sliced

Direction: Preparation Time: 10 minutes Servings: 6

- ✓ In a bowl, add all the ingredients except strawberries and mix until well combined.
- ✓ Transfer the mixture into an ice cream maker and process according to manufacturer's directions.
- ✓ Transfer the mixture into a bowl and freeze, covered for about 30-40 minutes or until desired consistency.
- ✓ Garnish with strawberry slices and serve. Meal Prep Tip: Line a cookie sheet with parchment paper. With a cookie scooper, place the yogurt portion onto the prepared cookie sheet.
- ✓ Freeze overnight. Remove from the freezer and transfer the frozen yogurt balls into an airtight container. Store in freezer up to 1 week. Remove from the freezer and set aside for 15-20 minutes before serving.

Nutrition: Calories 74 Total Fat 0.3 g Saturated Fat 0 g Cholesterol 4mg Total Carbs 5.6 g Sugar 4.9 g Fiber 0.1 g Sodium 58 mg Potassium 10 mg Protein 12 g

352) Spinach Sorbet

Ingredients:

- 3 cups fresh spinach, chopped
- 1 tablespoon fresh basil leaves
- ½ of avocado, peeled, pitted and chopped
- ¾ cup unsweetened almond milk 20 drops liquid stevia
- 1 teaspoon almonds, chopped very finely
- 1 teaspoon organic vanilla extract 1 cup ice cubes

Direction: Preparation Time: 15 minutes Servings: 4

- ✓ : In a blender, add all ingredients and pulse until creamy and smooth.
- ✓ Transfer into an ice cream maker and process according to manufacturer's directions. Transfer into an airtight container and freeze for at least 4-5 hours before serving.
- ✓ Meal Prep Tip: Transfer the sorbet into a shallow, flat container.
- ✓ With a plastic wrap, cover the ice cream and store in the back of the freezer.

Nutrition: Calories 70 Total Fat 5.9 g Saturated Fat 1.1 g Cholesterol 0 mg Total Carbs 3.6 g Sugar 0.4 g Fiber 2.4 g Sodium 53 mg Potassium 290 mg Protein 1.4 g

353) Avocado Mousse

Ingredients:

- 2 ripe Haas avocados, peeled, pitted and chopped roughly
- 1 teaspoon liquid stevia
- 1 teaspoon organic vanilla extract Pinch of salt

Direction: Preparation Time: 15 minutes Servings: 3

- ✓ In a high-speed blender, add all the ingredients and pulse until smooth.
- ✓ Transfer the pudding into a serving bowl. Cover the bowl and refrigerate to chill for at least 2 hours before serving.

Meal Prep Tip:

- ✓ Transfer the mousse into an airtight container.
- ✓ Cover the containers and refrigerate for about 1 day.

Nutrition: Calories 277 Total Fat 26.1 g Saturated Fat 5.5 g Cholesterol 0 mg Total Carbs 11.7 g Sugar 0.9 g Fiber 8 g Sodium 59 mg Potassium 652 mg Protein 2.6g

354) Strawberry Mousse

Ingredients:

- 1½ cups fresh strawberries, hulled
- 1 2/3 cups chilled unsweetened almond milk
- 2-3 drops liquid stevia
- 1 teaspoon organic vanilla extract

Direction: Preparation Time: 15 minutes Servings: 6

- ✓ In a food processor, add all the ingredients and pulse until smooth.
- ✓ Transfer into serving bowls and serve.

Meal Prep Tip:

- ✓ Transfer the mousse into an airtight container.
- ✓ Cover the containers and refrigerate for up to 3 days.

Nutrition: Calories 25 Total Fat 1.1g Saturated Fat 0.1 g Cholesterol 0 mg Total Carbs 3.4 g Sugar 1.9 g Fiber 1 g Sodium 50 mg Potassium 109 mg Protein 0.5 g

355) Blueberries Pudding

Ingredients:

- 1 small avocado, peeled, pitted and chopped
- 1 cup frozen blueberries
- ¼ teaspoon fresh ginger, grated freshly
- 1 teaspoon lime zest, grated finely
- 2 tablespoons fresh lime juice
- 10 drops liquid stevia
- 5 tablespoons filtered water

Direction: Preparation Time: 10 minutes Servings: 3

- ✓ In a blender, add all the ingredients and pulse till creamy and smooth.
- ✓ Transfer into serving bowls and serve.

Meal Prep Tip:

- ✓ Transfer the pudding into an airtight container.
- ✓ Cover the containers and refrigerate for up to 2 days.

Nutrition: Calories 166 Total Fat 13.3 g Saturated Fat 4.2.8 g Cholesterol 0 mg Total Carbs 13.1 g Sugar 5.2 g Fiber 5.8 g Sodium 4 mg Potassium 331 mg Protein 1.7 g

356) Raspberry Chia Pudding

Ingredients:

- 1½ cups unsweetened almond milk
- 1¼ cups fresh raspberries
- ½ cup chia seeds
- 1 tablespoon flax meal
- 3-4 drops liquid stevia
- 2 teaspoons organic vanilla extract

Direction: Preparation Time: 10 minutes Servings: 4

- ✓ : In a blender, add the almond milk and raspberries and pulse until smooth.
- ✓ Transfer the milk mixture into a large bowl.
- ✓ Add the remaining ingredients except raspberries and stir until well combined.
- ✓ Refrigerate to chill for at least 1 hour before serving.

Meal Prep Tip:

- ✓ Transfer the pudding into an airtight container.
- ✓ Cover the containers and refrigerate for about 1 day.

Nutrition: Calories 107 Total Fat 7.2 g Saturated Fat 0.5 g Cholesterol 0 mg Total Carbs 12.1 g Sugar 2 g Fiber 8.4 g Sodium 68 mg Potassium 246 mg Protein 4.2 g

357) Brown Rice Pudding

Ingredients:

- 2 cups low-fat milk 1/3 cup Erythritol 1½ teaspoons organic vanilla extract
- ¼ teaspoon ground cinnamon 1 egg 2 cups cooked brown rice

Direction: Preparation Time: 15 minutes Cooking Time: 30 minutes Servings: 4

- ✓ In a medium pan, add the milk, Erythritol, vanilla extract and cinnamon over medium-high heat and bring to a boil, stirring continuously. Remove from the heat.
- ✓ In a large bowl, add the egg and beat well. Slowly, add the hot milk mixture, a little bit at a time and beat until well combined. In the same pan, add the milk mixture and rice and
- ✓ Place the 2 cups of cooked rice into the pan used to cook the milk mixture and stir to combine.
- ✓ Place the pan over medium-high heat and bring to a boil, stirring continuously.
- ✓ Reduce heat to low and simmer for about 15-20 minutes, stirring after every 5 minutes. Remove from the heat and transfer into a bowl. With a wax paper, cover the top of pudding and refrigerate to chill before serving.

Meal Prep Tip:

- ✓ Transfer the pudding into an airtight container. Cover the containers and refrigerate for up to 2 days.

Nutrition: Calories 416 Total Fat 4.8 g Saturated Fat 1.6 g Cholesterol 47 mg Total Carbs 78 g Sugar 6 g Fiber 3.3 g Sodium 73 mg Potassium 455 mg Protein 12.5 g

358) Lemon Cookies

Ingredients: Preparation Time: 10 minutes Cooking Time: 12 minutes Servings: 6

- ¼ cup unsweetened applesauce 1 cup cashew butter 1 teaspoon fresh lemon zest, grated finely
- 2 tablespoons fresh lemon juice Pinch of sea salt

Direction:

- ✓ Preheat the oven to 350 degrees F. Line a large cookie sheet with parchment paper. In a food processor, add all ingredients and pulse until smooth. With a tablespoon, place the mixture onto prepared cookie sheet in a single layer. Bake for about 12 minutes or until golden brown. Remove from oven and place the cookie sheet onto a wire rack to cool for about 5 minutes.
- ✓ Carefully invert the cookies onto wire rack to cool completely before serving. Meal Prep Tip: Store these cookies in an airtight container, by placing parchment papers between the cookies to avoid the sticking. These cookies can be stored in the refrigerator for up to 2 weeks.

Nutrition: : Calories 257 Total Fat 21.9 g Saturated Fat 4.2 g Cholesterol 0 mg Total Carbs 13.1 g Sugar 1.2 g Fiber 1 g Sodium 47 mg Potassium 248 mg Protein 7.6 g

359) Yogurt Cheesecake

Ingredients:

- 2½ cups fat-free plain Greek yogurt
- 6-8 drops liquid stevia 3 egg whites
- 1/3 cup cacao powder
- ¼ cup arrowroot starch
- 1 teaspoon organic vanilla extract
- Pinch of sea salt

Direction: Preparation Time: 15 minutes Cooking Time: 35 minutes Servings: 8

- ✓ Preheat the oven to 35 degrees F. Grease a 9-inch cake pan.
- ✓ In a large bowl, add all ingredients and mix until well combined.
- ✓ Place the mixture into the prepared pan evenly. Bake for about 30-35 minutes. Remove from oven and let it cool completely.
- ✓ Refrigerate to chill for about 3-4 hours or until set completely.
- ✓ Cut into 8 equal sized slices and serve.

Meal Prep Tip:

- ✓ With foil pieces, wrap the cheesecake slices and refrigerate for about 1-3 days. Reheat in the microwave before serving.

Nutrition: Calories 74 Total Fat 0.9g Saturated Fat 0.4 g Cholesterol 2 mg Total Carbs 8.5 g Sugar 3 g Fiber 1.1 g Sodium 89 mg Potassium 21 mg Protein 9.5 g

360) Flourless Chocolate Cake

Ingredients:

- 1/2 Cup of stevia
- 12 Ounces of unsweetened baking chocolate
- 2/3 Cup of ghee
- 1/3 Cup of warm water
- ¼ Teaspoon of salt
- 4 Large pastured eggs
- 2 Cups of boiling water

Direction: Preparation time: 10 minutes
Cooking time: 45 minutes Yield: 6 Servings

- ✓ Line the bottom of a 9-inch pan of a spring form with a parchment paper.
- ✓ Heat the water in a small pot; then add the salt and the stevia over the water until wait until the mixture becomes completely dissolved.
- ✓ Melt the baking chocolate into a double boiler or simply microwave it for about 30 seconds.
- ✓ Mix the melted chocolate and the butter in a large bowl with an electric mixer.
- ✓ Beat in your hot mixture; then crack in the egg and whisk after adding each of the eggs.
- ✓ Pour the obtained mixture into your prepared spring form tray.
- ✓ Wrap the spring form tray with a foil paper.
- ✓ Place the spring form tray in a large cake tray and add boiling water right to the outside; make sure the depth doesn't exceed 1 inch.
- ✓ Bake the cake into the water bath for about 45 minutes at a temperature of about 350 F.
- ✓ Remove the tray from the boiling water and transfer to a wire to cool.
- ✓ Let the cake chill for an overnight in the refrigerator.
- ✓ Serve and enjoy your delicious cake!

Nutrition: Calories: 295| Fat: 26g | Carbohydrates: 6g | Fiber: 4g |Protein: 8g

361) Raspberry Cake With White Chocolate Sauce

Ingredients:

- 5 Ounces of melted cacao butter
- 2 Ounces of grass-fed ghee
- 1/2 Cup of coconut cream
- 1 Cup of green banana flour
- 3 Teaspoons of pure vanilla
- 4 Large eggs
- 1/2 Cup of as Lakanto Monk Fruit
- 1 Teaspoon of baking powder
- 2 Teaspoons of apple cider vinegar
- 2 Cup of raspberries
- For the white chocolate sauce:
- 3 and 1/2 ounces of cacao butter
- 1/2 Cup of coconut cream
- 2 Teaspoons of pure vanilla extract
- 1 Pinch of salt

Direction: Preparation time: 15 minutes
Cooking time: 60 minutes Yield: 5-6 Servings

- ✓ Preheat your oven to a temperature of about 280 degrees Fahrenheit.
- ✓ Combine the green banana flour with the pure vanilla extract, the baking powder, the coconut cream, the eggs, the cider vinegar and the monk fruit and mix very well.
- ✓ Leave the raspberries aside and line a cake loaf tin with a baking paper.
- ✓ Pour in the batter into the baking tray and scatter the raspberries over the top of the cake.
- ✓ Place the tray in your oven and bake it for about 60 minutes; in the meantime, prepare the sauce by
- ✓ Directions for sauce:
- ✓ Combine the cacao cream, the vanilla extract, the cacao butter and the salt in a saucepan over a low heat.
- ✓ Mix all your ingredients with a fork to make sure the cacao butter mixes very well with the cream.
- ✓ Remove from the heat and set aside to cool a little bit; but don't let it harden.
- ✓ Drizzle with the chocolate sauce.
- ✓ Scatter the cake with more raspberries.
- ✓ Slice your cake; then serve and enjoy it!

Nutrition: Calories: 323| Fat: 31.5g | Carbohydrates: 9.9g | Fiber: 4g |Protein: 5g

362) Ketogenic Lava Cake

Ingredients:

- 2 Oz of dark chocolate; you should at least use chocolate of 85% cocoa solids
- 1 Tablespoon of super-fine almond flour
- 2 Oz of unsalted almond butter
- 2 Large eggs

Direction: Preparation time: 10 minutes
Cooking time: 10 minutes Yield: 2 Servings

- ✓ Heat your oven to a temperature of about 350 Fahrenheit.
- ✓ Grease 2 heat proof ramekins with almond butter.
- ✓ Now, melt the chocolate and the almond butter and stir very well.
- ✓ Beat the eggs very well with a mixer.
- ✓
- ✓ Add the eggs to the chocolate and the butter mixture and mix very well with almond flour and the swerve; then stir.
- ✓ Pour the dough into 2 ramekins.
- ✓ Bake for about 9 to 10 minutes.
- ✓ Turn the cakes over plates and serve with pomegranate seeds!
- ✓

Nutrition: Calories: 459| Fat: 39g | Carbohydrates: 3.5g | Fiber: 0.8g |Protein: 11.7g

363) Ketogenic Cheese Cake

Ingredients:

- For the Almond Flour Cheesecake Crust:
- 2 Cups of Blanched almond flour
- 1/3 Cup of almond Butter
- 3 Tablespoons of Erythritol (powdered or granular)
- 1 Teaspoon of Vanilla extract
- For the Keto Cheesecake Filling:
- 32 Oz of softened Cream cheese
- 1 and ¼ cups of powdered erythritol
- 3 Large Eggs
- 1 Tablespoon of Lemon juice
- 1 Teaspoon of Vanilla extract

Direction: Preparation time: 15 minutes
Cooking time: 50 minutes Yield: 6 Servings

- ✓ Preheat your oven to a temperature of about 350 degrees F.
- ✓ Grease a spring form pan of 9" with cooking spray or just line its bottom with a parchment paper.
- ✓ In order to make the cheesecake rust, stir in the melted butter, the almond flour, the vanilla extract and the erythritol in a large bowl.
- ✓ The dough will get will be a bit crumbly; so press it into the bottom of your prepared tray.
- ✓ Bake for about 12 minutes; then let cool for about 10 minutes.
- ✓ In the meantime, beat the softened cream cheese and the powdered sweetener at a low speed until it becomes smooth.
- ✓ Crack in the eggs and beat them in at a low to medium speed until it becomes fluffy. Make sure to add one a time.
- ✓ Add in the lemon juice and the vanilla extract and mix at a low to medium speed with a mixer.
- ✓ Pour your filling into your pan right on top of the crust. You can use a spatula to smooth the top of the cake.
- ✓ Bake for about 45 to 50 minutes.
- ✓ Remove the baked cheesecake from your oven and run a knife around its edge.
- ✓ Let the cake cool for about 4 hours in the refrigerator.

Nutrition: Calories: 325| Fat: 29g | Carbohydrates: 6g | Fiber: 1g |Protein: 7g

364) Cake with Whipped Cream Icing

Ingredients:

- ¾ Cup Coconut flour
- ¾ Cup of Swerve Sweetener
- 1/2 Cup of Cocoa powder
- 2 Teaspoons of Baking powder
- 6 Large Eggs
- 2/3 Cup of Heavy Whipping Cream
- 1/2 Cup of Melted almond Butter
- For the whipped Cream Icing:
- 1 Cup of Heavy Whipping Cream
- ¼ Cup of Swerve Sweetener
- 1 Teaspoon of Vanilla extract
- 1/3 Cup of Sifted Cocoa Powder

Direction: Preparation time: 20 minutes
Cooking time: 25 minutes Yield: 7 Servings

- ✓ Pre-heat your oven to a temperature of about 350 F.
- ✓ Grease an 8x8 cake tray with cooking spray.
- ✓ Add the coconut flour, the Swerve sweetener; the cocoa powder, the baking powder, the eggs, the melted butter; and combine very well with an electric or a hand mixer.
- ✓ Pour your batter into the cake tray and bake for about 25 minutes.
- ✓ Remove the cake tray from the oven and let cool for about 5 minutes.
- ✓ For the Icing:
- ✓ Whip the cream until it becomes fluffy; then add in the Swerve, the vanilla and the cocoa powder.
- ✓ Add the Swerve, the vanilla and the cocoa powder; then continue mixing until your ingredients are very well combined.
- ✓ Frost your baked cake with the icing; then slice it; serve and enjoy your delicious cake!

Nutrition: Calories: 357| Fat: 33g | Carbohydrates: 11g | Fiber: 2g |Protein: 8g

365) Walnut-Fruit Cake

Ingredients:

- 1/2 Cup of almond butter (softened)
- ¼ Cup of so Nourished granulated erythritol
- 1 Tablespoon of ground cinnamon
- 1/2 Teaspoon of ground nutmeg
- ¼ Teaspoon of ground cloves
- 4 Large pastured eggs
- 1 Teaspoon of vanilla extract
- 1/2 Teaspoon of almond extract
- 2 Cups of almond flour
- 1/2 Cup of chopped walnuts
- ¼ Cup of dried of unsweetened cranberries
- ¼ Cup of seedless raisins

Direction:

- ✓ Preheat your oven to a temperature of about 350 F and grease an 8-inch baking tin of round shape with coconut oil.
- ✓ Beat the granulated erythritol on a high speed until it becomes fluffy.
- ✓ Add the cinnamon, the nutmeg, and the cloves; then blend your ingredients until they become smooth.
- ✓ Crack in the eggs and beat very well by adding one at a time, plus the almond extract and the vanilla.
- ✓ Whisk in the almond flour until it forms a smooth batter then fold in the nuts and the fruit.
- ✓ Spread your mixture into your prepared baking pan and bake it for about 20 minutes.
- ✓ Remove the cake from the oven and let cool for about 5 minutes.
- ✓ Dust the cake with the powdered erythritol.
- ✓ Serve and enjoy your cake!

Nutrition: Calories: 250| Fat: 11g | Carbohydrates: 12g | Fiber: 2g |Protein: 7g

366) Ginger Cake

Ingredients:

- 1/2 Tablespoon of unsalted almond butter to grease the pan
- 4 Large eggs
- ¼ Cup coconut milk
- 2 Tablespoons of unsalted almond butter
- 1 and 1/2 teaspoons of stevia
- 1 Tablespoon of ground cinnamon
- 1 Tablespoon of natural unweeded cocoa powder
- 1 Tablespoon of fresh ground ginger
- 1/2 Teaspoon of kosher salt
- 1 and 1/2 cups of blanched almond flour
- 1/2 Teaspoon of baking soda

Direction: Preparation time: 15 minutes
Cooking time: 20 minutes Yield: 9 Servings

- ✓ Preheat your oven to a temperature of 325 F.
- ✓ Grease a glass baking tray of about 8X8 inches generously with almond butter.
- ✓ In a large bowl, whisk all together the coconut milk, the eggs, the melted almond butter, the stevia, the cinnamon, the cocoa powder, the ginger and the kosher salt.
- ✓ Whisk in the almond flour, then the baking soda and mix very well.
- ✓ Pour the batter into the prepared pan and bake for about 20 to 25 minutes.
- ✓ Let the cake cool for about 5 minutes; then slice; serve and enjoy your delicious cake.

Nutrition: Calories: 175| Fat: 15g | Carbohydrates: 5g | Fiber: 1.9g |Protein: 5g

367) Ketogenic Orange Cake

Ingredients:

- 2 and 1/2 cups of almond flour
- 2 Unwaxed washed oranges
- 5 Large separated eggs
- 1 Teaspoon of baking powder
- 2 Teaspoons of orange extract
- 1 Teaspoon of vanilla bean powder
- 6 Seeds of cardamom pods crushed
- 16 drops of liquid stevia; about 3 teaspoons
- 1 Handful of flaked almonds to decorate

Direction: Preparation time: 10 minutes
Cooking time: 50 minutes Yield: 8 Servings

- ✓ Preheat your oven to a temperature of about 350 Fahrenheit.
- ✓ Line a rectangular bread baking tray with a parchment paper.
- ✓ Place the oranges into a pan filled with cold water and cover it with a lid.
- ✓ Bring the saucepan to a boil, then let simmer for about 1 hour and make sure the oranges are totally submerged.
- ✓ Make sure the oranges are always submerged to remove any taste of bitterness.
- ✓ Cut the oranges into halves; then remove any seeds; and drain the water and set the oranges aside to cool down.
- ✓ Cut the oranges in half and remove any seeds, then puree it with a blender or a food processor.
- ✓ Separate the eggs; then whisk the egg whites until you see stiff peaks forming.
- ✓ Add all your ingredients except for the egg whites to the orange mixture and add in the egg whites; then mix.
- ✓ Pour the batter into the cake tin and sprinkle with the flaked almonds right on top.
- ✓ Bake your cake for about 50 minutes.
- ✓ Remove the cake from the oven and set aside to cool for 5 minutes.
- ✓ Slice your cake; then serve and enjoy its incredible taste!

Nutrition: Calories: 164| Fat: 12g | Carbohydrates: 7.1 | Fiber: 2.7g |Protein: 10.9g

368) Lemon Cake

Ingredients:

- 2 Medium lemons
- 4 Large eggs
- 2 Tablespoons of almond butter
- 2 Tablespoons of avocado oil
- 1/3 cup of coconut flour
- 4-5 tablespoons of honey (or another sweetener of your choice)
- 1/2 tablespoon of baking soda

Direction: Preparation time: 20 minutes
Cooking time: 20 minutes Yield: 9 Servings

- ✓ Preheat your oven to a temperature of about 350 F.
- ✓ Crack the eggs in a large bowl and set two egg whites aside.
- ✓ Whisk the 2 whites of eggs with the egg yolks, the honey, the oil, the almond butter, the lemon zest and the juice and whisk very well together.
- ✓ Combine the baking soda with the coconut flour and gradually add this dry mixture to the wet ingredients and keep whisking for a couple of minutes.
- ✓ Beat the two eggs with a hand mixer and beat the egg into foam. Add the white egg foam gradually to the mixture with a silicone spatula.
- ✓ Transfer your obtained batter to tray covered with a baking paper.
- ✓ Bake your cake for about 20 to 22 minutes.
- ✓ Let the cake cool for 5 minutes; then slice your cake.
- ✓ Serve and enjoy your delicious cake!

Nutrition: Calories: 164| Fat: 12g | Carbohydrates: 7.1 | Fiber: 2.7g |Protein: 10.9g

369) Cinnamon Cake

Ingredients:

- For the Cinnamon Filling:
- 3 Tablespoons of Swerve Sweetener
- 2 Teaspoons of ground cinnamon
- For the Cake:
- 3 Cups of almond flour
- ¾ Cup of Swerve Sweetener
- ¼ Cup of unflavoured whey protein powder
- 2 Teaspoon of baking powder
- 1/2 Teaspoon of salt
- 3 large pastured eggs
- 1/2 Cup of melted coconut oil
- 1/2 Teaspoon of vanilla extract
- 1/2 Cup of almond milk
- 1 Tablespoon of melted coconut oil
- For the cream cheese Frosting:
- 3 Tablespoons of softened cream cheese
- 2 Tablespoons of powdered Swerve Sweetener
- 1 Tablespoon of coconut heavy whipping cream
- 1/2 Teaspoon of vanilla extract

Direction: Preparation time: 15 minutes Cooking time: 35 minutes Yield: 8 Servings

- ✓ Preheat your oven to a temperature of about 325 F and grease a baking tray of 8x8 inch.
- ✓ For the filling, mix the Swerve and the cinnamon in a mixing bowl and mix very well; then set it aside.
- ✓ For the preparation of the cake; whisk all together the almond flour, the sweetener, the protein powder, the baking powder, and the salt in a mixing bowl.
- ✓ Add in the eggs, the melted coconut oil and the vanilla extract and mix very well.
- ✓ Add in the almond milk and keep stirring until your ingredients are very well combined.
- ✓ Spread about half of the batter in the prepared pan; then sprinkle with about two thirds of the filling mixture.
- ✓ Spread the remaining mixture of the batter over the filling and smooth it with a spatula.
- ✓ Bake for about 35 minutes in the oven.
- ✓ Brush with the melted coconut oil and sprinkle with the remaining cinnamon filling.
- ✓ Prepare the frosting by beating the cream cheese, the powdered erythritol, the cream and the vanilla extract in a mixing bowl until it becomes smooth.
- ✓ Drizzle frost over the cooled cake.
- ✓ Slice the cake; then serve and enjoy your cake!

Nutrition: Calories: 222| Fat: 19.2g | Carbohydrates: 5.4g | Fiber: 1.5g |Protein: 7.3g

370) Chocolate & Raspberry Ice Cream

Ingredients:

- ¼ cup almond milk
- 2 egg yolks
- 2 tablespoons cornstarch
- ¼ cup honey
- ¼ teaspoon almond extract
- ⅛ teaspoon salt
- 1 cup fresh raspberries
- 2 oz. dark chocolate, chopped
- ¼ cup almonds, slivered and toasted

Direction: Preparation Time: 12 hours and 20 minutes Cooking Time: 0 minutes Servings: 8

- ✓ Mix almond milk, egg yolks, cornstarch and honey in a bowl.
- ✓ Pour into a saucepan over medium heat.
- ✓ Cook for 8 minutes.
- ✓ Strain through a sieve. Stir in salt and almond extract.
- ✓ Chill for 8 hours.
- ✓ Put into an ice cream maker.
- ✓ Follow manufacturer's directions.
- ✓ Stir in the rest of the ingredients.
- ✓ Freeze for 4 hours.

Nutrition: Calories 142 Total Fat 7 g Saturated Fat 2 g Cholesterol 70 mg Sodium 87 mg Total Carbohydrate 18 g Dietary Fiber 2 g Total Sugars 13 g Protein 3 g Potassium 150 mg

371) Mocha Pops

Ingredients:

- 3 cups brewed coffee
- ½ cup low calorie chocolate flavored syrup
- ¾ cup low fat half and half

Direction: Preparation Time: 4 minutes Cooking Time: 0 minutes Servings: 15

- ✓ Mix the ingredients in a bowl.
- ✓ Pour into popsicle molds. Freeze for 4 hours.

Nutrition: Calories 21 Total Fat 0 g Saturated Fat 0 g Cholesterol 1 mg Sodium 28 mg Total Carbohydrate 4 g Dietary Fiber 0 g Total Sugars 3 g Protein 0 g Potassium 450 mg

372) Fruit Kebab

Ingredients:

- 3 apples
- ¼ cup orange juice
- 1 ½ lb. watermelon
- ¾ cup blueberries

Direction: Preparation Time: 30 minutes Cooking Time: 0 minutes Servings: 12

- ✓ Use a star-shaped cookie cutter to cut out stars from the apple and watermelon.
- ✓ Soak the apple stars in orange juice.
- ✓ Thread the apple stars, watermelon stars and blueberries into skewers.
- ✓ Refrigerate for 30 minutes before serving.

Nutrition: Calories 52 Total Fat 0 g Saturated Fat 0 g Cholesterol 0 mg Sodium 1 mg Total Carbohydrate 14 g Dietary Fiber 2 g Total Sugars 10 g Protein 1 g Potassium 134 mg

373) Salad Preparation

Ingredients:

- 8 oz. light cream cheese 6 oz. Greek yogurt 1 tablespoon honey
- 1 teaspoon orange zest
- 1 teaspoon lemon zest
- 1 orange, sliced into sections
- 3 kiwi fruit, peeled and sliced
- 1 mango, cubed 1 cup blueberries

Direction: Time: 5 minutes Cooking Time: 0 minute Servings: 6

- ✓ Beat cream cheese using an electric mixer. Add yogurt and honey.
- ✓ Beat until smooth. Stir in the orange and lemon zest. Toss the fruits to mix.
- ✓ Divide in glass jars. Top with the cream cheese mixture.

Nutrition: Calories 131 Total Fat 3 g Saturated Fat 2 g Cholesterol 9 mg Sodium 102 mg Total Carbohydrate 23 g Dietary Fiber 3 g Total Sugars 18 g Protein 5 g Potassium 234 mg

MORE RECIPES

374) Chili Chicken Wings

Ingredients:
- 2 lbs chicken wings
- 1/8 tsp. paprika
- 1/2 cup coconut flour
- 1/4 tsp. garlic powder
- 1/4 tsp. chili powder

Direction: Preparation Time: 10 minutes
Cooking Time: 1 hour 10 minutes **Servings:** 4

- ✓ Preheat the oven to 400 F/ 200 C.
- ✓ In a mixing bowl, add all ingredients except chicken wings and mix well.
- ✓ Add chicken wings to the bowl mixture and coat well and place on a baking tray.
- ✓ Bake in preheated oven for 55-60 minutes.
- ✓ Serve and enjoy.

Nutrition: Calories 440 Fat 17.1 g, Carbs 1.3 g, Sugar 0.2 g, Protein 65.9 g, Cholesterol 202 mg

375) Garlic Chicken Wings

Ingredients:
- 12 chicken wings
- 2 garlic clove, minced
- 3 tbsp. ghee
- 1/2 tsp. turmeric
- 2 tsp. cumin seeds

Direction: Preparation Time: 10 minutes
Cooking Time: 55 minutes
Servings: 6

- ✓ Preheat the oven to 425 F/ 215 C.
- ✓ In a large bowl, mix together 1 teaspoon cumin, 1 tbsp. ghee, turmeric, pepper, and salt.
- ✓ Add chicken wings to the bowl and toss well.
- ✓ Spread chicken wings on a baking tray and bake in preheated oven for 30 minutes.
- ✓ Turn chicken wings to another side and bake for 8 minutes more.
- ✓ Meanwhile, heat remaining ghee in a pan over medium heat.
- ✓ Add garlic and cumin to the pan and cook for a minute.
- ✓ Remove pan from heat and set aside.
- ✓ Remove chicken wings from oven and drizzle with ghee mixture/
- ✓ Bake chicken wings 5 minutes more.
- ✓ Serve and enjoy.

Nutrition: Calories 378 Fat 27.9 g, Carbs 11.4 g, Sugar 0 g, Protein 19.7 g, Cholesterol 94 mg

376) Spinach Cheese Pie

Ingredients:
- 6 eggs, lightly beaten
- 2 boxes frozen spinach, chopped
- 2 cup cheddar cheese, shredded
- 15 oz. cottage cheese
- 1 tsp. salt

Direction: Preparation Time: 10 minutes
Cooking Time: 40 minutes **Servings:** 8

- ✓ Preheat the oven to 375 F/ 190 C.
- ✓ Spray an 8*8-inch baking dish with cooking spray and set aside.
- ✓ In a mixing bowl, combine together spinach, eggs, cheddar cheese, cottage cheese, pepper, and salt.
- ✓ Pour spinach mixture into the prepared baking dish and bake in preheated oven for 10 minutes.
- ✓ Serve and enjoy.

Nutrition: Calories 229 Fat 14 g, Carbs. 5.4 g, Sugar 0.9 g, Protein 21 g, Cholesterol 157 mg

377) Tasty Harissa Chicken

Ingredients:
- 1 lb. chicken breasts, skinless and boneless
- 1/2 tsp. ground cumin
- 1 cup harissa sauce
- 1/4 tsp. garlic powder
- 1/2 tsp. kosher salt

Direction: Preparation Time: 10 minutes
Cooking Time: 4 hours 10 minutes **Servings:** 4

- ✓ Season chicken with garlic powder, cumin, and salt.
- ✓ Place chicken to the slow cooker.
- ✓ Pour harissa sauce over the chicken.
- ✓ Cover slow cooker with lid and cook on low for 4 hours.
- ✓ Remove chicken from slow cooker and shred using a fork.
- ✓ Return shredded chicken to the slow cooker and stir well.
- ✓ Serve and enjoy.

Nutrition: Calories 232 Fat 9.7 g, Carbs 1.3 g, Sugar 0.1 g, Protein 32.9 g, Cholesterol 101 mg

378) Roasted Balsamic Mushrooms

Ingredients:
- 8 oz. mushrooms, sliced
- 1/2 tsp. thyme
- 2 tbsp. balsamic vinegar
- 2 tbsp. extra virgin olive oil
- 2 onions, sliced

Direction: Preparation Time: 10 minutes
Cooking Time: 50 minutes **Servings:** 4

- ✓ Preheat the oven to 375 F/ 190 C.
- ✓ Line baking tray with aluminum foil and spray with cooking spray and set aside.
- ✓ In a mixing bowl, add all ingredients and mix well.
- ✓ Spread mushroom mixture onto a prepared baking tray.
- ✓ Roast in preheated oven for 45 minutes.
- ✓ Season with pepper and salt.
- ✓ Serve and enjoy.

Nutrition: Calories 96 Fat 7.2 g, Carbohydrates 7.2 g, Sugar 3.3 g, Protein 2.4 g, Cholesterol 0 mg

379) Roasted Cumin Carrots

Ingredients:

- 8 carrots, peeled and cut into 1/2 inch thick slices
- 1 tsp. cumin seeds
- 1 tbsp. olive oil
- 1/2 tsp. kosher salt

Direction: Preparation Time: 10 minutes
Cooking Time: 45 minutes **Servings:** 4

- ✓ Preheat the oven to 400 F/ 200 C.
- ✓ Line baking tray with parchment paper.
- ✓ Add carrots, cumin seeds, olive oil, and salt in a large bowl and toss well to coat.
- ✓ Spread carrots on a prepared baking tray and roast in preheated oven for 20 minutes.
- ✓ Turn carrots to another side and roast for 20 minutes more.
- ✓ Serve and enjoy.

Nutrition: Calories 82 Fat 3.6 g, Carbohydrates 12.2 g, Sugar 6 g, Protein 1.1 g, Cholesterol 0 mg

380) Tasty & Tender Brussels Sprouts

Ingredients:

- 1 lb. Brussels sprouts, trimmed cut in half
- ¼ cup balsamic vinegar
- 1 onion, sliced
- 1 tbsp. olive oil

Direction: Preparation Time: 10 minutes
Cooking Time: 35 minutes **Servings:** 4

- ✓ Add water in a saucepan and bring to boil.
- ✓ Add Brussels sprouts and cook over medium heat for 20 minutes. Drain well.
- ✓ Heat oil in a pan over medium heat.
- ✓ Add onion and cook until softened. Add sprouts and vinegar and stir well and cook for 1-2 minutes.
- ✓ Serve and enjoy.

Nutrition: Calories 93 Fat 3.9 g, Carbohydrates 13 g, Sugar 3.7 g, Protein 4.2 g, Cholesterol 0 mg

381) Sautéed Veggies

Ingredients:

- 1/2 cup mushrooms, sliced
- 1 zucchini, diced
- 1 squash, diced
- 2 1/2 tsp. southwest seasoning
- 3 tbsp. olive oil

Direction: Preparation Time: 10 minutes
Cooking Time: 15 minutes **Servings:** 4

- ✓ In a medium bowl, whisk together southwest seasoning, pepper, olive oil, and salt.
- ✓ Add vegetables to a bowl and mix well to coat.
- ✓ Heat pan over medium-high heat.
- ✓ Add vegetables in the pan and sauté for 5-7 minutes.
- ✓ Serve and enjoy.

Nutrition: Calories 107, Fat 10.7 g, Carbs 3.6 g, Sugar 1.5 g, Protein 1.2 g, Cholesterol 0 mg

382) Mustard Green Beans

Ingredients:

- 1 lb. green beans, washed and trimmed
- 1 tsp. whole grain mustard
- 1 tbsp. olive oil
- 2 tbsp. apple cider vinegar
- 1/4 cup onion, chopped

Direction: Preparation Time: 10 minutes
Cooking Time: 20 minutes **Servings:** 4

- ✓ Steam green beans in the microwave until tender.
- ✓ Meanwhile, in a pan heat olive oil over medium heat.
- ✓ Add the onion in a pan sauté until softened.
- ✓ Add water, apple cider vinegar, and mustard in the pan and stir well.
- ✓ Add green beans and stir to coat and heat through.
- ✓ Season green beans with pepper and salt.
- ✓ Serve and enjoy.

Nutrition: Calories 71 Fat 3.7 g, Carbohydrates 8.9 g, Sugar 1.9 g, Protein 2.1 g, Cholesterol 0 mg

383) Zucchini Fries

Ingredients:

- 1 egg
- 2 medium zucchini, cut into fries shape
- 1 tsp. Italian herbs
- 1 tsp. garlic powder
- 1 cup parmesan cheese, grated

Direction: Preparation Time: 10 minutes
Cooking Time: 40 minutes **Servings:** 4

- ✓ Preheat the oven to 425 F/ 218 C.
- ✓ Spray a baking tray with cooking spray and set aside.
- ✓ In a small bowl, add egg and lightly whisk it.
- ✓ In a separate bowl, mix together spices and parmesan cheese.
- ✓ Dip zucchini fries in egg then coat with parmesan cheese mixture and place on a baking tray.
- ✓ Bake in preheated oven for 25-30 minutes. Turn halfway through.
- ✓ Serve and enjoy.

Nutrition: Calories 184 Fat 10.3 g, Carbs 3.9 g, Sugar 2 g, Protein 14.7 g, Cholesterol 71 mg

384) Broccoli Nuggets

Ingredients:

- 2 cups broccoli florets
- 1/4 cup almond flour
- 2 egg whites
- 1 cup cheddar cheese, shredded
- 1/8 tsp. salt

Direction: Preparation Time: 10 minutes
Cooking Time: 25 minutes **Servings:** 4

- ✓ Preheat the oven to 350 F/ 180 C.
- ✓ Spray a baking tray with cooking spray and set aside.
- ✓ Using potato masher breaks the broccoli florets into small pieces.
- ✓ Add remaining ingredients to the broccoli and mix well.
- ✓ Drop 20 scoops onto baking tray and press lightly into a nugget shape.
- ✓ Bake in preheated oven for 20 minutes.
- ✓ Serve and enjoy.

Nutrition: Calories 148 Fat 10.4 g, Carbs 3.9 g, Sugar 1.1 g, Protein 10.5 g, Cholesterol 30 mg

385) Zucchini Cauliflower Fritters

Ingredients:

- 2 medium zucchini, grated and squeezed
- 3 cups cauliflower florets
- 1 tbsp. coconut oil
- 1/4 cup coconut flour
- 1/2 tsp. sea salt

Direction: Preparation Time: 10 minutes
Cooking Time: 15 minutes **Servings:** 4

- ✓ Steam cauliflower florets for 5 minutes.
- ✓ Add cauliflower into the food processor and process until it looks like rice.
- ✓ Add all ingredients except coconut oil to the large bowl and mix until well combined.
- ✓ Make small round patties from the mixture and set aside.
- ✓ Heat coconut oil in a pan over medium heat.
- ✓ Place patties in a pan and cook for 3-4 minutes on each side.
- ✓ Serve and enjoy.

Nutrition: Calories 68 Fat 3.8 g, Carbs 7.8 g, Sugar 3.6 g, Protein 2.8 g, Cholesterol 0 mg

386) Roasted Chickpeas

Ingredients:

- 15 oz. can chickpeas, drained, rinsed and pat dry
- 1/2 tsp. paprika
- 1 tbsp. olive oil
- 1/2 tsp. pepper
- 1/2 tsp. salt

Direction: Preparation Time: 10 minutes
Cooking Time: 30 minutes **Servings:** 4

- ✓ Preheat the oven to 450 F/ 232 C.
- ✓ Spray a baking tray with cooking spray and set aside.
- ✓ In a large bowl, toss chickpeas with olive oil, paprika, pepper, and salt.
- ✓ Spread chickpeas on a prepared baking tray and roast in preheated oven for 25 minutes. Stir every 10 minutes.
- ✓ Serve and enjoy.

Nutrition: Calories 158 Fat 4.8 g, Carbs 24.4 g, Sugar 0 g, Protein 5.3 g, Cholesterol 0 mg

387) Peanut Butter Mousse

Ingredients:

- 1 tbsp. peanut butter
- 1 tsp. vanilla extract
- 1 tsp. stevia
- 1/2 cup heavy cream

Direction: Preparation Time: 10 minutes
Cooking Time: 10 minutes **Servings:** 2

- ✓ Add all ingredients into the bowl and whisk until soft peak forms.
- ✓ Spoon into the serving bowls and enjoy.

Nutrition: Calories 157 Fat 15.1 g, Carbohydrates 5.2 g, Sugar 3.6 g, Protein 2.6 g, Cholesterol 41 mg

388) Coffee Mousse

Ingredients:

- 4 tbsp. brewed coffee
- 16 oz. cream cheese, softened
- 1/2 cup unsweetened almond milk
- 1 cup whipping cream
- 2 tsp. liquid stevia

Direction: Preparation Time: 10 minutes
Cooking Time: 20 minutes **Servings:** 8

- ✓ Add coffee and cream cheese in a blender and blend until smooth.
- ✓ Add stevia, and milk and blend again until smooth.
- ✓ Add cream and blend until thickened.
- ✓ Pour into the serving glasses and place in the refrigerator.
- ✓ Serve chilled and enjoy.

Nutrition: Calories 244 Fat 24.6 g, Carbs 2.1 g, Sugar 0.1 g, Protein 4.7 g,

VEGETARIAN

389) Baked Beans

Ingredients:

- ¼ pound dry lima beans, soaked overnight and drained
- ¼ pound dry red kidney beans, soaked overnight and drained
- 1¼ tablespoons oive oil 1 small onion, chopped
- 4 garlic cloves, minced 1 teaspoon dried thyme, crushed
- ½ teaspoon ground cumin
- ½ teaspoon red pepper flakes, crushed
- ¼ teaspoon paprika
- 1 tablespoon balsamic vinegar
- 1 cup homemade tomato puree
- 1 cup low-sodium vegetable broth
- Ground black pepper, as required
- 2 tablespoons fresh parsley, chopped

Direction: Preparation Time: 15 minutes Cooking Time: 2 hours 10 minutes Servings: 4

- ✓ In a large pan of the boiling water, add the beans over high heat and bring to a boil.
- ✓ Now, reduce the heat to low and simmer, covered for about 1 hour. Remove from the heat and drain the beans well.
- ✓ Preheat the oven to 325 degrees F. In a large ovenproof pan, heat the oil over medium heat and cook the onion for about 8-9 minutes, stirring frequently.
- ✓ Add the garlic, thyme and red spices and sauté for about 1 minute.
- ✓ Add the cooked beans and remaining ingredients and immediately remove from the heat.
- ✓ Cover the pan and transfer into the oven. Bake for about 1 hour. Serve with the garnishing of cilantro.

Meal Prep Tip:

- ✓ Transfer the beans mixture into a large bowl and set aside to cool. Divide the mixture into 4 containers evenly. Cover the containers and refrigerate for 1-2 days. Reheat in the microwave before serving.

Nutrition: Calories 136 Total Fat 4.3 g Saturated Fat 0.9 g Cholesterol 0 mg Total Carbs 19 g Sugar 4.7 g Fiber 4.6 g Sodium 112 mg Potassium 472 mg Protein 5.7 g Spicy

390) Grains Combo

Ingredients:

- : ¾ cup amaranth 1 cup quinoa, rinsed
- ¼ cup wild rice
- 4¼ cups filtered water
- 2 teaspoons ground cumin
- ½ teaspoon paprika Salt, as required
- 1¼ cups boiled chickpeas
- 2 medium carrots, peeled and grated
- 1 garlic clove, minced
- Ground black pepper, as required

Direction: Preparation Time: 15 minutes Cooking Time: 35 minutes Servings: 6

- ✓ In a large pan, add the amaranth, quinoa, wild rice, water and spices over medium-high heat and bring to a boil.
- ✓ Now, reduce the heat to medium-low and simmer, covered for about 20-25 minutes.
- ✓ Stir in remaining ingredients and simmer for about 3-5 minutes. Serve hot.
- ✓

Meal Prep Tip:

- ✓ Transfer the grains mixture into a large bowl and set aside to cool. Divide the mixture into 6 containers evenly.
- ✓ Cover the containers and refrigerate for 1 day. Reheat in the microwave before serving.

Nutrition: Calories 365 Total Fat 5.6 g Saturated Fat 0.6 g Cholesterol 0 mg Total Carbs 64 g Sugar 5.8 g Fiber 12 g Sodium 58 mg Potassium 686 mg Protein 16.4 g

391) Black Beans

Ingredients:

- 4 cups filtered water
- 1½ cups dried black beans, soaked for
- 8 hours and drained
- ½ teaspoon ground turmeric
- 3 tablespoons olive oil
- 1 small onion, chopped finely
- 1 green chili, chopped
- 1 (1-inch) piece fresh ginger, minced
- 2 garlic cloves, minced
- 1-1½ tablespoons ground coriander
- 1 teaspoon ground cumin
- ½ teaspoon cayenne pepper Sea salt, as required
- 2 medium tomatoes, chopped finely
- ½ cup fresh cilantro, chopped

Direction: Preparation Time: 15 minutes Cooking Time: 1½ hours Servings: 6

- ✓ In a large pan, add water, black beans and turmeric and bring to a boil on high heat.
- ✓ Now, reduce the heat to low and simmer, covered for about 1 hour or till desired doneness of beans. Meanwhile, in a skillet, heat the oil over medium heat and sauté the onion for about 4-5 minutes.
- ✓ Add the green chili, ginger, garlic, spices and salt and sauté for about 1-2 minutes. Stir in the tomatoes and cook for about 10 minutes, stirring occasionally.
- ✓ Transfer the tomato mixture into the pan with black beans and stir to combine.
- ✓ Increase the heat to medium-low and simmer for about 15-20 minutes. Stir in the cilantro and simmer for about 5 minutes.
- ✓ Serve hot.

Meal Prep Tip:

- ✓ Transfer the beans mixture into a large bowl and set aside to cool. Divide the mixture into 6 containers evenly. Cover the containers and refrigerate for 1-2 days. Reheat in the microwave before serving.

Nutrition: Calories 160 Total Fat 8 g Saturated Fat 1 g Cholesterol 0 mg Total Carbs 17.9 g Sugar 2.4 g Fiber 6.2 g Sodium 50 mg Potassium 343 mg Protein 6 g

392) Lentils Chili

Ingredients:

- 2 teaspoons olive oil
- 1 large onion, chopped 3 medium carrot, peeled and chopped
- 4 celery stalks, chopped 2 garlic cloves, minced
- 1 jalapeño pepper, seeded and chopped
- ½ tablespoon dried thyme, crushed 1 tablespoon chipotle chili powder
- ½ tablespoon cayenne pepper
- 1½ tablespoons ground coriander
- 1½ tablespoons ground cumin 1 teaspoon ground turmeric
- Ground black pepper, as required
- 1 tomato, chopped finely
- 1 pound lentils, rinsed
- 8 cups low-sodium vegetable broth
- 6 cups fresh spinach
- ½ cup fresh cilantro, chopped

Direction: Preparation Time: 15 minutes Cooking Time: 2 hours 20 minutes Servings: 8

- ✓ : In a large pan, heat the oil over medium heat and sauté the onion, carrot and celery for about 5 minutes.
- ✓ Add the garlic, jalapeño pepper, thyme and spices and sauté for about 1 minute.
- ✓ Add the tomato paste, lentils and broth and bring to a boil.
- ✓ Now, reduce the heat to low and simmer for about 2 hours.
- ✓ Stir in the spinach and simmer for about 3-5 minutes. Stir in cilantro and remove from the heat.
- ✓ Serve hot.

Meal Prep Tip:

- ✓ Transfer the chili into a large bowl and set aside to cool. Divide the chili into 8 containers evenly.
- ✓ Cover the containers and refrigerate for 1-2 days. Reheat in the microwave before serving.

Nutrition: Calories 259 Total Fat 2.3 g Saturated Fat 0.3 g Cholesterol 0 mg Total Carbs 41 g Sugar 3.6 g Fiber 19 g Sodium 118 mg Potassium 856 mg Protein 18.2 g

393) Quinoa in Tomato

Ingredients:

- 2 tablespoons olive oil
- 1 cup quinoa, rinsed
- 1 green bell pepper, seeded and chopped
- 1 medium onion, chopped finely
- 3 garlic cloves, minced
- 2½ cups filtered water
- 2 cups tomatoes, crushed finely
- 1 teaspoon red chili powder
- ¼ teaspoon ground cumin
- ¼ teaspoon garlic powder
- Ground black pepper, as required

Direction: Sauce Preparation Time: 15 minutes Cooking Time: 40 minutes Servings: 4

- ✓ In a large pan, heat the oil over medium-high heat and cook the quinoa, onion, bell pepper and garlic for about 5 minutes, stirring frequently.
- ✓ Stir in the remaining ingredients and bring to a boil.
- ✓ Now, reduce the heat to medium-low.
- ✓ Cover the pan tightly and simmer for about 30 minutes, stirring occasionally. Serve hot.

Meal Prep Tip:

- ✓ Transfer the quinoa mixture into a large bowl and set aside to cool.
- ✓ Divide the chili into 4 containers evenly.
- ✓ Cover the containers and refrigerate for 1-2 days. Reheat in the microwave before serving.

Nutrition: Calories 260 Total Fat 10 g Saturated Fat 1.4 g Cholesterol 0 mg Total Carbs 36.9 g Sugar 5.2 g Fiber 5.4 g Sodium 16 mg Potassium 575 mg Protein 7.7 g

394) Barley Pilaf

Ingredients:

- ½ cup pearl barley
- 1 cup low-sodium vegetable broth
- 2 tablespoons olive oil, divided
- 2 garlic cloves, minced finely
- ½ cup onion, chopped
- ½ cup eggplant, sliced thinly
- ½ cup green bell pepper, seeded and chopped
- ½ cup red bell pepper, seeded and chopped
- 2 tablespoons fresh cilantro, chopped
- 2 tablespoons fresh mint leaves, chopped

Direction: Preparation Time: 20 minutes Cooking Time: 1 hour 5 minutes Servings: 4

- ✓ In a pan, add the barley and broth over medium-high heat and bring to a boil. Immediately, reduce the heat to low and simmer, covered for about 45 minutes or until all the liquid is absorbed. In a large skillet, heat 1 tablespoon of oil over high heat and sauté the garlic for about 1 minute.
- ✓ Stir in the cooked barley and cook for about 3 minutes. Remove from heat and set aside. In another skillet, heat remaining oil over medium heat and sauté the onion for about 5-7 minutes.
- ✓ Add the eggplant and bell peppers and stir fry for about 3 minutes. Stir in the remaining ingredients except walnuts and cook for about 2-3 minutes. Stir in barley mixture and cook for about 2-3 minutes.
- ✓ Serve hot.

Meal Prep Tip:

- ✓ Transfer the pilaf into a large bowl and set aside to cool. Divide the pilaf into 4 containers evenly. Cover the containers and refrigerate for 1 day. Reheat in the microwave before serving.

Nutrition: Calories 168 Total Fat 7.4 g Saturated Fat 1.1 g Cholesterol 0 mg Total Carbs 23.5 g Sugar 1.9 g Fiber 5 g Sodium 22 mg Potassium 164 mg Protein 3.6 g

395) Baked Veggies Combo

Ingredients:

- 2 large zucchinis, sliced
- 1 large yellow squash, sliced
- 3 cups fresh broccoli florets
- 1-pound fresh asparagus, trimmed
- 2 garlic cloves, minced
- 1 tablespoon fresh rosemary, minced
- 1 tablespoon fresh thyme, minced
- ½ teaspoon ground cumin
- ½ teaspoon red pepper flakes, crushed
- ¼ teaspoon cayenne pepper
- 2 tablespoons olive oil
- Salt, as required

Direction: Preparation Time: 15 minutes Cooking Time: 40 minutes Servings: 8

- ✓ Preheat the oven to 400 degrees F. Line 2 large baking sheets with aluminum foil. In a large bowl, add all ingredients and toss to coat well.
- ✓ Divide the vegetables mixture onto prepared baking sheets and spread in a single layer.
- ✓ Roast for about 35-40 minutes. Remove from oven and serve.

Meal Prep Tip:

- ✓ Remove from oven and set the veggies aside to cool completely.
- ✓ Transfer the veggie mixture into 8 containers and refrigerate for 2-3 days.
- ✓ Reheat in microwave before serving.

Nutrition: Calories 77 Total Fat 4 g Saturated Fat 0.6 g Cholesterol 0 mg Total Carbs 9.4 g Sugar 3.8 g Fiber 3.8 g Sodium 45 mg Potassium 554 mg Protein 3.8 g

396) Mixed Veggie Salad

Ingredients:

For Dressing:
- 1/3 cup olive oil ½ cup fresh lemon juice
- 1 tablespoon fresh ginger, grated
- 2 teaspoons mustard 4-6 drops liquid stevia
- ¼ teaspoon salt

For Salad:
- 2 avocados, peeled, pitted and chopped
- 2 tablespoons fresh lemon juice
- 2 cups fresh baby spinach, torn
- 2 cups small broccoli florets
- 1 cup red cabbage, shredded
- 1 cup purple cabbage, shredded
- 2 large carrots, peeled and grated
- 1 small orange bell pepper, seeded and sliced into matchsticks
- 1 small yellow bell pepper, seeded and sliced into matchsticks
- ½ cup fresh parsley leaves, chopped
- 1 cup walnuts, chopped

Direction: Preparation Time: 20 minutes Servings: 8

- ✓ For dressing: in a food processor, add all ingredients and pulse until well combined. In a large bowl, add the avocado slices and drizzle with lemon juice.
- ✓ Add the remaining vegetables and mix. Place the dressing and toss to coat well.
- ✓ Serve immediately.

Meal Prep Tip:
- ✓ Transfer dressing into a small jar and refrigerate for 1 day. In 8 containers, divide avocado and remaining vegetables.
- ✓ Refrigerate for 1 day. Before serving, drizzle each portion with dressing and serve.

Nutrition: Calories 314 Total Fat 28.1 g Saturated Fat 4 g Cholesterol 0 mg Total Carbs 14.1 g Sugar 4.3g Fiber 6.9 g Sodium 113 mg Potassium 642 mg Protein 6.8 g

397) Tofu with Brussels Sprout

Ingredients:

- 1 tablespoon olive oil, divided
- 8 ounces extra-firm tofu, drained, pressed and cut into slices
- 2 garlic cloves, chopped
- 1/3 cup pecans, toasted and chopped
- 1 tablespoon unsweetened applesauce
- ¼ cup fresh cilantro, chopped
- ¾ pound Brussels sprouts, trimmed and cut into wide ribbons

Direction: Preparation Time: 15 minutes Cooking Time: 15 minutes Servings: 4

- ✓ In a skillet, heat ½ tablespoon of the oil over medium heat and sauté the tofu and for about 6-7 minutes or until golden brown.
- ✓ Add the garlic and pecans and sauté for about 1 minute. Add the applesauce and cook for about 2 minutes.
- ✓ Stir in the cilantro and remove from heat. Transfer tofu into a plate and set aside In the same skillet, heat the remaining oil over medium-high heat and cook the Brussels sprouts for about 5 minutes.
- ✓ Stir in the tofu and remove from the heat. Serve immediately.

Meal Prep Tip:
- ✓ Remove the tofu mixture from heat and set aside to cool completely.
- ✓ In 4 containers, divide the tofu mixture evenly and refrigerate for about 2 days. Reheat in microwave before serving.

Nutrition: Calories 204 Total Fat 15.5 g Saturated Fat 1.8 g Cholesterol 0 mg Total Carbs 11.5 g Sugar 3 g Fiber 4.8 g Sodium 27 mg Potassium 468 mg Protein 9.9 g

398) Beans, Walnuts & Veggie Burgers

Ingredients:

- ½ cup walnuts
- 1 carrot, peeled and chopped
- 1 celery stalk, chopped
- 4 scallions, chopped
- 5 garlic cloves, chopped
- 2¼ cups cooked black beans
- 2½ cups sweet potato, peeled and grated
- ½ teaspoon red pepper flakes, crushed
- ¼ teaspoon cayenne pepper
- Salt and ground black pepper, as required

Direction: Preparation Time: 20 minutes Cooking Time: 25 minutes Servings: 8

- ✓ Preheat the oven to 400 degrees F. Line a baking sheet with parchment paper. In a food processor, add walnuts and pulse until finely ground. Add the carrot, celery, scallion and garlic and pulse until chopped finely.
- ✓ Transfer the vegetable mixture into a large bowl. In the same food processor, add beans and pulse until chopped. Add 1½ cups of sweet potato and pulse until a chunky mixture forms.
- ✓ Transfer the bean mixture into the bowl with vegetable mixture. Stir in the remaining sweet potato and spices and mix until well combined.
- ✓ Make 8 patties from mixture. Arrange the patties onto prepared baking sheet in a single layer. Bake for about 25 minutes. Serve hot.

Meal Prep Tip:
- ✓ Remove the burgers from oven and set aside to cool completely. Store these burgers in an airtight container, by placing parchment papers between the burgers to avoid the sticking.
- ✓ These burgers can be stored in the freezer for up to 3 weeks. Before serving, thaw the burgers and then reheat in microwave.

Nutrition: Calories 177 Total Fat 5 g Saturated Fat 0.3 g Cholesterol 0 mg Total Carbs 27.6 g Sugar 5.3 g Fiber 7.6 g Sodium 205 mg Potassium 398 mg Protein 8 g

DIABETIC AIR FRYER

399) Hard Boiled Eggs

Ingredients:

6 eggs (right out of the fridge)

Direction: Time: 22 minutes | Servings: 6

- ✓ Fix the wire rack of your air fryer inside the basket.
- ✓ Arrange the eggs on top of the wire rack.
- ✓ Allow the eggs to cook in the air fryer for 16 minutes and temperature to 250 F.
- ✓ Withdraw the cooked eggs and place them into an ice water bath to stop the cooking.
- ✓ Peel the cooked eggs and serve.

400) Breakfast Egg Rolls

Ingredients:

- 12 egg roll wrappers:
- Filling ingredients:
- 6 eggs, scrambled
- 3 cups frozen hash browns
- 8 strips bacon
- 1 cup shredded cheese
- For the sauce:
- ½ cup ketchup
- 1 tbsp hot sauce (Sriracha)
- ½ cup maple syrup

Direction: Time: 40 minutes | Servings: 12

- ✓ Get a skillet and cook the eggs in it.
- ✓ Set aside the cooked eggs and allow to cool.
- ✓ Get a skillet and brown the hash browns in it. Set aside and allow to cool too.
- ✓ Crisp the bacon in another skillet or the oven and cut into small pieces.
- ✓ Make your egg rolls by filling each wrapper with some of the filling ingredients (at the center). Brush the edges of the wrapper using a small amount of water to help it stick.
- ✓ Set the heat to medium-high and heat a skillet containing about 3 inches of vegetable oil.
- ✓ Divide the egg rolls into batches, fry each batch while turning halfway through.
- ✓ Remove when they are crispy and golden brown on both sides.
- ✓ Line a plate with paper towels and place the fried egg rolls into it to catch the excess warm.
- ✓ To prepare the dipping sauce, make a mixture of the ketchup and the hot sauce.
- ✓ Serve warm alongside the dipping sauce.

401) Scrambled Eggs

Ingredients:

- 4 large eggs
- Salt and ground black pepper
- 2 slices whole meal bread

Direction: Time: 12 minutes | Servings: 2

- ✓ Ensure that your bread is harder like toast by warming it up for 3 minutes at 390 F.
- ✓ Crack your eggs into a bowl, and stir before adding the seasoning.
- ✓ Transfer the mixture into the baking pan inside the air fryer. Allow to cook at 360 F for 2 minutes, and then an additional 4 minutes at 360 F.
- ✓ Pour the scrambled eggs over the whole meal toast.
- ✓ Serve.

402) Lemon Dill Scallops

Ingredients:

- 1 lb scallops
- 2 tsp olive oil
- 1 tsp dill, chopped
- 1 tbsp fresh lemon juice
- Pepper Salt

Direction: Time: 15 minutes - Serve: 4

- ✓ Add scallops into the bowl and toss with oil, dill, lemon juice, pepper, and salt.
- ✓ Add scallops into the air fryer basket and cook at 360 F for 5 minutes.
- ✓ Serve and enjoy.

403) Herb Mushrooms

Ingredients:

- 10 mushrooms, stems remove
- 1 tbsp dill, chopped
- 1 tbsp olive oil
- 1 tbsp parmesan cheese, grated
- ½ tbsp oregano
- ½ tsp dried basil
- Salt

Direction: Time: 22 minutes - Serve: 2

- ✓ Add mushrooms into the bowl and toss with oil, oregano, basil and salt.
- ✓ Add mushrooms into the air fryer basket and cook at 360 F for 6 minutes.
- ✓ Add dill and cheese and toss well and cook for 6 minutes more.
- ✓ Serve and enjoy.

404) Omelette with Cheese And Onion

Ingredients:

- 2 eggs
- Ground black pepper to taste
- Soy sauce to taste
- Cooking spray
- 1 medium onion-sliced Cheddar cheese- grated

Direction: Time: 25 minutes | Servings: 1

- ✓ Get a clean bowl and crack open the eggs in it.
- ✓ Add the pepper and soy sauce (as seasoning).
- ✓ Spritz some cooking spray lightly into the pan.
- ✓ Transfer the sliced onions in the oiled pan at air fry for 8-10 minutes at 360 F.
- ✓ Withdraw when the onion is softened.
- ✓ Transfer the egg mixture into the pan, and add bits of Cheddar Cheese.
- ✓ Air fry until the eggs are fully cooked – about 3 to 5 minutes.
- ✓ Serve.

405) Radish Hash Browns

Ingredients:

- 1 lb radishes, washed and cut off roots
- 1 tbsp olive oil
- 1/2 tsp paprika
- 1/2 tsp onion powder
- 1/2 tsp garlic powder
- 1 medium onion
- 1/4 tsp pepper
- 3/4 tsp sea salt

Direction: Time: 23 minutes Serve: 4

- Slice onion and radishes using a mandolin slicer.
- Add sliced onion and radishes in a large mixing bowl and toss with olive oil.
- Transfer onion and radish slices in air fryer basket and cook at 360 F for 8 minutes.
- Shake basket twice.
- Return onion and radish slices in a mixing bowl and toss with seasonings.
- Again, cook onion and radish slices in air fryer basket for 5 minutes at 400 F. Shake basket halfway through.
- Serve and enjoy.

406) Spinach Frittata

Ingredients:

- 3 eggs
- 1 cup spinach, chopped
- 1 small onion, minced
- 2 tbsp mozzarella cheese, grated
- Pepper Salt

Direction: Time: 13 minutes - Serve: 1

- Preheat the air fryer to 350 F.
- Spray air fryer pan with cooking spray.
- In a bowl, whisk eggs with remaining ingredients until well combined.
- Pour egg mixture into the prepared pan and place pan in the air fryer basket.
- Cook frittata for 8 minutes or until set.
- Serve and enjoy.

407) Omelette Frittata with Cheese and Mushrooms

Ingredients:

- 3 eggs, lightly beaten
- 2 tbsp cheddar cheese, shredded
- 2 tbsp heavy cream
- 2 mushrooms, sliced
- 1/4 small onion, chopped
- 1/4 bell pepper, diced
- Pepper Salt

Direction: Time: 16 minutes - Serve: 2

- In a bowl, whisk eggs with cream, vegetables, pepper, and salt.
- Preheat the air fryer to 400 F.
- Pour egg mixture into the air fryer pan.
- Place pan in air fryer basket and cook for 5 minutes.
- Add shredded cheese on top of the frittata and cook for 1 minute more.
- Serve and enjoy.

408) Asparagus Frittata

Ingredients:

- 6 eggs
- 10 asparagus, chopped
- 1/4 cup half and half 2 tsp butter, melted
- 1 cup mozzarella cheese, shredded
- pepper and salt

Direction: Time: 20 minutes - Serve: 4

- Toss asparagus with melted butter and add into the air fryer basket.
- Cook asparagus at 350 F for 5 minutes. Shake basket twice.
- Meanwhile, in a bowl, whisk together eggs, half and half, pepper, and salt.
- Transfer cook asparagus into the air fryer baking dish.
- Pour egg mixture over mushrooms and asparagus.
- Place dish in the air fryer and cook at 350 F for 5 minutes or until eggs are set.
- Slice and serve.

409) Breakfast Jalapeno Muffins

Ingredients:

- 5 eggs
- 1/3 cup coconut oil, melted
- 2 tsp baking powder
- 3 tbsp erythritol
- 3 tbsp jalapenos, sliced
- 1/4 cup unsweetened coconut milk
- 2/3 cup coconut flour
- 3/4 tsp sea salt

Direction: Time: 25 minutes - Serve: 8

- Preheat the air fryer to 325 F.
- In a large bowl, stir together coconut flour, baking powder, erythritol, and sea salt.
- Stir in eggs, jalapenos, coconut milk, and coconut oil until well combined.
- Pour batter into the silicone muffin molds and place into the air fryer basket.
- Cook muffins for 15 minutes.
- Serve and enjoy.

410) Mushroom and Spinach Frittata

Ingredients:

- 1 cup egg whites
- 1 cup spinach, chopped
- 2 mushrooms, sliced
- 2 tbsp parmesan cheese, grated
- Salt and Pepper

Direction: Time: 23 minutes - Serve: 1

- Spray pan with cooking spray and heat over medium heat.
- Add mushrooms and sauté for 2-3 minutes.
- Add spinach and cook for 1-2 minutes or until wilted.
- Transfer mushroom spinach mixture into the air fryer pan.
- Whisk egg whites in a mixing bowl until frothy. Season with a pinch of salt and pepper.
- Pour egg white mixture into the spinach and mushroom mixture and sprinkle with parmesan cheese.
- Place pan in air fryer basket and cook frittata at 350 F for 8 minutes.
- Slice and serve.

411) Avocado Egg Rolls

Ingredients:

- 2 ripe avocados, roughly chopped
- 8 egg roll wrappers
- 1 tomato, peeled and chopped
- Salt and black pepper to taste

Direction: Time: 15 minutes - 4 Servings

- ✓ Place the avocados, tomato, salt, and black pepper in a bowl.
- ✓ Mash with a fork until somewhat smooth.
- ✓ Divide the mixture between the egg wrappers.
- ✓ Fold the edges in and over the filling, roll up tightly, and seal the wrappers with a bit of water.
- ✓ Arrange them on the greased frying basket.
- ✓ Spray the rolls with cooking spray and Bake for 10 minutes at 350 F, turning halfway through until crispy and golden.
- ✓ Serve

412) Air Fryer Eggs (Perfect)

Ingredients:

- 6 large eggs
- Salt and black pepper to taste

Direction: Time: 20 minutes - 6 Servings

- ✓ Preheat the air fryer to 270 F.
- ✓ Lay the eggs in the basket (or in a muffin tray) and cook for 10 minutes for runny or 15 minutes for hard.
- ✓ Using tongs, place the eggs in a bowl with cold water to cool for 5 minutes.
- ✓ When cooled, remove the shells, cut them in half, and sprinkle with salt and pepper.
- ✓ Serve.

413) Bacon and Eggs

Ingredients:

- 8 back bacon
- 4 large eggs
- Salt and ground black pepper to taste
- Fresh chives
- optional 4 ramekins

Direction: Time: 15 minutes | Servings: 4

- ✓ Eject the ramekins and add the bacon around the sides and the bottom, such that the overlapping is same as when making a pastry over an apple pie.
- ✓ Crack an egg into the center of each of the ramekin.
- ✓ Allow the ramekin to cook the air fryer for 360 F for 13 minutes.
- ✓ Add pepper and salt as seasonings, alongside fresh chives.
- ✓ Serve.

414) Breakfast Soufflé

Ingredients:

- Red chili pepper
- Parsley
- 2 eggs, beaten
- 2 tbsp cream (light)

Direction: Time: 25 minutes | Servings: 2

- ✓ Chop your chili and parsley into fine pieces.
- ✓ Get a bowl and place the eggs, alongside the cream, parsley, and pepper.
- ✓ Stir.
- ✓ Pour the egg mixture into the dishes until half-filled.
- ✓ Allow baking for 8 minutes at 390 F.
- ✓ If you prefer the Soufflés Baveux soft, cook for only 5 minutes.
- ✓ Serve.

415) Whole 30 Air fryer Muffins

Ingredients:

- 3 handfuls leftover cooked vegetables
- 3 oz plain granola
- 2 oz coconut milk
- 1 tbsp coriander Handful fresh
- thyme thinly diced
- Salt and ground black pepper to taste

Direction: Time: 45 minutes | Servings: 2

- ✓ Get a mixing bowl and in it, add your cooked leftover vegetables.
- ✓ Whizz your plain granola in a blender until you have an appearance of breadcrumbs.
- ✓ Combine the vegetables with the granola, coconut milk, and the seasoning.
- ✓ Mix thoroughly and shape into balls.
- ✓ Allow cooking for 20 minutes in the air fryer at 360 F.
- ✓ Serve.

416) Bacon Egg Muffins

Ingredients:

- 12 eggs
- 2 tbsp fresh parsley, chopped
- 1/2 tsp mustard powder
- 1/3 cup heavy cream
- 2 green onion, chopped
- 4 oz cheddar cheese, shredded
- 8 bacon slices, cooked and crumbled
- Pepper Salt

Direction: Time: 30 minutes - Serve: 12

- ✓ Preheat the air fryer to 350 F.
- ✓ In a mixing bowl, whisk together eggs, mustard powder, heavy cream, pepper, and salt.
- ✓ Divide cheddar cheese, onions, and bacon into the silicone muffin molds.
- ✓ Now pour egg mixture into the silicone muffin molds and place in the air fryer basket.
- ✓ Cook muffins for 20 minutes.
- ✓ Serve and enjoy.

417) Sausage Cheese Mix

Ingredients:
- 8 eggs, lightly beaten
- 1 cup coconut milk
- 1 cup mozzarella cheese, shredded
- 1 cup cheddar cheese, shredded
- 10 oz sausage, cooked and crumbled
- Pepper Salt

Direction: Time: 30 minutes - Serve: 4

- In a bowl, add all ingredients and stir until well combined.
- Transfer bowl mixture into the air fryer baking pan and place into the air fryer.
- Cook at 380 F for 20 minutes. Serve and enjoy.

418) Kale Omelet

Ingredients:
- 3 eggs, lightly beaten
- 1 tbsp parsley, chopped
- 1 tbsp basil, chopped
- 3 tbsp kale, chopped
- 3 tbsp cottage cheese, crumbled
- Pepper Salt

Direction: Time: 20 minutes - Serve: 1

- Spray air fryer baking dish with cooking spray.
- In a bowl, whisk eggs with pepper and salt.
- Add remaining ingredients into the egg and stir to combine.
- Pour egg mixture into the prepared dish and place into the air fryer.
- Cook at 330 F for 10 minutes.
- Serve and enjoy.

419) Super Easy Crispy Bacon

Ingredients:

slices back bacon

Direction: Time: 8 minutes | Servings: 4

- Ensure that your air fryer is preheated to 360 F.
- Carefully put four slices of back bacon into the air fryer's basket
- Allow each side to cook for 2-3 minutes.
- Serve.

420) French Toast

Ingredients:
- Butter
- 4 slices bread
- 2 eggs
- ½ tsp cinnamon

Direction: Time: 10 minutes | Servings: 2

- After adding butter to both sides of the bread, cut it into sticks or strips.
- Combine the cinnamon with whisked eggs.
- Spritz some cooking oil into the basket of air fryer.
- Dip the bread sticks into the egg mixture and transfer it into the basket of the air fryer.
- Set the air fryer to 360 F and allow to cook for 3 minutes.
- Change to the other side and cook for an extra 2 minutes.
- Serve.

421) French Toast Sticks

Ingredients:
- 1 tsp ground cinnamon
- 1 tsp vanilla extract
- 1 tbsp butter, melted
- 2 large eggs, beaten
- 1/3 cup milk
- 4 slices day-old bread, cut into thirds
- 1 tsp confectioners' sugar, or to taste

Direction: Time: 25 minutes | Servings: 12

- Ensure that your Air Fryer is preheated to 360 F.
- Combine the cinnamon, vanilla extract, butter, eggs, and milk in a mixing bowl.
- After lining the air fryer basket with parchment paper, dip each bread piece into the milk mixture and place in the basket.
- Ensure that there are spaces between them, and divide into batches if there is the need to.
- place in the basket containing the bread.
- Allow to cook for 6 minutes, and change to the other side, and cook for an extra 3 minutes.
- Sprinkle each stick with confectioner's sugar.
- Serve.

422) French Toast Sticks (Ver.2)

Ingredients:
- 4 slices slightly stale thick bread, such as Texas toast
- 2 eggs, lightly beaten
- 1 tsp cinnamon
- 1 tsp vanilla extract
- 1 pinch ground nutmeg, optional
- ¼ cup milk

Direction: Cooking Time: 25 minutes | Servings: 2

- Ensure that your Air Fryer is preheated to 360 F.
- Make sticks out of the slice of bread by cutting each slice into three.
- Trim a piece of parchment paper into a size that fits the base of the air fryer basket.
- In a mixing bowl, combine eggs, cinnamon, vanilla extract, nutmeg, and milk and mix thoroughly.
- Dip each piece of bread into the mixture.
- Remove when the piece is well submerged and shake to get rid of the excess egg mixture.
- Transfer the coated piece into the air fryer basket.
- Maintain a single layer in the basket, and divide into batches if necessary.
- Allow each batch to cook for 5 minutes each per side.
- Serve.

423) Mushroom Leek Frittata

Ingredients:
- 6 eggs
- 6 oz mushrooms, sliced
- 1 cup leeks, sliced
- Salt

Direction: Time: 42 minutes - Serve: 4

- Preheat the air fryer to 325 F.
- Spray air fryer baking dish with cooking spray and set aside.
- Heat another pan over medium heat.
- Spray pan with cooking spray.
- Add mushrooms, leeks, and salt in a pan sauté for 6 minutes.
- Break eggs in a bowl and whisk well.
- Transfer sautéed mushroom and leek mixture into the prepared baking dish.
- Pour egg over mushroom mixture.
- Place dish in the air fryer and cook for 32 minutes.
- Serve.

424) French Toast Sticks With Berries

Ingredients:

- 4 (1½ -oz) whole-grain bread slices
- 2 large eggs, beaten and wisked
- 1 tsp vanilla extract
- ¼ cup packed light brown sugar, divided
- ¼ cup 2% reduced-fat milk
- ½ tsp ground cinnamon
- 2/3 cup flax seed meal Cooking spray
- 2 cups sliced fresh strawberries
- 8 tsp pure maple syrup, divided
- 1 tsp powdered sugar

Direction: Time: 1 hour | Servings: 4

- ✓ Make four long sticks out of each bread slice.
- ✓ Combine whisked eggs, vanilla, one tablespoon brown sugar, milk, and cinnamon into a shallow dish.
- ✓ Get another shallow dish and combine flax seed meal alongside three tablespoons of brown sugar.
- ✓ Dip the pieces of bread in the egg mixture until they are slightly soaked while allowing the excess to drip off.
- ✓ Dredge the soaked piece in the flaxseed mixture, ensuring that the coating is uniform.
- ✓ Apply some cooking spray to coat the bread pieces also.
- ✓ Transfer the coated bread pieces into the air fryer basket, arranging them in a single layer and leaving space between each.
- ✓ Allow to cook for 10 minutes at 375 F or until they are crunchy and golden brown.
- ✓ Turn them over halfway through cooking.
- ✓ Place four sticks on each plate, topped with ½ cup strawberries, two teaspoons maple syrup, as well as a sprinkle of powdered sugar.
- ✓ Serve immediately.

425) Breakfast Egg Muffins

Ingredients:

- 6 eggs
- 1 lb ground pork sausage
- 3 tbsp onion, minced
- 1/2 red pepper, diced
- 1 cup egg whites
- 1/2 cup mozzarella cheese
- 1 cup cheddar cheese

Direction: Time: 30 minutes - Serve: 12

- ✓ Preheat the air fryer to 325 F.
- ✓ Brown sausage over medium-high heat until meat is no pink.
- ✓ Divide red pepper, cheese, cooked sausages, and onion into each silicone muffin mold.
- ✓ In a large bowl, whisk together egg whites, egg, pepper, and salt.
- ✓ Pour egg mixture into each muffin mold and place into the air fryer basket in batches.
- ✓ Cook muffins in the air fryer for 20 minutes.
- ✓ Serve and enjoy.

426) Cheese Pie

Ingredients:

- 8 eggs
- 1/2 cups heavy whipping cream
- 1 lb cheddar cheese, grated
- Pepper Salt

Direction: Time: 26 minutes - Serve: 4

- ✓ Preheat the air fryer to 325 F.
- ✓ In a bowl, whisk together cheese, eggs, whipping cream, pepper, and salt.
- ✓ Spray air fryer baking dish with cooking spray.
- ✓ Pour egg mixture into the prepared dish and place in the air fryer basket.
- ✓ Cook for 16 minutes or until the egg is set.
- ✓ Serve and enjoy.

427) Spinach Egg Breakfast

Ingredients:

- 3 eggs
- 1/4 cup coconut milk
- 1/4 cup parmesan cheese, grated
- 4 oz spinach, chopped
- 3 oz cottage cheese

Direction: Time: 30 minutes - Serve: 4

- ✓ Preheat the air fryer to 350 F.
- ✓ Add eggs, milk, half parmesan cheese, and cottage cheese in a bowl and whisk well.
- ✓ Add spinach and stir well.
- ✓ Pour mixture into the air fryer baking dish.
- ✓ Sprinkle remaining half parmesan cheese on top.
- ✓ Place dish in the air fryer and cook for 20 minutes.
- ✓ Serve.

428) Parmesan Breakfast Casserole

Ingredients:

- 5 eggs
- 2 tbsp heavy cream
- 3 tbsp chunky tomato sauce
- 2 tbsp parmesan cheese, grated

Direction: Time: 30 minutes - Serve: 3

- ✓ Preheat the air fryer to 325 F.
- ✓ In mixing bowl, combine together cream and eggs.
- ✓ Add cheese and tomato sauce and mix well
- ✓ Spray air fryer baking dish with cooking spray.
- ✓ Pour mixture into baking dish and place in the air fryer basket.
- ✓ Cook for 20 minutes.
- ✓ Serve and enjoy.

429) Vegetable Quiche

Ingredients:
- 8 eggs
- 1 cup coconut milk
- 1 cup tomatoes, chopped
- 1 cup zucchini, chopped
- 1 tbsp butter
- 1 onion, chopped
- 1 cup Parmesan cheese, grated
- 1/2 tsp pepper
- 1 tsp salt

Direction: Time: 34 minutes - Serve: 6

- ✓ Preheat the air fryer to 370 F.
- ✓ Melt butter in a pan over medium heat then add onion and sauté until onion lightly brown.
- ✓ Add tomatoes and zucchini to the pan and sauté for 4-5 minutes.
- ✓ Transfer cooked vegetables into the air fryer baking dish.
- ✓ Beat eggs with cheese, milk, pepper, and salt in a bowl.
- ✓ Pour egg mixture over vegetables in a baking dish.
- ✓ Place dish in the air fryer and cook for 24 minutes or until eggs are set.
- ✓ Slice and serve.

430) Tomato Mushroom Frittata

Ingredients:
- 1 cup egg whites
- 1/4 cup tomato, sliced
- 2 tbsp coconut milk
- 2 tbsp chives, chopped
- 1/4 cup mushrooms, sliced
- Pepper Salt

Direction: Time: 25 minutes - Serve: 2

- ✓ Preheat the air fryer to 320 F.
- ✓ In a bowl, whisk together all ingredients.
- ✓ Spray air fryer baking pan with cooking spray.
- ✓ Pour egg mixture into the prepared pan and place in the air fryer.
- ✓ Cook frittata for 15 minutes.
- ✓ Serve and enjoy.

431) Breakfast Egg Tomato

Ingredients:
- 2 eggs
- 2 large fresh tomatoes
- 1 tsp fresh parsley
- Pepper Salt

Direction: Time: 34 minutes - Serve: 2

- ✓ Preheat the air fryer to 325 F.
- ✓ Cut off the top of a tomato and spoon out the tomato innards.
- ✓ Break the egg in each tomato and place in air fryer basket and cook for 24 minutes.
- ✓ Season with parsley, pepper, and salt.
- ✓ Serve and enjoy.

432) Healthy Mix Vegetables

Ingredients:
- ½ cup mushrooms, sliced
- 1 onion, sliced
- ½ cup zucchini, sliced
- ½ cup squash, sliced
- ½ cup baby carrot
- 1 cup cauliflower florets
- 1 cup broccoli florets
- ¼ cup parmesan cheese
- 1 tsp red pepper flakes
- 1 tbsp garlic, minced
- 1 tbsp olive oil
- ¼ cup vinegar
- ¼ tsp pepper
- ½ tsp salt

Direction: Time: 30 minutes - Serve: 4

- ✓ Preheat the air fryer to 400 F.
- ✓ In a bowl, mix together oil, vinegar, garlic, pepper, red pepper flakes, and salt.
- ✓ Add vegetables into the bowl and toss to coat.
- ✓ Transfer vegetable mixture into the air fryer basket and cook for 16 minutes.
- ✓ Shake basket halfway through.
- ✓ Sprinkle with cheese and cook for 1-2 minutes more.
- ✓ Serve and enjoy.

433) Broccoli Frittata

Ingredients:
- 3 eggs 1/2 cup bell pepper, chopped
- 1/2 cup broccoli florets
- 2 tbsp parmesan cheese, grated
- 1/4 tsp garlic powder
- 1/4 tsp onion powder
- 2 tbsp coconut milk
- Pepper Salt

Direction: Time: 27 minutes - Serve: 2

- ✓ Spray air fryer baking dish with cooking spray.
- ✓ Place bell peppers and broccoli in the prepared baking dish.
- ✓ Cook broccoli and bell pepper in the air fryer at 350 F for 7 minutes.
- ✓ In a bowl, whisk together eggs, milk, and seasoning.
- ✓ Once veggies are cooked then pour egg mixture over vegetables and sprinkle cheese on top.
- ✓ Cook frittata in the air fryer for 10 minutes.
- ✓ Serve and enjoy.

434) Tasty Salsa Chicken

Ingredients:
- 1 lb chicken thighs, boneless and skinless
- 1 cup salsa
- Pepper Salt

Direction: Preparation Time: 40 minutes - Serve: 4

- ✓ Preheat the air fryer to 350 F.
- ✓ Place chicken thighs into the air fryer baking dish and season with pepper and salt.
- ✓ Top with salsa.
- ✓ Place in the air fryer and cook for 30 minutes.
- ✓ Serve and enjoy.

435) Perfect Breakfast Frittata

Ingredients:
- 2 large eggs
- 1 tbsp bell peppers, chopped
- 1 tbsp spring onions, chopped
- 1 sausage patty, chopped
- 1 tbsp butter, melted
- 2 tbsp cheddar cheese
- Pepper Salt

Direction: Time: 20 minutes - Serve: 2
- ✓ Add sausage patty in air fryer baking dish and cook in air fryer 350 F for 5 minutes.
- ✓ Meanwhile, in a bowl whisk together eggs, pepper, and salt.
- ✓ Add bell peppers, onions and stir well. Pour egg mixture over sausage patty and stir well.
- ✓ Sprinkle with cheese and cook in the air fryer at 350 F for 5 minutes.
- ✓ Serve and enjoy.

436) Buttery Scallops

Ingredients:
- 1 lb jumbo scallops
- 1 tbsp fresh lemon juice
- 2 tbsp butter, melted

Direction: Time: 18 minutes - Serve: 2
- ✓ Preheat the air fryer to 400 F.
- ✓ In a small bowl, mix together lemon juice and butter.
- ✓ Brush scallops with lemon juice and butter mixture and place into the air fryer basket.
- ✓ Cook scallops for 4 minutes.
- ✓ Turn halfway through.
- ✓ Again brush scallops with lemon butter mixture and cook for 4 minutes more.
- ✓ Turn halfway through.
- ✓ Serve and enjoy.

437) Sausage Egg Cups

Ingredients:
- 1/4 cup egg beaters
- 1/4 sausage, cooked and crumbled
- 4 tsp jack cheese, shredded
- 1/4 tsp garlic powder
- 1/4 tsp onion powder
- 4 tbsp spinach, chopped
- Pepper Salt

Direction: Time: 20 minutes - Serve: 2
- ✓ In a bowl, whisk together all ingredients until well combined.
- ✓ Pour batter into the silicone muffin molds and place in the air fryer basket.
- ✓ Cook at 330 F for 10 minutes.
- ✓ Serve and enjoy.

438) Cheese Stuff Peppers

Ingredients:
- 8 small bell pepper, cut the top of peppers
- 3.5 oz feta cheese, cubed
- 1 tbsp olive oil 1 tsp Italian seasoning
- 1 tbsp parsley, chopped
- 1/4 tsp garlic powder
- Pepper Salt

Direction: Time: 13 minutes - Serve: 8
- ✓ In a bowl, toss cheese with oil and seasoning.
- ✓ Stuff cheese in each bell peppers and place into the air fryer basket.
- ✓ Cook at 400 F for 8 minutes.
- ✓ Serve and enjoy.

439) Roasted Pepper Salad

Ingredients:
- 4 bell peppers
- 2 oz rocket leaves
- 2 tbsp olive oil
- 4 tbsp heavy cream
- 1 lettuce head, torn
- 1 tbsp fresh lime juice
- Pepper Salt

Direction: Time: 20 minutes - Serve: 4
- ✓ Add bell peppers into the air fryer basket and cook for 10 minutes at 400 F.
- ✓ Remove peppers from air fryer and let it cool for 5 minutes.
- ✓ Peel cooked peppers and cut into strips and place into the large bowl.
- ✓ Add remaining ingredients into the bowl and toss well.
- ✓ Serve.

440) Breakfast Casserole Delicious

Ingredients:
- 4 eggs
- 7 oz spinach, chopped
- 3 bacon slices, chopped
- 8 grape tomatoes, halved
- 1 garlic clove, minced
- 8 mushrooms, sliced
- Pepper Salt

Direction: Time: 30 minutes - Serve: 4
- ✓ Spray air fryer baking dish with cooking spray and set aside.
- ✓ Add all ingredients into the large bowl and whisk until well combined.
- ✓ Pour bowl mixture into the prepared baking dish.
- ✓ Place dish in the air fryer and cook at 400 F for 20 minutes.
- ✓ Serve.

441) Huevos Rancheros

Ingredients:

- 4 large eggs
- ¼ teaspoon kosher salt
- ¼ cup masa harina (corn flour)
- 1 teaspoon olive oil
- ¼ cup warm water
- ½ cup salsa
- ¼ cup crumbled queso fresco or feta cheese

Direction: Time: 45 minutes | Serves 4

- ✓ Crack the eggs into a baking pan, season with the kosher salt, and bake at 330°F (166°C) for 3 minutes.
- ✓ Pause the fryer, gently scramble the eggs, and bake for 2 more minutes.
- ✓ Remove the eggs from the fryer, keeping the fryer on, and set the eggs aside to slightly cool. (Clean the baking pan before making the tortillas.)
- ✓ Increase the temperature to 390°F (199°C).
- ✓ In a medium bowl, combine the masa harina, olive oil, and ¼ teaspoon of kosher salt by hand, then slowly pour in the water, stirring until a soft dough forms.
- ✓ Divide the dough into 4 equal balls, then place each ball between 2 pieces of parchment paper and use a pie plate or a rolling pin to flatten the dough.
- ✓ Spray the baking pan with nonstick cooking spray, then place one flattened tortilla in the pan and air fry for 5 minutes.
- ✓ Repeat this process with the remaining tortillas.
- ✓ Remove the tortillas from the fryer and place on a serving plate, then top each tortilla with the scrambled eggs, salsa, and cheese before serving.
- ✓ Yummy

442) Flourless Broccoli Cheese Quiche

Ingredients:

- 1 large broccoli
- 3 large carrots
- 1 tsp thyme
- 1 tsp parsley
- Salt and ground black pepper to taste
- 2 large eggs
- 5 oz whole milk
- 1 large tomato
- 4 oz cheddar cheese grated
- 1 oz feta cheese

Direction: Time: 55 minutes | Servings: 2

- ✓ Chop up your broccoli into florets.
- ✓ Then dice your peeled carrots and combine it with the broccoli in a food steamer.
- ✓ Allow cooking until soft (for about 20 minutes).
- ✓ Get a measuring cup, and in it, combine all the seasonings, and crack the eggs into it as well.
- ✓ Mix thoroughly before adding the milk gradually until the mixture is pale.
- ✓ After steaming, drain the vegetables and use it to line the base of your quiche dish.
- ✓ Layer with the tomatoes and then add your cheese on top.
- ✓ Pour the liquid over and then add a little bit more cheese on top.
- ✓ Transfer the liquid into the fryer and allow to cook for 20 minutes at 360 F.
- ✓ Serve.

443) Asparagus Cheese Strata

Ingredients:

- asparagus spears, cut into 2-inch pieces
- 2 slices whole-wheat bread, cut into ½-inch cubes
- 4 eggs
- 3 tbls whole milk
- ½ cup grated Havarti or Swiss cheese
- 2 tablespoons chopped flat-leaf parsley
- Pinch salt
- Freshly ground black pepper, to taste

Direction: Time: 30 minutes | Serves 4-6

- ✓ Place the asparagus spears and 1 tablespoon water in a baking pan and place in the air fryer basket.
- ✓ Bake at 330°F (166°C) for 3 to 5 minutes or until crisp and tender.
- ✓ Remove the asparagus from the pan and drain it.
- ✓ Spray the pan with nonstick cooking spray.
- ✓ Arrange the bread cubes and asparagus into the pan and set aside.
- ✓ In a medium bowl, beat the eggs with the milk until combined.
- ✓ Add the cheese, parsley, salt, and pepper.
- ✓ Pour into the baking pan. Bake for 11 to 14 minutes or until the eggs are set and the top starts to brown.
- ✓ Serve

444) Almond Crunch Granola

Ingredients:

- ⅓ cups
- ⅔ cup rolled oats
- ⅓ cup unsweetened shredded coconut
- ⅓ cup sliced almonds
- 1 teaspoon canola oil
- 2 teaspoons honey
- ¼ teaspoon kosher salt

Direction: Time: 8 to 10 minutes | Makes 1

- ✓ In a medium bowl, combine the rolled oats, shredded coconut, sliced almonds, canola oil, honey, and kosher salt.
- ✓ Place a small piece of parchment paper on the bottom of a baking pan, then pour the mixture into the pan and distribute it evenly.
- ✓ Bake at 360°F (182°C) for 5 minutes, pause the fryer to gently stir the granola, and bake for 3 more minutes.
- ✓ Remove the granola from the fryer and allow to cool in the pan on a wire rack for 5 minutes, then transfer the granola to a serving plate to cool completely before serving.
- ✓ Enjoy

Tips:

- ✓ (It becomes crunchier as it cools. Store the granola in an airtight container for up to 2 weeks.)

445) Breakfast Burrito

Ingredients:

- 2 hard-boiled egg whites, chopped
- 1 hard-boiled egg, chopped
- 1 avocado, peeled, pitted, and chopped
- 1 red bell pepper, chopped
- 3 tablespoons low-sodium salsa,
- additional for serving(optional):
- 1 (1.2-ounce / 34-g) slice low-sodium, low-fat American cheese, torn into pieces
- 4 low-sodium whole-wheat flour tortillas

Direction: Time: 13 to 15 minutes | Serves 4

- ✓ In a medium bowl, thoroughly mix the egg whites, egg, avocado, red bell pepper, salsa, and cheese.
- ✓ Place the tortillas on a work surface and evenly divide the filling among them.
- ✓ Fold in the edges and roll up.
- ✓ Secure the burritos with toothpicks if necessary.
- ✓ Put the burritos in the air fryer basket.
- ✓ Air fry at 390°F (199°C) for 3 to 5 minutes, or until the burritos are light golden brown and crisp.
- ✓ Serve with more salsa if desired

446) Pumpkin Oatmeal with Raisins

Ingredients:

- 1 cup rolled oats
- 2 tablespoons raisins
- ¼ teaspoon ground cinnamon
- Pinch of kosher salt
- ¼ cup pumpkin purée
- 2 tablespoons pure maple syrup
- 1 cup low-fat milk

Direction: Time: 10 minutes | Makes 3 cups

- ✓ In a medium bowl, combine the rolled oats, raisins, ground cinnamon, and kosher salt, then stir in the pumpkin purée, maple syrup, and low-fat milk.
- ✓ Spray a baking pan with nonstick cooking spray, then pour the oatmeal mixture into the pan and bake at 300°F (149°C) for 10 minutes.
- ✓ Remove the oatmeal from the fryer and allow to cool in the pan on a wire rack for 5 minutes
- ✓ Serve

447) Mushroom and Black Bean Burrito

Ingredients:

- 2 tablespoons canned black beans, rinsed and drained
- ¼ cup sliced baby portobello mushrooms
- 1 teaspoon olive oil
- Pinch of kosher salt
- 1 large egg
- 1 slice low-fat Cheddar cheese
- 1 (8-inch) whole grain flour tortilla
- Hot sauce (optional)

Direction: Time: 15 minutes | Serves 1

- ✓ Spray a baking pan with nonstick cooking spray, then place the black beans and baby portobello mushrooms in the pan, drizzle with the olive oil, and season with the kosher salt.
- ✓ Bake at 360°F (182°C) for 5 minutes, then pause the fryer to crack the egg on top of the beans and mushrooms.
- ✓ Bake for 8 more minutes or until the egg is cooked as desired.
- ✓ Pause the fryer again, top the egg with cheese, and bake for 1 more minute.
- ✓ Remove the pan from the fryer, then use a spatula to place the bean mixture on the whole grain flour tortilla.
- ✓ Fold in the sides and roll from front to back.
- ✓ Serve warm with the hot sauce on the side (if using).

448) Yogurt Raspberry Cake

Ingredients:

- ½ cup whole wheat pastry flour
- ⅛ teaspoon kosher salt
- ¼ teaspoon baking powder
- ½ cup whole milk vanilla yogurt
- 2 tablespoons canola oil
- 2 tablespoons pure maple syrup
- ¾ cup fresh raspberries

Direction: Time: 18 minutes | Makes 4 slices

- ✓ In a large bowl, combine the whole wheat pastry flour, kosher salt, and baking powder, then stir in the whole milk vanilla yogurt, canola oil, and maple syrup and gently fold in the raspberries.
- ✓ Spray a baking pan with nonstick cooking spray, then pour the cake batter into the pan and bake at 300°F (149°C) for 8 minutes.
- ✓ Remove the cake from the fryer and allow to cool in the pan on a wire rack for 10 minutes before cutting and serving.

449) Turkey Egg Casserole

Ingredients:

- 12 eggs
- 2 tomatoes, chopped
- 1 cup spinach, chopped
- ½ sweet potato, cubed
- 1 tsp chili powder
- 1 tbsp olive oil
- 1 lb ground turkey
- Pepper Salt

Direction: Time: 35 minutes - Serve: 6

- ✓ In a bowl, whisk eggs with pepper, chili powder, and salt until well combined.
- ✓ Add spinach, sweet potato, tomato, and turkey and stir well.
- ✓ Pour egg mixture into the air fryer baking dish and place in the air fryer.
- ✓ Cook at 350 F for 25 minutes.
- ✓ Serve.

450) Mixed Berry Dutch Pancake

Ingredients:

- 2 egg whites
- 1 egg
- ½ cup whole-wheat pastry flour
- ½ cup 2% milk
- 1 teaspoon pure vanilla extract
- 1 tablespoon unsalted butter, melted
- 1 cup sliced fresh strawberries
- ½ cup fresh blueberries
- ½ cup fresh raspberries

Direction: time: 26 to 28 minutes | Serves 4

- In a medium bowl, use an eggbeater or hand mixer to quickly mix the egg whites, egg, pastry flour, milk, and vanilla until well combined.
- Use a pastry brush to grease the bottom of a baking pan with the melted butter.
- Immediately pour in the batter and put the baking pan in the fryer.
- Bake at 330°F (166°C) for 12 to 16 minutes, or until the pancake is puffed and golden brown.
- Remove the pan from the air fryer; the pancake will fall.
- Top with the strawberries, blueberries, and raspberries.
- Serve immediately.

451) Jalapeño Potato Hash

Ingredients:

- 2 large sweet potatoes
- ½ small red onion, cut into large chunks
- 1 green bell pepper, cut into large chunks
- 1 jalapeño pepper, seeded and sliced
- ½ teaspoon kosher salt
- ¼ teaspoon freshly ground black pepper,
- extra for serving:
- 1 teaspoon olive oil
- 1 large egg.

Direction: Time: 30 minutes | Makes 4 cups

- poached Cook the sweet potatoes on high in the microwave until softened but not completely cooked (3 to 4 minutes), then set aside to cool for 10 minutes.
- Remove the skins from the sweet potatoes, then cut the sweet potatoes into large chunks.
- In a large bowl, combine the sweet potatoes, red onion, green bell pepper, jalapeño pepper, kosher salt, black pepper, and olive oil, tossing gently.
- Spray the air fryer basket with nonstick cooking spray, then pour the mixture into the basket and air fry at 360°F (182°C) for 8 minutes.
- Pause the fryer to shake the basket, then air fry for 8 more minutes or until golden brown.
- Remove the hash from the fryer, place on a plate lined with a paper towel, and allow to cool for 5 minutes, then add the poached egg, sprinkle black pepper on top.
- Serve

452) Bacon and Egg Sandwiches

Ingredients:

- 2 large eggs
- ¼ teaspoon kosher salt, divided
- ¼ teaspoon freshly ground black pepper, divided
- plus extra for serving:
- 2 slices Canadian bacon
- 2 slices American cheese
- 2 whole grain English muffins, sliced in half

Direction: Time: 10 minutes | Makes 2 sandwiches

- Spray two 3-inch ramekins with nonstick cooking spray, then crack one egg into each ramekin and add half the kosher salt and half the black pepper to each egg.
- Place the ramekins in the fryer basket and bake at 360°F (182°C) for 5 minutes.
- Pause the fryer and top each partially cooked egg with a slice of Canadian bacon and a slice of American cheese.
- Bake for 3 more minutes or until the cheese has melted and the egg yolk has just cooked through.
- Remove the ramekins from the fryer and allow to cool on a wire rack for 2 to 3 minutes, then flip the eggs, bacon, and cheese out onto English muffins and sprinkle some black pepper on top.
- Serve

453) Spinach and Tomato Egg Cup

Ingredients:

- 2 egg whites, beaten
- 2 tablespoons chopped tomato
- 2 tablespoons chopped spinach
- Pinch of kosher salt
- Red pepper flakes (optional)

Direction: Time: 10 minutes | Serves 1

- Spray a 3-inch ramekin with nonstick cooking spray, then combine the egg whites, tomato, spinach, kosher salt, and red pepper flakes (if using) in the ramekin.
- Place the ramekin in the air fryer basket and bake at 300°F (149°C) for 10 minutes or until the eggs have set.
- Remove the ramekin from the fryer and allow to cool on a wire rack for 5 minutes before serving.

454) Egg Muffins with Bell Pepper

Ingredients:

- 4 large eggs
- ½ bell pepper, finely chopped
- 1 tablespoon finely chopped red onion
- ¼ teaspoon kosher salt
- ¼ teaspoon freshly ground black pepper,
- extra for serving:
- 2 tablespoons shredded Cheddar cheese

Direction: Time: 10 minutes | Serves 2

- In a large bowl, whisk together the eggs, then stir in the bell pepper, red onion, kosher salt, and black pepper.
- Spray two 3-inch ramekins with nonstick cooking spray, then pour half the egg mixture into each ramekin and place the ramekins in the fryer basket.
- Bake at 390°F (199°C) for 8 minutes.
- Pause the fryer, sprinkle 1 tablespoon of shredded Cheddar cheese on top of each cup, and bake for 2 more minutes.
- Remove the ramekins from the fryer and allow to cool on a wire rack for 5 minutes, then turn the omelet cups out on plates and sprinkle some black pepper on top
- serve

455) Tomato and Spinach Egg Cup

Ingredients:

- 2 egg whites, beaten
- 2 tablespoons chopped tomato
- 2 tablespoons chopped spinach
- Pinch of kosher salt
- Red pepper flakes (optional)

Direction: Time: 10 minutes | Serves 1

- ✓ Spray a 3-inch ramekin with nonstick cooking spray, then combine the egg whites, tomato, spinach, kosher salt, and red pepper flakes (if using) in the ramekin.
- ✓ Place the ramekin in the air fryer basket and bake at 300ºF (149ºC) for 10 minutes or until the eggs have set.
- ✓ Remove the ramekin from the fryer and allow to cool on a wire rack for 5 minutes
- ✓ Serve

456) Egg and Cheese Pockets

Ingredients:

- 1 large egg, beaten
- Pinch of kosher salt
- ½ sheet puff pastry
- 1 slice Cheddar cheese, divided into 4 pieces

Direction: Time: 35 minutes | Makes 4 pockets

- ✓ Pour the egg into a baking pan, season with the kosher salt, and bake at 330ºF (166ºC) for 3 minutes.
- ✓ Pause the fryer, gently scramble the egg, and bake for 2 more minutes.
- ✓ Remove the egg from the fryer, keeping the fryer on, and set the egg aside to slightly cool.
- ✓ Roll the puff pastry out flat and divide into 4 pieces.
- ✓ Place a piece of Cheddar cheese and ¼ of the egg on one side of a piece of pastry, fold the pastry over the egg and cheese, and use a fork to press the edges closed.
- ✓ Repeat this process with the remaining pieces.
- ✓ Place 2 pockets in the fryer and bake for 15 minutes or until golden brown.
- ✓ Repeat this process with the other 2 pockets.
- ✓ Remove the pockets from the fryer and allow to cool on a wire rack for 5 minutes
- ✓ Serve

457) Leftovers Bubble and Squeak

Ingredients:

- leftover vegetables (mash veggie bake, sprouts, cabbage, stuffing,
- 1 tbsp mixed herbs
- 1 tsp tarragon Salt and ground black pepper to taste
- 2 oz Cheddar cheese, shredded
- 1 medium onion, peeled and sliced
- 2 medium eggs, beaten
- 4 slices turkey breast

Direction: Cooking Time: 30 minutes | Servings: 4

- ✓ Get a large mixing bowl, and in it, place the leftovers, breaking them into small bits to facilitate blending.
- ✓ To the mixture, add the seasoning, cheese, onions, and eggs. Chop up the turkey and add it to the bowl and mix thoroughly using the hands.
- ✓ Transfer the mixture into ramekins or a baking dish and then into the air fryer.
- ✓ Allow cooking for 25 minutes at 360 F.
- ✓ Remove when it is bubbling on top. Serve.

458) Baked Mini Spinach Quiches

Ingredients:

- 4 cupcake moulds or small ramekins that fit inside the air fryer
- For the dough: 8 oz flour 3 oz butter 1 egg, beaten
- 2 tbsp milk Salt and ground black pepper to taste
- Filling: 1 small onion 1 tbsp olive oil 8 oz spinach 1 egg, beaten 8 oz cottage cheese (unsalted)

Direction: Cooking Time: 40 minutes | Servings: 4

- ✓ Combine all the ingredients for the dough in a food processor. Add a pinch of salt and blend until you have a ball of dough.
- ✓ Transfer the dough onto a worktop and using your hands, knead until the dough is smooth.
- ✓ Allow the kneaded dough to refrigerate for 15 minutes. Transfer the finely chopped onion into the pan containing the already-heated oil. Fry until the onion is translucent, then add the spinach and allow to fry for about 1 or 2 minutes or until when the spinach is wilted.
- ✓ Get a clean bowl and whisk the egg, adding the cottage cheese. Get rid of the excess water in the spinach by squeezing, then chop the squeezed spinach and add to the cheese mixture.
- ✓ Make four halves out of the dough, and roll each into a round that is large enough to cover the base of the molds.
- ✓ Line the molds with the dough, and fill each with the spinach mixture.
- ✓ Ensure that your air fryer is preheated to 360 F. Transfer the quiche(s) into the air fryer basket and slide it in. Allow cooking for 15 minutes.
- ✓ Serve the quiches either cold or lukewarm.

459) Cheesy Garlic Bread

Ingredients:

- 2 dinner rolls
- ½ cup grated Parmesan cheese
- 2 tbsp butter, melted
- 2 tbsp garlic and herb seasoning, or more to taste

Direction: Cooking Time: 20 minutes | Servings: 2

- ✓ Into each roll, cut a crisscross that almost reaches the base, while leaving the bottom crusts untouched.
- ✓ Fill all the holes with Parmesan cheese. Use melted butter to paint the tops of the rolls, and sprinkle garlic seasoning also.
- ✓ Ensure that your air fryer is preheated to 350 F.
- ✓ Transfer the rolls in the air fryer basket, and allow to cook for 5 minutes, or until you have the cheese melted.

460) Fried Ravioli

Ingredients:

- 1 (9-oz) box cheese ravioli, store-bought or meat ravioli
- 1 cup buttermilk
- 2 cups Italian-style bread crumbs
- 1 tsp olive oil 1 (14-oz) jar marinara sauce
- ¼ cup Parmesan cheese, shredded

Direction: ooking Time: 12 minutes | Servings: 6

- ✓ Dip the ravioli in buttermilk. Combine breadcrumbs and the olive oil, and press the ravioli into the breadcrumbs.
- ✓ Transfer the breaded ravioli into a preheated air fryer or baking paper
- ✓ Allow cooking for 5 minutes at 200 F.
- ✓ Serve while warm alongside marinara sauce for dipping and cheese for topping.

461) Fast Food Hot Dogs

Ingredients:

- 2 hot dogs 2 hot dog buns
- 2 tbsp of grated cheese, optional

Direction: Cooking Time: 12 minutes | Servings: 2

- ✓ Ensure that your air fryer is preheated at 390 F for about 4 minutes.
- ✓ Cook the two hot dogs in the air fryer for about 5 minutes, and remove.
- ✓ Transfer the hot dog into a bun, and you may add cheese. Return the dressed hot dog into the air fryer, and allow to cook for an extra 2 minutes.

462) Taco Dogs

Ingredients:

- 2 jumbo hot dogs
- 1 tsp taco seasoning mix
- 2 hot dog buns
- 1/3 cup guacamole
- 4 tbsp salsa
- 6 pickled jalapeno slices

Direction: Cooking Time: 17 minutes | Servings: 2

- ✓ Ensure that your air fryer is preheated at 390 F for at least four minutes.
- ✓ Make five slits into each hot dog, and rub ½ teaspoon taco seasoning over each hot dog.
- ✓ Allow the hot dogs to cook in the air fryer for about 5 minutes, before placing them in bus and back into the air fryer basket.
- ✓ This time around, cook until the buns are toasted and hot dogs crisp.
- ✓ This takes about 4 minutes or more.
- ✓ Top the hot dogs with guacamole, salsa, and jalapenos – all in equal amounts.

463) Pizza Dogs

Ingredients:

- 2 hot dogs
- 4 slices pepperoni, halved
- ½ cup pizza sauce
- 2 hot dog buns
- ¼ cup shredded mozzarella cheese
- 2 tsp sliced olives

Direction: Cooking Time: 17 minutes | Servings: 2

- ✓ Ensure that your air fryer is preheated to 200°C.
- ✓ Cut four slits into each hot dog, and place them into the basket of the air fryer.
- ✓ Allow cooking for 3 minutes before withdrawing onto a cutting board using tongs.
- ✓ Put a pepperoni half in each of the slits in the hot dogs. Divide the pizza sauce between the buns, and fill with the olives, hot dogs, and mozzarella cheese.
- ✓ Place the hot dogs in the basket of the air fryer and allow to cook, again.
- ✓ Remove when the cheese is melted, and the buns appear crisp – this takes about 2 minutes.

464) Pizza with Salami and Mushrooms

Ingredients:

- 4 oz flour
- 1 tsp instant yeast
- Salt to taste
- ½ tbsp olive oil
- 2 oz tomato sauce
- ½ ball of mozzarella, sliced thinly
- 2-3 mushrooms, sliced
- 2 oz salami, in strips
- 2 tsp dried oregano
- 2 tbsp Parmesan cheese, grated Freshly ground black pepper
- Handful of arugula
- Small pizza pan, 7 – inch diameter, buttered

Direction: Cooking Time: 30 minutes | Servings: 1

- ✓ Combine the flour and yeast with a pinch of salt, water (2-3 oz), and olive oil. Mix to form a smooth dough ball, and knead until you have an elastic and flexible dough.
- ✓ Ensure that your air fryer is preheated to 390 F.
- ✓ Flour your work surface, and on it, roll out the dough to an 7 - inch round, and put the same in the pizza pan. Form a crust by folding the excess edge of the dough inward.
- ✓ Spread the tomato sauce evenly over the dough, and on top of the sauce, add the mozzarella slices.
- ✓ Ensure even distribution of the mushrooms and the salami over the cheese. Add some sprinkles of oregano, Parmesan cheese, pepper, and arugula on the pizza.
- ✓ Transfer the pizza pan into the air fryer basket, and bake the pizza until golden brown – it takes about 12 minutes. You may use ready-to-use pizza dough for faster but same results.

465) Amazing XXL burger

Ingredients:

- 2 burgers (beef) 2 burger buns
- Mayonnaise to taste
- Ketchup to taste Lollo rosso lettuce
- 1 tomato, sliced
- 1 red onion, chopped
- 2 slices cheddar cheese Garden cress

Direction: Cooking Time: 15 minutes | Servings: 1

- ✓ Ensure that your air fryer is preheated when cooking the meat. Set the burgers in the air fryer and allow to cook at 390 F for five minutes.
- ✓ Cut the bread buns along the center to produce the needed two bottom halves and a top half.
- ✓ Add some mayonnaise on one bottom half, and some ketchup on the other.
- ✓ Combine the lettuce, the sliced tomatoes, and the chopped onions, and add the mixture to the bottoms.
- ✓ Open the air fryer, and add the cheddar cheese on the burgers. Allow cooking for 2 minutes at 390 F.
- ✓ After putting the hamburger together, and strengthen it with a cocktail stick.

466) Quick Blend Mexican Chicken Burgers

Ingredients:

- 3 tbsp smoked paprika 1 tbsp mustard powder
- 1 jalapeno pepper 1 tsp cayenne pepper
- 1 tbsp thyme, dried
- 1 tbsp oregano, dried
- Salt and ground black pepper to taste
- 1 small cauliflower
- 1 large egg, beaten
- 4 chicken breasts skin and bones removed

Direction: Cooking Time: 40 minutes | Servings: 4

- ✓ Ensure that your air fryer is preheated to 360 F. Combine your seasonings and the cauliflower in a blender and blend until you have the appearance of breadcrumbs.
- ✓ Take away ¾ of the blended cauliflower mixture and add it to the mixing bowl. Set aside. Get a separate bowl and add your beaten egg. Set aside also.
- ✓ Now add the chicken breasts into the blender, and alongside ¼ of the cauliflower and seasoning mixture, add some extra pepper and salt and blend.
- ✓ Remove the mixture from the blender and make it into burger shapes.
- ✓ You may add some extra cauliflower crumbs if the binding is not strong enough. Roll each burger in the cauliflower crumbs, roll in the egg, and the cauliflower crumbs again.
- ✓ After rolling and dipping all the burgers, arrange them on a baking mat and allow to cook in the air fryer at 360 F for 2 minutes.
- ✓ After 2 minutes, change the sides and allow to cook for an extra 10 minutes.
- ✓ This is to ensure that both sides are tasty and crispy. Serve the burger alongside pickles, crisps, and coleslaw.

467) Chicken Spiedie Recipe

Ingredients:

- 2 chicken breasts 1 large lemon 4 garlic cloves, thinly-sliced
- 1 tbsp basil 2 tbsp oregano Fresh mint
- Salt and ground black pepper to taste
- 1 tbsp olive oil
- Homemade bread rolls
- Homemade mayonnaise Skewers

Direction: Cooking Time: 40 minutes | Servings: 4

- ✓ The first step is to marinate your chicken.
- ✓ To marinate, dice your chicken into big-sized chunks and set them aside in a mixing bowl.
- ✓ Squeeze the juice from the lemon into the same bowl, and the peeled and thinly-sliced garlic also.
- ✓ Then add seasoning and the olive oil. Mix thoroughly with the hands and ensure the chicken is well coated.
- ✓ Now fill the skewers with the chicken and keep them in the fridge overnight. The next step is to make the bread.
- ✓ Gather four bread rolls into the air fryer and allow them to cook at 365 F for 15 minutes.
- ✓ Withdraw the cooked bread rolls and cook the chicken too, at 365 F for 15 minutes.
- ✓ Fill the bread rolls with the stewed chicken, adding some homemade mayonnaise in the process. Serve.

468) Simple Grilled American Cheese Sandwich

Ingredients:

- 2-3 slices cheddar cheese
- 2 slices sandwich bread
- 2 tsp Butter

Direction: Cooking Time: 12 minutes | Servings: 1

- ✓ With the cheese between the bread slices, spread the butter to the outside of both slices of bread.
- ✓ Transfer the buttered bread into the air fryer and allow to cook for 8 minutes at 370 F.
- ✓ After 4 minutes, flip the bread, and allow to cook for the next 4 minutes.
- ✓ Note that you can use any type of cheese you want and may stuff with tomatoes if that's your preference.

469) Fried Pizza Sticks

Ingredients:

- 12 egg roll wrappers
- 36 slices pepperoni
- 12 pieces string cheese
- Oil for frying Marinara sauce for dipping

Direction: Cooking Time: 15 minutes | Servings: 6

- ✓ The first step is to lay an egg roll wrapper out flat. On the wrapper, lay three pieces of pepperoni, towards the center on the diagonal.
- ✓ Now, lay a mozzarella stick on top of the pepperoni.
- ✓ Fold the corners of the egg wrapper down over the cheese, and then fold one or both larger corners down over the cheese.
- ✓ Once folded, start rolling the folded cheese until you have used up the entire wrapper.
- ✓ Add drops of water to hold the edges shut.
- ✓ Do the same for the other 11 mozzarella sticks. Transfer the wrapped mozzarella sticks into a deep frying pan containing an already heated oil.
- ✓ Now fry the wrapped cheese for about a minute or until there is a golden brown color on both sides.
- ✓ Serve while hot, alongside marinara sauce for dipping.

470) Five Cheese Pull Apart Bread

Ingredients:

- 1 oz goats cheese 1 oz Cheddar cheese 1 oz Mozzarella cheese 1 oz Edam cheese 1 oz soft cheese
- 4 oz butter Salt and ground black pepper to taste 2 tsp chives 2 tsp garlic puree 1 large bread loaf

Direction: Cooking Time: 20 minutes | Servings: 2

- ✓ The hard cheese should be grated into four separate piles and set aside. Get a clean saucepan and place it on medium heat.
- ✓ Melt the butter in the saucepan, and add the pepper, salt, chives, and the garlic. Allow the mixture to cook for another 2 minutes while mixing. Set aside.
- ✓ Make little slits into the bread with the aid of a sharp bread knife.
- ✓ Cover each slit wholes with garlic butter until every slit is well covered.
- ✓ Then cover all the slits with soft cheese – to ensure the lovely creamy taste in the end. Add a little goat's cheese and a little cheddar into every other slit.
- ✓ Add the Edam and Mozzarella to those that have not been filled.
- ✓ Transfer them into the air fryer and allow to cook for 4 minutes at 360 F or until you have melted cheese and warm bread. Serve.

471) Grilled Cheese

Ingredients:

- 2 slices of bread I used GF bread Butter
- 1 slice of cheese

Direction: Cooking Time: 12 minutes | Servings: 1

- ✓ Add butter generously to one side of each of the slices of bread, however, avoid too much butter.
- ✓ Add the folded cheese in-between the bread slices, while ensuring that the buttered side is facing out.
- ✓ Avoid letting the cheese hang outside the bread; otherwise, it will burn in the air fryer. If you want to grill, set the air fryer temperature to 360 F and the timer to 8 minutes.
- ✓ Flip the bread after 5 minutes. Allow to cool and serve. Juicy Lucy

472) Cheese Burger

Ingredients:

- 1 onion 0.5 lb minced beef
- 1 tsp mixed herbs
- Salt and ground black pepper to taste
- 4 oz cheddar cheese

Direction: Cooking Time: 25 minutes | Servings: 2

- ✓ Ensure that your air fryer is preheated to 360 F.
- ✓ Dice the onion and set it aside. Get a large mixing bowl, and in it, combine minced beef, seasoning, and the onion. Mix the combination thoroughly.
- ✓ Roll the mixture into four even-sized balls and transfer them to the chopping board.
- ✓ Squash the burgers until you have very thin pieces. In-between two of the burgers, add half of the cheese and merge them so that there is a burger, then the cheese and then the second burger.
- ✓ Repeat the process for the third and fourth burger, ensuring that the cheese is well hidden in each. Transfer the burgers (two at a time) into the air fryer and allow cooking for 15 minutes at 360 F. Withdraw the burgers from the air fryer and see if the cheese has melted in the center.
- ✓ Also, place a knife or cake tester through it to confirm if they are well cooked. If the juices run clear, it means the burgers are cooked, and if not, return them into the air fryer and cook for an extra 10 minutes at 360 F Serve the cooked burger in a burger bun alongside garnish.

473) Chicken Burgers

Ingredients:

- 1 lb chicken, minced Salt and ground black pepper to taste
- 1 tbsp oregano
- 4 oz wholemeal breadcrumbs
- 2 oz mozzarella cheese

Direction: Cooking Time: 25 minutes | Servings: 4

- ✓ With the minced chicken in a mixing bowl, add salt, pepper, and oregano, alongside ¾ of the breadcrumbs.
- ✓ Mix thoroughly to ensure that the seasoning is well coated. Mold the mixture into burger shapes. Roll each burger in the remaining breadcrumbs first, then in the cheese
- ✓ . In each case, ensure that the bottom, top, and the sides are entirely coated. Transfer the coated burger into the air fryer and allow cooking at 360 F for 18 minutes.
- ✓ Withdraw cooked burger and serve in bread buns alongside salad and mayonnaise.

474) Chicken Avocado Burgers

Ingredients:

- 14 oz avocado, peeled
- 14 oz chicken, minced
- 1 tbsp mexican seasoning

Direction: Cooking Time: 15 minutes | Servings: 2

- ✓ Slice the peeled avocado and cut three slices into small cubes.
- ✓ Keep the rest aside as whole slices.
- ✓ Transfer the minced chicken into a mixing bowl, and add the chunks of avocado alongside the Mexican seasoning.
- ✓ After mixing the contents of the bowl above thoroughly, form the mixture into chicken burger patty shapes.
- ✓ Transfer the burger into the air fryer and allow to cook for 12 minutes at 360 F for 12 minutes.
- ✓ To get that ideal Mexican meal, serve the burger alongside potato wedges.

475) Veggie Burgers

Ingredients:

- 7 oz carrots 2 lb cauliflower
- 1 lb sweet potato
- 1 cup warm water
- 1 cup chickpeas
- 2 cups wholemeal breadcrumbs 1 tbsp basil
- 1 tbsp mixed herbs
- Salt and ground black pepper to taste
- 1 cup grated mozzarella cheese

Direction: Cooking Time: 35 minutes | Servings: 6

- ✓ Chop the peeled vegetables. Then transfer them into the bottom of the Instant Pot.
- ✓ Add a cup of warm water and close the lid on the instant pot. Set the valve to sealing and allow the vegetables to cook for 10 minutes on manual.
- ✓ After 10 minutes, withdraw the vegetables and squeeze out the excess water after draining with the aid of a tea towel.
- ✓ Ensure that the vegetables are very dry. Combine the chickpeas and the vegetables.
- ✓ Mash together. Add the breadcrumbs and mix thoroughly, and add the seasonings. Make the mixture into veggie burger shapes.
- ✓ Roll the burgers in the grated cheese, ensuring that the cheese covers everywhere.
- ✓ Transfer the veggie burgers into the air fryer and allow cooking at 360 F for 10 minutes. After this first round of cooking, change the temperature to 390 F and cook again for 5 minutes extra.
- ✓ This ensures that the veggie burger gets that crusty texture. Serve while warm, in bread buns or alongside a salad, or both.

476) Cauliflower Veggie Burger Recipe

Ingredients:

- 2 lbs cauliflower
- Salt and ground black pepper to taste
- 1 tsp mustard powder
- 2 tsp garlic puree 1 tsp mixed spice
- 2 tsp thyme 2 tsp chives
- 2 tsp parsley 3 tsp coconut oil
- ½ cup oats
- 1 cup bread crumbs ¼ desiccated coconut
- 3 tbsp plain flour 1 small egg beaten
- 2 cups herby bread crumbs

Direction: Cooking Time: 50 minutes | Servings: 8

- ✓ Chop up the cauliflower into florets. Steam the florets for 25 minutes in the soup maker.
- ✓ Drain the cauliflower and retain it in the soup maker. With the aid of a vegetable knife, dice the cauliflower so that you have very tiny pieces of cauliflower.
- ✓ To the diced cauliflower, add salt, pepper, mustard and a teaspoon of garlic puree. Blend this mixture for a couple of minutes and drain the blend over the sink.
- ✓ Transfer the cauliflower into a tea towel, and use the same in squeezing out any excess water. You may stop when it appears like a bread dough. Get a clean bowl and in it, combine the cauliflower with salt, pepper, the remaining seasoning, extra garlic puree, and coconut oil.
- ✓ Mix them thoroughly. Then add the oats, a cup of bread crumbs and the desiccated coconut. Again, mix thoroughly.
- ✓ Dip your hands in flour to ensure that you don't sick to the burgers. Now, shape the mixture above into burgers.
- ✓ Roll the shaped burgers in the flour, and then the egg, and finally the herby breadcrumbs. Transfer the rolled burgers into the air fryer. Set the temperature to 360 F and allow to cook for 10 minutes.
- ✓ Flip and cook the other side for an extra 10 minutes.
- ✓ Withdraw and serve alongside salad garnish and a burger bun.

477) Falafel Burger

Ingredients:

- 1 tbsp oregano 1 tbsp parsley
- 1 tbsp coriander
- Salt and ground black pepper to taste
- 1 tbsp garlic puree
- 1 small lemon
- 14 oz can chickpeas 1 small red onion
- 4 tbsp soft cheese 1 oz hard cheese
- 1 oz feta cheese
- 5 oz gluten free oats
- 3 tbsp Greek yoghurt

Direction: Cooking Time: 20 minutes | Servings: 2

- ✓ Combine all the seasonings, garlic, lemon rind, drained chickpeas, and red onion in the food processor or blender. Blend until you have a coarse mixture – don't allow them to smoothen up.
- ✓ Transfer the blended mixture into a bowl, add half of the soft cheese, the hard cheese, and the feta.
- ✓ Mold the mixture into burger shapes. Roll the burgers in the gluten-free oats until the chickpea mixture isn't visible anymore.
- ✓ Transfer the rolled burgers into the air fryer's baking pan and allow to cook at 360 F for 8 minutes. To make the burger sauce, combine the soft cheese, salt, pepper, and the Greek
- ✓ Yoghurt in a clean mixing bowl. Mix thoroughly until you have a fluffy mixture, then add the juice of the last lemon and mix again.
- ✓ Place the falafel burger inside the homemade buns with garnish. Then load it up with your burger sauce. Serve and enjoy.

478) Vegan Lentil Burgers

Ingredients:

- 10 oz gluten free oats
- 4 oz black beluga lentils
- 4 vegan burger buns
- 4 oz white cabbage
- 1 large onion peeled and diced
- 1 large carrot peeled and grated 1 tsp cumin
- 1 tbsp garlic puree
- Salt and ground black pepper to taste
- Handful fresh basil cleaned and chopped

Direction: Cooking Time: 45 minutes | Servings: 4

- ✓ The first step is to transfer the gluten-free oats in the blender and blend until it appears like a flower.
- ✓ Get a clean saucepan and place the lentils in it. Pour water until the lentils are submerged.
- ✓ Then cook on medium heat for about 45 minutes. While cooking put the vegetables into the Instant
- ✓ Pot and allow to steam for 5 minutes with the steam function.
- ✓ Remove the water from the lentils and transfer them in a bowl alongside the oats, steamed vegetables, and seasonings.
- ✓ Make the mixture into burger shapes.
- ✓ Transfer the burgers into the air fryer, set the temperature to 360 F and the timer to 30 minutes.
- ✓ Serve the cooked burgers alongside vegan mayonnaise and salad garnish.

479) Spanakopita Bites

Ingredients:

- 1 (10-oz) pkg. baby spinach leaves 2 tbsp water
- 1/8 tsp cayenne pepper
- ¼ tsp kosher salt
- ¼ tsp black pepper 1 tsp dried oregano 1 large egg white
- 1 tsp lemon zest (from 1 lemon)
- 2 tbsp finely grated Parmesan cheese
- ¼ cup 1% low-fat cottage cheese
- 1 oz feta cheese, crumbled (about 1/4 cup)
- 4 (13- x 18-inch) sheets frozen phyllo dough, thawed
- 1 tbsp olive oil Cooking spray

Direction: Cooking Time: 50 minutes | Servings: 8

- In a large cooking pot, combine spinach and enough water and cook over high heat. Stir often while cooking, for 5 minutes, or until wilted. Drain the spinach and allow cooling for 10 minutes.
- To get rid of excess moisture, press firmly using a paper towel. Get a clean medium bowl, and in it, mix the cayenne pepper, salt, black pepper, oregano, egg white, zest,
- Parmesan cheese, spinach, cottage cheese, feta cheese until you have a smooth mixture. Spread one phyllo sheet on the work surface and brush lightly with oil using a pastry brush.
- Add another sheet of phyllo and brush with oil again.
- Following the same procedure, add two more layers of oiled sheets to make four.
- Start working from the long side, cut the stack of phyllo sheets into eight strips, each with 2¼ inches of width.
- Cut the eight strips into a half, crosswise, giving 16 x 2¼ inches of width strips.
- Place each tablespoon of filling onto one short end of each strip.
- Fold one corner over the filling, thus creating a triangle. Keep folding back and forth until you get to the end of the strip, and by then, you must have created a triangle-shaped phyllo packet.
- Coat the air fryer basket mildly using the cooking spray. Arrange eight packets of the phyllo, seam side down, in the basket. Spray the tops with cooking oil and allow cooking till 375 F for about 12 minutes or until you have crispy and deep golden brown phyllo packets.
- Turn the packets to the other side halfway through cooking. Do the same for the uncooked phyllo packets. Serve at room temperature or while warm.

480) Fried Calzones

Ingredients:

- 1 tsp olive oil
- ¼ cup red onion, finely chopped
- 3 cups baby spinach leaves
- 1/3 cup shredded rotisserie chicken breast
- 1/3 cup lower-sodium marinara sauce
- 6 oz fresh prepared whole-wheat pizza dough
- 1½ oz pre-shredded part-skim mozzarella cheese (about 6 tbsp) Cooking spray

Direction: Cooking Time: 30 minutes | Servings: 2

- Get a medium-sized non-stick skillet and in it, heat the oil over medium-high. Toss in the onions, and cook while stirring occasionally.
- Stop cooking when the onions are tender – this takes about 2 minutes.
- Now toss in the spinach, and allow to cook until wilted, while covering the skillet. This takes about 1.5 minutes.
- Withdraw the pan from the heat and stir in the chicken and the marinara sauce.
- Halve the dough into four and roll each piece on a lightly floured surface to form a circle of 6 inches.
- Place 1/4th of the spinach mixture over half of each dough circle, and top with 1/4th of the cheese.
- Form half-moons by folding the dough over the filling, and crimp the edges to seal.
- Transfer the calzones into the air fryer basket and allow cooking for 12 minutes at 325 F, or until you have the golden-brown dough.
- Turn the calzones to the other side after the first 8 minutes. Serve.

481) Reuben Calzones

Ingredients:

- g spray 1 tube (13.8 oz) refrigerated pizza crust
- 4 slices Swiss cheese
- 1 cup sauerkraut, rinsed and well drained
- ½ lb sliced cooked corned beef Thousand Island salad dressing

Direction: Cooking Time: 30 minutes | Servings: 6

- Ensure that your air fryer is preheated to 400 F.
- Drizzle some cooking spray over the air fryer basket. Prepare a lightly floured surface, and on it, unroll the pizza crust dough while patting into a 12-inches square.
- Cut the dough into four squares. Layer a slice of the cheese, 1/4th of the sauerkraut, and the corned beef diagonally over half of each square to within 0.5 inches of edges.
- Form a triangle by folding one corner over filling to the opposite corner.
- Seal by pressing the edges with your fork.
- Arrange two calzones in a single layer in the sprayed air fryer basket.
- Allow cooking for about 8-12 minutes or until the calzones are golden brown.
- Turn the sides after 4-6 minutes of cooking.
- When fully cooked, withdraw and keep warm while preparing the other calzones. Serve alongside salad dressing.

482) Popcorn

Ingredients:

- 3 tbsp corn kernels, dried Spray avocado oil (Substitutes: safflower oil; coconut oil; peanut oil)
- Sea salt and ground black pepper to taste Garnish:
- 2 tbsp nutritional yeast Dried chives

Direction: Cooking Time: 30 minutes | Servings: 6

- ✓ Ensure that your air fryer is set to 390F. In the air fryer basket, arrange the kernels gently and light-spray some coconut or avocado oil.
- ✓ You may line the tray sides with aluminum foil – this ensures that the popped popcorn does not escape the basket.
- ✓ Return the air fryer basket into the air fryer and allow cooking for 15 minutes.
- ✓ Pay close attention to the cooking kernels to ensure that they do not burn.
- ✓ At the sound of popping sounds, monitor closely until they do not pop anymore – or until the 15 minutes lapses. Withdraw the basket immediately and transfer the contents into a large bowl.
- ✓ Spray the cooked kernels with some avocado or coconut oil. Dust with garnish according to your preference. Serve warm or at room temperature.

483) Mexican-Style Corn on the Cob

Ingredients:

- 4 ears fresh corn (about
- 1½ lbs), shucked Cooking spray
- 1½ tbsp unsalted butter
- 1 tsp lime zest
- 2 tsp chopped garlic 1 tbsp fresh juice (from 1 lime)
- ½ tsp black pepper
- 2 tbsp chopped fresh cilantro
- ½ tsp kosher salt

Direction: Cooking Time: 25 minutes | Servings: 4

- ✓ Coat your corn mildly with some cooking spray before placing in the air fryer basket following a single layer. Allow cooking at 400 F until the corn is tender or mildly charred – this takes about 14 minutes.
- ✓ Turn the corn over after the first 7 minutes of cooking.
- ✓ While cooking the corn, get a small bowl that is suitable for microwaving and in it, combine the butter, lime zest, garlic, and lime juice.
- ✓ Set the microwave to 'high' and microwave the mixture until the butter is melted and the fragrance of the garlic obvious – this takes about 30 seconds.
- ✓ Transfer the corn on a platter, and pour the butter mixture on it.
- ✓ Add sprinkles of pepper, cilantro, and salt to taste. Serve immediately.

484) Salt and Vinegar Chickpeas

Ingredients:

- 1 (15 oz) can chickpeas, drained and rinsed
- 1 cup white vinegar
- ½ tsp sea salt
- 1 tbsp olive oil

Direction: Cooking Time: 55 minutes | Servings: 2

- ✓ Get a clean small saucepan, and in it, combine chickpeas and vinegar. Bring to a simmer over high heat.
- ✓ Once simmering, withdraw and allow to stand for 30 minutes. Drain the chickpeas and get rid of all loose skins. Ensure that your air fryer is preheated to 390 F.
- ✓ With the chickpeas spread evenly in the air fryer basket, allow cooking for about 4 minutes or until the chickpeas dry out.
- ✓ Move the dried chickpeas into a heat-proof bowl.
- ✓ Drizzle with sea salt and oil and stir to coat evenly.
- ✓ Place the coated chickpeas into the air fryer again and allow cooking for about 8 minutes.
- ✓ Endeavor to shake the basket at 2 or 3 minutes intervals. Withdraw once you have lightly browned chickpeas. Serve instantly.

485) Curry Chickpeas

Ingredients:

- 1 (15-oz) can no-salt-added chickpeas (garbanzo beans), drained and rinsed (about
- 1½ cups) 2 tbsp olive oil
- 2 tbsp red wine vinegar
- ¼ tsp ground coriander
- ¼ tsp plus 1/8 tsp ground cinnamon
- ¼ tsp ground cumin
- 2 tsp curry powder
- ½ tsp ground turmeric Thinly sliced fresh cilantro
- ½ tsp Aleppo pepper
- ¼ tsp kosher salt

Direction: Cooking Time: 35 minutes | Servings: 4

- ✓ Smash the chickpeas mildly in a medium bowl with your hands. Remove the chickpea skins. Pour over the oil and vinegar into the chickpeas.
- ✓ Stir to coat evenly, and add coriander, cinnamon, cumin, curry powder and turmeric. Stir the mixture gently to combine.
- ✓ In the air fryer basket, arrange the chickpeas in a single layer and allow cooking at 400 F for about 15 minutes or until the chickpeas are crispy
- ✓ Ensure that you shake the chickpeas after the first 7 or 8 minutes of cooking.
- ✓ Move the cooked chickpeas into a bowl, while sprinkling the cilantro, Aleppo pepper, and salt – toss to coat.

486) Buffalo-Ranch Chickpeas

Ingredients:

- 1 (15 oz) can chickpeas, drained and rinsed
- 2 tbsp Buffalo wing sauce
- 1 tbsp dry ranch dressing mix

Direction: Cooking Time: 35 minutes | Servings: 2

- ✓ Ensure that your air fryer is preheated to 350 F.
- ✓ After lining your baking sheet with paper towels, spread the chickpeas over the lined paper towels.
- ✓ Cover the chickpeas with another layer of paper towels, and press gently to drain any excess moisture.
- ✓ Place the chickpeas in a bowl and pour in the wing sauce. Stir the mixture to combine.
- ✓ Add ranch dressing powder and mix well to combine.
- ✓ Arrange the air fryer in an even layer in the air fryer basket.
- ✓ Allow cooking for 8 minutes. Stop, shake, and cook for an extra 5 minutes, shake again, and cook for 5 minutes more, and shake again for the last time, before cooking for the final 2 minutes.
- ✓ Set aside the cooked chickpeas for about 5 minutes to allow cooling. Serve immediately.

487) Baja Fish Taco Recipe

Ingredients:

- 1 red onion 1 large mango
- 7 oz fresh cod fillet
- Salt and ground black pepper to taste
- 2 tbsp coriander 1 tbsp cumin
- 8 tbsp mexican seasoning
- 2 medium eggs
- 1 tbsp garlic puree
- 2 tbsp quark
- 4 limes
- 5 oz gluten free oats
- 4 homemade tortilla wraps

Direction: Cooking Time: 40 minutes | Servings: 4

- ✓ After peeling the red onion and mango, chop them into small pieces and set aside.
- ✓ Clean and cut the fresh cod into pieces that can be bitten easily.
- ✓ Add salt and pepper generously, alongside half of the coriander.
- ✓ Get a large mixing bowl, and in it, combine all the seasonings and the other half of the coriander.
- ✓ Also, add ¾ of the red onion chopped earlier, the eggs, and the garlic.
- ✓ Mix well to combine. Toss in the quark, and stir in the juice, and the rind of 3 out of 4 limes.
- ✓ Mix thoroughly again to form a smooth batter.
- ✓ Place ¾ of the oats in a blender and blend until you have a mixture like fine breadcrumbs.
- ✓ Combine the blend with unblended oats and mix well before tossing in the fresh cod. Ensure that the fresh cod is well coated in the oats mixture.
- ✓ Transfer the battered cod pieces into the air fryer grill pan, and allow cooking for 10 minutes at 365 F.
- ✓ Withdraw and shake, before allowing to cook for an additional 3 minutes at 390 F.
- ✓ Toss in the cooked fish into the just cooked wraps. Add the mango and red onion mixture as the toppings. Add some lime juice from the remaining lime as seasoning, alongside salt and pepper. Serve.

488) Lighten up Empanadas

Ingredients:

- 1 tbsp olive oil
- 3 oz lean ground beef
- ¼ cup white onion, chopped
- 3 oz cremini mushrooms, chopped
- 6 pitted green olives, chopped
- ¼ tsp ground cumin
- 2 tsp garlic, chopped
- ¼ tsp paprika
- 1/8 tsp ground cinnamon ½ cup tomatoes, chopped
- 8 square gyoza wrappers 1 large egg, lightly beaten

Direction: Cooking Time: 50 minutes | Servings: 2

- ✓ Get a clean medium skillet and pour in some oil. Heat over medium-high.
- ✓ Toss in beef and onion, and allow cooking while stirring to crumble. Stop cooking after 3 minutes or when the beef and onion start browning. Add the mushrooms, and continue cooking while stirring occasionally.
- ✓ Stop cooking after 6 minutes or when the mushrooms are appearing brown. Now toss in the olives, cumin, garlic, paprika, and cinnamon, cook until the mushrooms are very soft and devoid of moisture – this will take about 3 minutes.
- ✓ Add the tomatoes and cook further for a minute while stirring intermittently.
- ✓ Transfer the filling into a clean bowl and set aside to cool for about 5 minutes. On your work surface, carefully arrange four gyoza wrappers.
- ✓ At the center of each wrapper, pour about 1.5 tablespoons filling. Now brush the wrapper's edges with egg and fold each over. Seal by pinching the edges.
- ✓ Do the same for the other wrappers and filling. Arrange four empanadas in your air fryer basket following a single layer.
- ✓ Allow cooking at 400 F for 7 minutes or until nicely browned.
- ✓ Do the same for the other empanadas.

489) Whole-Wheat Pizzas

Ingredients:

- 2 whole-wheat pita rounds
- ¼ cup lower-sodium marinara sauce
- 1 cup baby spinach leaves (1 oz)
- 1 oz pre-shredded part-skim mozzarella cheese (about ¼ cup)
- 1 small garlic clove, thinly sliced
- 1 small plum tomato, cut into 8 slices
- ¼ oz shaved Parmigiano-Reggiano cheese (about 1 tbsp)

Direction: Cooking Time: 20 minutes | Servings: 2

- ✓ Lay out your pita bread.
- ✓ Spread the marina sauce evenly over the side facing upwards.
- ✓ Add half of the spinach leaves, cheeses, garlic, and tomato slices as toppings.
- ✓ Transfer each pita into the air fryer basket, and allow cooking at 350 F for about 4-5 minutes or until you have melted cheese.
- ✓ Do the same for other pitas.

490) Hot Dogs

Ingredients:

- 4 hot dog buns
- 4 hot dogs

Direction: Cooking Time: 15 minutes | Servings: 4

- ✓ Ensure that your air fryer is preheated to 390 F.
- ✓ Move your buns into the air fryer basket and allow cooking for 2 minutes.
- ✓ Withdraw the cooked buns to a plate
- ✓ Replace the buns with the hot dogs, and allow cooking for 3 minutes.
- ✓ Withdraw and place in the same plate as the buns. Serve.

491) Crunchy Corn Dog Bites

Ingredients:

- 2 uncured all-beef hot dogs
- 12 craft sticks or bamboo skewers
- ½ cup (about 2 1/8 oz.) all-purpose flour
- 2 large eggs, lightly beaten
- 1½ cups cornflakes cereal, finely crushed
- Cooking spray 8 tsp yellow mustard

Direction: Cooking Time: 45 minutes | Servings: 4

- ✓ After slicing your hotdog in half, lengthwise, proceed to cut each half into three equal pieces.
- ✓ Find a bamboo skewer or a craft stick into one end of each piece of hot dog. Get a clean shallow dish and place the flour in it. In another shallow dish, place the lightly beaten eggs. In the third shallow dish, place the crushed cornflakes.
- ✓ Now dredge the hot dogs in the flour (shake to get rid of excess flour), then dip in the egg (allowing excess egg mixture to drip off), and finally dredge in cornflakes (press mildly to make the cornflakes adhere).
- ✓ Coat your air fryer basket with little cooking spray.
- ✓ Arrange six corn dog bites in the basket, and spray the top lightly with the cooking spray.
- ✓ Allow cooking for 10 minutes at 375 F or until the corn dog bites over halfway through cooking.
- ✓ Do the same for the other corn dog bites.
- ✓ Serve immediately by placing three corn dog bites per plate, and adding two teaspoons of mustard.

492) Crispy Veggie Quesadillas

Ingredients:

- 4 (6-inch) sprouted whole-grain flour tortillas
- 1 cup reduced-fat sharp Cheddar cheese, shredded
- 1 cup sliced red bell pepper
- 1 cup no-salt-added canned black beans, drained and rinsed
- 1 cup sliced zucchini Cooking spray
- 1 tsp lime zest plus
- 1 tbsp fresh juice (from 1 lime)
- 2 oz plain 2% reduced-fat Greek yogurt
- ¼ tsp ground cumin 2 tbsp chopped fresh cilantro
- ½ cup drained refrigerated pico de gallo

Direction: Cooking Time: 45 minutes | Servings: 4

- ✓ With your tortillas on the work surface, sprinkle two tablespoons shredded cheese over half of each tortilla.
- ✓ Add cheese on each tortilla, alongside ¼ cup each red pepper slices, black beans, and zucchini slices.
- ✓ Sprinkle the unused ½ cup cheese evenly over the tortilla.
- ✓ Now form half-moon shaped quesadillas by folding the tortillas.
- ✓ Use some of the cooking sprays to coat the quesadillas mildly.
- ✓ Finally, secure the coated quesadillas with toothpicks. Into the already sprayed air fryer basket, add two quesadillas gently and allow cooking at 400 F until you have golden brown and slightly crispy tortillas.
- ✓ By then, the cheese will be melted and vegetables a bit tender.
- ✓ This should take about 10 minutes. Ensure that you change the side after 5 minutes of cooking.
- ✓ Do the same for the other quesadillas. Meanwhile, combine the lime juice, yogurt, and cumin in a small bowl and stir together. Serve by cutting each quesadilla into wedges, and sprinkle a little cilantro on it.
- ✓ Finally, add a tablespoon of cumin cream alongside two tablespoons of pico de gallo.

493) Homemade Sausage Rolls

Ingredients:

- 4 oz butter
- 8 oz plain flour
- 1 tsp parsley, dried
- Salt and ground black pepper to taste
- 1 tbsp olive oil
- 1 tsp mustard
- 11 oz sausage meat
- 1 medium egg beaten

Direction: Cooking Time: 50 minutes | Servings: 4

- ✓ The first step is to make your pastry. Combine the butter, flour, and the seasoning into a mixing bowl.
- ✓ Using the rubbing-in method, rub the fat into the flour until the mixture looks like breadcrumbs.
- ✓ Stir in the olive oil and little water bit by bit, while mixing into a flaky dough.
- ✓ While incorporating the pastry together, knead it until it becomes very smooth. On your worktop, roll out the smooth pastry and make a square shape.
- ✓ Rub the mustard into the pastry, either with your fingers or a teaspoon
- ✓ Move the sausage meat to the center, before brushing the edges of the pastry with egg. Roll up the sausage rolls.
- ✓ Divide the rolled up portions into portions. Brush all sides and tops of the sausage rolls with more eggs.
- ✓ Use a knife to cut off the top of the sausage rolls to allow some breathing space.
- ✓ Allow cooking in the air fryer for 20 minutes at 320 F. Increase the heat to 390 F and allow cooking for an additional 5 minutes to ensure that you have a crunchy pastry. Serve.

494) Feta Cheese Dough Balls

Ingredients:

- Leftover pizza dough get the recipe here
- 1 tbsp Greek yoghurt
- 2 oz soft cheese 1 tsp mustard
- 1 tsp garlic puree 1 tbsp olive oil
- 2 tsp rosemary
- Salt and ground black pepper to taste
- 2 oz feta cheese

Direction: Cooking Time: 25 minutes | Servings: 8

- ✓ After removing it from the fridge, allow the pizza dough acclimatize to the room temperature so that working with it is easy.
- ✓ Combine the dough with some flour and knead for a while. This makes the dough soft and gives it the local dough feel. Set aside. In a clean mixing bowl, combine all the ingredients, except the feta and the dough.
- ✓ Mix thoroughly to form a creamy paste.
- ✓ Make eight equal sized pieces from the dough and flatten each piece out like a pancake.
- ✓ Top each flat piece with about 1/3 teaspoon of the ingredients mix.
- ✓ Now, add a little square of feta and seal it up. Repeat the same process for the other seven flatten pieces, so that you have 8 top nice little balls. Now transfer them into the air fryer and allow cooking for 10 minutes at 360 F.
- ✓ Reduce the heat to 320 F and allow cooking for an additional 5 minutes.

495) Flourless Crunchy Cheese Straws

Ingredients:

- 4 oz gluten free oats
- 1 large cauliflower
- 1 large egg
- 6 oz cheddar cheese
- 1 red onion peeled and thinly diced
- 1 tsp mustard
- 1 tsp mixed herbs
- Salt and ground black pepper to taste

Direction: Cooking Time: 50 minutes | Servings: 8

- ✓ Blitz your oats in a food processor until you have the appearance of fine breadcrumbs.
- ✓ Place your cauliflower florets in the steamer and allow to steam for 20 minutes.
- ✓ Immediately after steaming, drain and allow the florets to cool.
- ✓ Get rid of all excess water by squeezing out using a clean pillowcase.
- ✓ Divide the cauliflower into two, and move the half into a separate bowl, alongside the other ingredients.
- ✓ Mix well to form a dough and if necessary add some more cauliflower to ensure even combination.
- ✓ Twist the mixture into straw strips and move them into the air fryer baking mat.
- ✓ Allow cooking for 10 minutes at 360 F. Switch sides and allow cooking for another 10 minutes at 360 F. Serve.

496) Baked Camembert Cheese with Soldiers

Ingredients:

- 1 camembert
- 2 slices bread

Direction: Cooking Time: 20 minutes | Servings: 2

- ✓ Move your camembert, in a clean, sturdy container, into the air fryer.
- ✓ Allow cooking for 15 minutes at 360 F while shaking at 5-minute intervals.
- ✓ . This ensures that the cheese melts evenly.
- ✓ With about 2 minutes to the completion of the cooking, make the toast and then cut them into soldiers.
- ✓ Once the cheese is ready, rip the top layer off. Serve.

497) Low-Fat Mozzarella Cheese Sticks and marinara sauce

Ingredients:

- Salt and ground black pepper to taste
- 1 cup Italian breadcrumbs
- 1 egg ½ cup flour
- 10 pieces mozzarella string cheese
- 1 cup marinara sauce

Direction: Cooking Time: 30 minutes | Servings: 5

- ✓ Add salt and pepper to the breadcrumbs to taste. Into three different bowls, place the eggs, breadcrumbs, and the flour.
- ✓ Now dip each string of cheese in the flour, egg, and breadcrumbs respectively. To harden the sticks, freeze them for about an hour.
- ✓ This ensures that the cheese doesn't lose its stick shape while frying.
- ✓ To avoid the items getting a stick, season your air fryer before every use. You may use the coconut oil and a cooking brush to apply the seasoning.
- ✓ Set your air fryer to 400 F.
- ✓ Add the sticks to the fryer and allow cooking for 8 minutes. Withdraw the basket and flip each stick using thongs, while avoiding distorting the shapes.
- ✓ You may use your hands if the sticks are not too hot. Cook for 8 minutes more.
- ✓ After the timer goes off, retain the sticks in the air fryer pan for 5 minutes before withdrawing them from the pan. If any of the sticks leak some cheese on the outside, correct the shape of such sticks after it must have cooled. Serve with marinara sauce.

498) Homemade Mozzarella Sticks (ver. 2)

Ingredients:

- 3 oz gluten free oats
- 2 tbsp Italian seasoning
- 1 tbsp garlic powder
- 1 tsp basil
- 4 oz mozzarella
- Salt and ground black pepper to taste
- 1 medium egg

Direction: Cooking Time: 8 minutes | Servings: 6

- ✓ Combine the gluten free oats alongside all the seasonings in your blender and allow blending until you have a mixture like coarse breadcrumbs – this takes about 5 seconds.
- ✓ Dry the mozzarella by patting it with a clean tea towel or kitchen towel.
- ✓ Apply salt and pepper to season the mozzarella before cutting into stick pieces.
- ✓ Get a clean small dish and beat the egg into it. Set aside
- ✓ Get a larger mixing dish and transfer the blended oat mixture into it.
- ✓ Place the sticks of mozzarella in the oats mixture, then the egg, and finally into the oats mixture again.
- ✓ Transfer the coated sticks into the air fryer's baking pan.
- ✓ Allow cooking at 350 F for 3 minutes. Add some ketchup before serving.

499) Fried Mozzarella Sticks

Ingredients:

- Batter: ½ sp salt
- 1 tsp garlic powder
- ½ cup water
- ¼ cup all-purpose flour
- 5 tbsp cornstarch
- 1 tbsp cornmeal Coating:
- 1 cup panko bread crumbs
- ¼ tsp onion powder
- ½ tsp garlic powder
- ½ tsp parsley flakes
- ½ tsp ground black pepper
- ½ tsp salt ¼ tsp oregano, dried
- ¼ tsp basil, dried
- 5 oz mozzarella cheese, cut into
- ½ -inch strips
- 1 tbsp all-purpose flour, or as needed
- Cooking spray

Direction: Cooking Time: 1 hour 40 minutes | Servings: 4

- ✓ Get a clean shallow bowl and in it combine salt, garlic powder, water, flour, cornstarch, and cornmeal.
- ✓ Mix until you have the consistency of a pancake batter. You may add or remove ingredients to get the correct consistency.
- ✓ Get another wide, shallow bowl, and in it, combine panko, onion powder, garlic powder, parsley, pepper, salt, oregano and basil. Stir thoroughly.
- ✓ Coat the mozzarella sticks with flour, lightly one after the other. Place the coated stick in the batter and toss in the panko mixture.
- ✓ Remove when the stick is fully coated, and transfer to the baking sheet. With the sticks arranged in a single layer, allow them to freeze for at least an hour.
- ✓ Ensure that your air fryer is preheated to 400 F. Arrange the mozzarella sticks in a row in the air fryer basket, and spray lightly with cooking spray.
- ✓ Allow cooking for 6 minutes.
- ✓ After 6 minutes, flip the sticks using thongs, and resume cooking until the sticks are golden brown – or about 7-9 minutes.

500) Feta Triangles

Ingredients:

- 1 egg yolk
- 2 tbsp flat-leafed parsley, finely chopped
- 4 oz feta 1 green onion, finely sliced into rings
- Freshly ground black pepper
- 5 sheets of frozen filo pastry, defrosted

Direction: Cooking Time: 30 minutes | Servings: 3

- ✓ Get a clean bowl and in it, beat the egg and combine it with parsley, feta, and green onion. Season to taste with pepper.
- ✓ Make three strips out of each sheet of filo pastry. Take a full teaspoon of the feta mixture and place on the underside of a strip of pastry.
- ✓ Form a triangle by folding the pastry over the filling, after which you fold the strip zigzag until you have all the filling wrapped up in a triangle of pastry.
- ✓ Do the same for other strips. Ensure that your air fryer is preheated to 390 F.
- ✓ With little oil, brush the triangles lightly, before arranging them in the basket – 5 at a time.
- ✓ With the basket in the air fryer, allow baking for 3 minutes or until the feta triangles are golden brown.
- ✓ Do the same for other feta triangles. Serve the baked triangles in a platter.

501) Cheese and Onion Nuggets

Ingredients:

- 2 spring onion
- 7 oz Edam cheese
- 2 tbsp Kyle's mayonnaise
- Salt and ground black pepper to taste
- 1 tbsp thyme 1 tbsp coconut oil
- ¼ short crust pastry
- 1 small egg, beaten

Direction: Cooking Time: 20 minutes | Servings: 8

- ✓ Dice the cleaned spring onion into thin pieces.
- ✓ Grate the cheese.
- ✓ Combine the onion, mayonnaise, salt, pepper, dried thyme, and coconut oil in a medium mixing bowl.
- ✓ Mix thoroughly and make the mixture into eight small balls. Keep the balls in the fridge for an hour.
- ✓ Make eight nugget shapes out of your short crust pastry. Ensure that there are no gaps by sealing it up.
- ✓ With the aid of a pastry brush, brush the egg over the pastry.
- ✓ This gives them an eggy glow when cooked.
- ✓ Allow the egg to cook in the air fryer at 356 F for 12 minutes. Serve warm with the cheese still melting.

502) Airfryer Cheese and Bacon Fries

Ingredients:

- 2 medium potatoes, peeled
- 2 tsp olive oil
- 4 bacon rashers
- Salt and ground black pepper to taste
- 1 oz cheddar cheese, grated

Direction: Cooking Time: 25 minutes | Servings: 2 I

- ✓ Ensure that your air fryer is preheated to 360 F. Dice the peeled potatoes and transfer them into the air fryer.
- ✓ Sprinkle a teaspoon of olive oil over them.
- ✓ Allow cooking at 360 F for 10 minutes.
- ✓ Dice the fat-free bacon into bits, and add them to the cooked potatoes in the air fryer.
- ✓ . Allow the combination to cook for another 5 minutes.
- ✓ Shake and add another teaspoon of olive oil.
- ✓ Resume cooking for another 2 minutes but at a higher temperature of 390 F.
- ✓ Withdraw and sprinkle with pepper, salt, and the grated cheese. Serve.

503) Roasted Pepper Rolls

Ingredients:

- 2 medium-sized red, yellow and/or orange bell peppers,
- halved Filling as desired Tapas forks

Direction: Cooking Time: 40 minutes | Servings: 8

- ✓ Ensure that your air fryer is preheated to 390 F. In the air fryer basket, place the bell peppers and allow cooking for 10 minutes.
- ✓ The peppers will be roasted until they have slightly charred skin. Divide the peppers into two by cutting lengthwise. Remove the skin and the seeds.
- ✓ Apply your preferred filling in coating the bell pepper pieces. Roll them up, starting from the narrowest end.
- ✓ Use tapas forks to secure the rolls, before placing them in a platter.
- ✓ Fillings: Anchovy with Capers Empty a tin of anchovy fillets, and chop the fillets into fine bits.
- ✓ Combine the anchovy fillets with one crushed clove of garlic, two tablespoons of finely chopped parsley, some freshly ground black pepper, and two tablespoons of finely chopped capers.
- ✓ Mix. Feta with green onion Combine the crumbled 100g Greek Feta cheese with one thinly sliced green onion, alongside two teaspoons finely chopped oregano, and mix well. Tuna with Red Onion Empty one tin of tuna in olive oil, and combine with freshly ground black pepper, salt, two tablespoons of capers, one tablespoon of grated lemon peel, and one finely chopped red onion.

504) Mini Peppers with Goat Cheese

Ingredients:

- 8 mini or snack peppers
- 1 tsp freshly ground black pepper
- ½ tbsp olive oil
- 4 oz soft goat cheese, in eight pieces

Direction: Cooking Time: 20 minutes | Servings: 8

- ✓ Ensure that your air fryer is preheated to 390 F.
- ✓ Get rid of the membrane, seeds, and the caps of the mini peppers. In a deep mixing dish, combine the Italian herbs, the olive oil, and the pepper.
- ✓ Place the pieces of goat cheese in the mixture one after the other. Withdraw and transfer each piece into each of the mini pepper.
- ✓ Arrange the goat cheese-filled mini peppers in the basket, placing them next to each other.
- ✓ Return the basket into the air fryer. Allow baking for 8 minutes, or until you have the cheese all melted.
- ✓ Serve the mini peppers by placing them in small dishes. They are best eaten as snacks or appetizers.

505) Mini Frankfurters in Pastry

Ingredients:

- 1 tin of mini frankfurters (approx. 22 frankfurters)
- 4 oz ready-made puff pastry (chilled or frozen, defrosted) 1 tbsp fine mustard

Direction: Cooking Time: 35 minutes | Servings: 3

- ✓ Ensure that your air fryer is preheated to 390 F.
- ✓ Drain the sausages very well, on a layer of kitchen paper before dabbing them dry.
- ✓ Make strips of 2 x 0.5 inch out of the puff pastry, and coat each strip with a thin layer of mustard.
- ✓ Roll each sausage into a strip of pastry, spirally.
- ✓ Divide the rolled sausages into two.
- ✓ Transfer half into the air fryer basket and allow baking for 10 minutes or until they are golden brown.
- ✓ Do the same for the other half. Serve the sausages in a platter, alongside a small dish of mustard.

506) Mini Quiche Wedges

Ingredients:

- 4 oz (frozen or chilled) ready-made pie crust dough (pâte brisée)
- ½ tbsp oil
- 3 tbsp whipping cream
- 1½ oz Parmesan cheese, grated
- 1 egg Freshly ground black pepper to taste
- Salt to taste Filling as desired
- 2 small pie moulds of 4 inch

Direction: Cooking Time: 20 minutes | Servings: 6

- ✓ Ensure that your air fryer is preheated to 390 F.
- ✓ Make two rounds of 6 inch from the dough.
- ✓ Grease the molds lightly using oil and line them with the dough.
- ✓ Apply some force along the edges of the dough.
- ✓ Combine the cream, cheese, and the beaten egg in a bowl. Season with pepper and salt to taste
- ✓ Transfer the mixture into the molds and add the filling.
- ✓ Put only one mold in the air fryer basket and allow baking for 12 minutes or until it is golden brown.
- ✓ Do the same for the other quiches. Withdraw the quiches from the molds and cut each into six wedges.
- ✓ Serve the pieces warm or at room temperature.

507) Air fryer Pizza Hut Bread Sticks

Ingredients:

- 1/3 homemade pizza dough
- 2 tbsp desiccated coconut
- 1 tsp garlic puree
- 1 oz cheddar cheese Bread seeds, optional
- 1 tsp parsley
- Salt and ground black pepper to taste

Direction: Cooking Time: 30 minutes | Servings: 2

- ✓ Melt the coconut in a small pan until it becomes a liquid – preferably on medium heat.
- ✓ Pour in your seasonings alongside the garlic puree.
- ✓ Mix well. Shape your pizza dough into a thick rectangular shape.
- ✓ Coat it evenly with your garlic oil using a baking brush. Add some sprinkles of desiccated coconut oil on the top until it covers the garlic oil entirely.
- ✓ Add some additional sprinkles of cheddar cheese, and finally some bread seeds.
- ✓ Allow cooking in the air fryer for 10 minutes at 355 F. Set the temperature to 390 F and allow cooking for a further 5 minutes or until the pizza is crispy and nice on the outside, and hot in the middle.
- ✓ Chop the well-cooked pizza into fingers and serve.

508) Healthy Flapjacks Recipe

Ingredients:

- 4 oz butter
- 10 oz gluten free oats
- 4 oz brown sugar
- 2 tbsp honey

Direction: Cooking Time: 20 minutes | Servings:

- ✓ Place the baking pan on top of the air fryer grill pan and ensure that it slots in place inside the air fryer.
- ✓ Dice the butter into quarters and transfer them onto the baking pan.
- ✓ Allow cooking for 2 minutes at 360 F or until you have the butter melted.
- ✓ Blend the gluten-free oats in the blender until they appear like breadcrumbs.
- ✓ Combine the brown sugar and the honey, and finally the oats.
- ✓ Mix well with a fork until you have a smooth mixture.
- ✓ Allow cooking for 10 minutes at 320 F.
- ✓ Raise the temperature to 360 F and allow cooking for an extra 5 minutes.
- ✓ Withdraw and serve.

509) Air Fryer Chewy Granola Bars

Ingredients:

- 10 oz gluten free oats
- 1 oz brown sugar
- 1 tsp vanilla essence
- 1 tsp cinnamon
- 1 tbsp olive oil
- 3 tbsp honey
- 2 oz melted butter
- 1 medium apple, peeled and cooked
- Handful raisins

Direction: Cooking Time: 20 minutes | Servings: 6

- ✓ After blending the gluten-free oats into a smooth mixture, toss in the other dry ingredients.
- ✓ Combine the wet ingredients into the baking pan of the air fryer. Stir well using a small wooden spoon.
- ✓ Transfer the dry ingredients from the blender into the baking pan. Mix thoroughly with a fork.
- ✓ Toss in the raisins and press down the mixture into the baking pan, until it is all level. Allow cooking for 10 minutes at 320 F.
- ✓ Raise the temperature to 360 F and cook for an extra 5 minutes.
- ✓ Withdraw and transfer into the freezer for about 5 minutes or until it stiffens up. Cut into chewy sizes. Serve your granola bars.

510) Roasted Corn

Ingredients:

- 4 fresh ears of corn
- 2 to 3 tsp vegetable oil
- Salt and ground black pepper to taste

Direction: Cooking Time: 25 minutes | Servings: 2

- ✓ After getting rid of the husks from the corn, wash them and pat them dry.
- ✓ If your basket is too small for the corn, you would have to cut it.
- ✓ Add some drizzles of vegetable oil over the corn until the oil covers the corn well.
- ✓ Add some salt and pepper to season to taste.
- ✓ Allow cooking for 10 minutes at 400 F.

511) Banana Chips

Ingredients:

- 3-4 raw bananas
- ½ tsp salt
- ½ tsp turmeric powder
- 1 tsp oil
- ½ tsp chaat masala

Direction: Cooking Time: 35 minutes | Servings 2-3

- ✓ After peeling the bananas, keep them. Combine salt, turmeric powder, and water, and in this mixture, cut the bananas into slices.
- ✓ This ensures that the banana doesn't turn black and retains its nice yellow color.
- ✓ Retain the banana slices in the mixture for about 5 to 10 minutes.
- ✓ Withdraw the chips from the mixture and dry. Then add some oil on the chips – this ensures that they do not stick while in the air fryer.
- ✓ Ensure that your air fryer is preheated to 360 F for 5 minutes.
- ✓ Place the chips in the air fryer basket and allow air frying for 15 minutes at 360 F. Add chat masala and salt. Keep the chips in an airtight jar, and serve instantly.

512) Corn Tortilla Chips

Ingredients:
- 8 corn tortillas
- 1 tbsp olive oil
- Salt and ground black pepper to taste

Direction: Cooking Time: 10 minutes | Servings: 4

- ✓ Ensure that your air fryer is preheated to 390 F.
- ✓ With the aid of your knife, make triangles out of your corn tortillas, and brush each triangle with olive oil.
- ✓ Divide the whole tortillas into two – transfer the first batch into the wire basket.
- ✓ Allow air frying for 3 minutes.
- ✓ Do the same for the second batch. Add sprinkles of salt and serve.

513) Bacon Cashews

Ingredients:
- 3 cups raw cashews
- 2 tbsp blackstrap molasses
- 3 tbsp liquid smoke
- 2 tsp salt

Direction: Cooking Time: 15 minutes | Servings: 12

- ✓ Get a large bowl and in it, combine all the ingredients and coat the cashews generously and evenly with the mixture.
- ✓ Transfer the coated cashews into the air fryer basket, and allow cooking for 8-10 minutes at 350 F.
- ✓ While cooking, shake the basket at intervals of 2 minutes – this ensures that the cashews cook evenly.
- ✓ Be extra careful at the last 2 minutes and shake/check consistently to avoid burning the cashews.
- ✓ Allow the cooked cashews to cool to room temperature – this takes about 15 minutes.
- ✓ Then transfer the cool cashews into an airtight storage container and serve.

514) Pumpkin Seeds

Ingredients:
- 1½ cups pumpkin seeds from a large whole pumpkin
- Olive oil
- 1 tsp smoked paprika
- 1½ tsp salt

Direction: Cooking Time: 1 hour 15 minutes minutes

- ✓ After cutting the pumpkin open, use your spoon to scrape out the contents inside. Remove the seeds from the flesh, and rinse the seeds with cold water.
- ✓ Boil two quarts of salted water, and toss in the pumpkin seeds. Allow the seeds to boil for 10 minutes.
- ✓ Then withdraw the seeds, drain them, and spread on paper towels for at least 20 minutes or until they are dry. Ensure that your air fryer is preheated to 350 F.
- ✓ Combine olive oil, smoked paprika and salt into a bowl. Toss the seeds into the mixture, before moving them into the air fryer basket. Allow the seeds to air fry for 35 minutes, while shaking the basket consistently while cooking.
- ✓ Stop cooking when the seeds are crispy and slightly browned.
- ✓ Do not serve or store the seeds in a bag or air-tight container until they are cool. Serve as a snack or as toppings for yogurt or salad.

515) Spiced Nuts

Ingredients:
- 1 packet stevia Pinch cayenne pepper, optional
- ½ tbsp cinnamon
- 1 tbsp egg white
- 1 cup nuts (walnuts, pecans and almonds)

Direction: Cooking Time: 40 minutes | Servings: 8

- ✓ Ensure that your air fryer is preheated to 300 F.
- ✓ Get a small bowl and in it, combine the stevia, cayenne pepper, and cinnamon.
- ✓ Keep the mixture.
- ✓ Get another bowl and in it, mix the egg whites with the nuts.
- ✓ Now, combine the spices mixture and the egg white mixture. Transfer the new mixture into the air fryer basket.
- ✓ Set the timer to 10 minutes and allow the mixture to bake. After the first 10 minutes, stir and allow the mixture bake for an extra 10 minutes.
- ✓ Serve the nuts when they are completely cool.

516) Salted Nuts

Ingredients:
- ½ cup whole almonds
- ½ cup whole cashews
- ½ cup fox nuts / makhana, optional
- 1 tsp ghee Vegans can use olive oil or canola oil
- Salt and ground black pepper to taste

Note:
- You may choose the nuts of your choice like pecans or walnuts, or macadamia etc.
- You may air fry these together as a mix or separate.

Direction: Cooking Time: 15 minutes | Servings: 1

- ✓ Ensure that your air fryer is preheated to 350 F for 2 minutes.
- ✓ Put all the nuts in a bowl, and add one teaspoon of melted ghee.
- ✓ With your hands, rub the nuts with the melted ghee, and transfer them into the air fryer.
- ✓ Allow them to air fry for 6 minutes. After 4 minutes, withdraw the basket and toss the nuts well.
- ✓ Return them into the basket and resume air frying for the remaining 2 minutes. In the end, you will have nice and pinkish nuts.
- ✓ If your preference is a darker rich color, extend the air frying time by 2 minutes.
- ✓ Withdraw the fried nuts and transfer them into a steel or glass bowl. Do not use plastic bowls, please. Add sprinkles of black pepper and salt, then toss well. Serve.

517) Low Carb Roasted Nuts

Ingredients:
- 2 cups pecan halves
- 1 tbsp butter, ghee, or oil
- 1-2 tsp of ground pink Himalayan

Direction: Cooking Time: 20 minutes | Servings: 2-3

- ✓ Ensure that your air fryer is preheated to 390 F for about 5 minutes.
- ✓ Melt your ghee or butter, or oil. Add some salt.
- ✓ Add some pecan halves into the melted butter and stir until the pecan are entirely coated.
- ✓ Transfer into the air fryer and allow air-frying for 4-6 minutes at 390 F or until the nuts are toasty.
- ✓ While frying, toss at 2 minutes interval.
- ✓ Withdraw and serve.

518) Frugal Cheesy Homemade Garlic Bread

Ingredients:

- 10 inch homemade pizza dough
- 5 oz cream cheese
- 5 oz butter
- 1 tsp garlic puree
- 1 tsp parsley
- Salt and ground black pepper to taste

Direction: Cooking Time: 30 minutes | Servings: 4

- ✓ Roll out your pizza dough and prepare it for topping.
- ✓ Add a layer of soft cheese on your base. Melt your butter in a pan on medium heat. Stop when you have a nice and runny liquid.
- ✓ Pour the melted butter into the garlic puree, salt, parsley, and pepper.
- ✓ Place the garlic butter mixture such that it forms a layer on top of the cream cheese.
- ✓ Transfer the layered dough into the oven.
- ✓ Allow cooking for 20 minutes at 355 F. Serve.

519) Budget Friendly Air fryer Mini Cheese Scones

Ingredients:

- 6 oz self raising flour
- 1 oz butter
- 1 tsp chives
- 1 tsp mustard
- Salt and ground black pepper to taste
- 3 oz cheddar cheese
- 1 medium egg 1 tbsp whole milk

Direction: Cooking Time: 35 minutes | Servings: 10

- ✓ Ensure that your air fryer is preheated to 355 F.
- ✓ Combine the flour and butter in a large mixing bowl.
- ✓ Mix until the mixture appears like fine breadcrumbs.
- ✓ Then toss in your seasonings, alongside 2 oz worth of the cheddar cheese.
- ✓ Mix thoroughly, again.
- ✓ Add the egg and milk, and mix again, preferably with your hands.
- ✓ Continue until the mixture appears like soft dough. To achieve the desired softness, you may add some more milk.
- ✓ Roll out until you have a thickness of ½ inch, then divide into ten equal pieces.
- ✓ Place some of the leftover cheese in the middle of each piece, and shape them into balls.
- ✓ You will have a lovely melted cheese center if done properly. Transfer the mini scones into the air fryer.
- ✓ Allow cooking for 20 minutes at 355 F. Slice the cooked scones in half, and place some butter in the center of each slice. Serve.

520) Bruschetta Recipe

Ingredients:

- 1 medium tomato Salt and ground black pepper to taste 1 tbsp oregano
- 3 tbsp olive oil 1 tbsp garlic puree 1 oz Italian cheese Fresh basil Medium Ciabatta

Direction: Cooking Time: 10 minutes | Servings: 4

- ✓ Dice the fresh tomato into thin small pieces. Season to taste with salt, pepper, and oregano.
- ✓ Get a small mixing bowl and in it combine the olive oil and the garlic puree, alongside the seasonings.
- ✓ Mix and set aside. Slice the ciabatta into medium-sized pieces and brush one side with the garlic mixture above with the aid of a pastry brush.
- ✓ Allow the ciabatta pieces cook in the air fryer grill pan for 4 minutes at 360 F, with the oil sides facing down.
- ✓ Turn the pieces to the other side using your thongs, and decorate the other side with cheese, tomatoes, and the fresh basil respectively.
- ✓ Allow the pieces to cook again for 2 minutes but at 390 F. Serve while warm.

521) Two Ingredient Croutons

Ingredients:

- 2 slices wholemeal bread
- 1 tbsp olive oil

Direction: Cooking Time: 15 minutes | Servings: 8

- ✓ Cut your bread slices into chunks of medium sizes.
- ✓ Transfer the chunks into the air fryer and add the olive oil.
- ✓ Allow cooking for 8 minutes at 390 F.
- ✓ Serve as a snack or over your soup.

522) Vegan Croutons

Ingredients:

- 2 heaping cups of cubed baguette (or your preferred bread), cut in
- 1 inch pieces
- 2 tsp extra virgin olive oil
- 2 tsp lemon juice
- ½ tsp dried basil
- ½ tsp granulated garlic
- ½ tsp dried oregano
- Salt and ground black pepper to taste

Direction: Cooking Time: 15 minutes | Servings: 2

- ✓ Get a clean large mixing bowl, and in it, add the cubed baguette, drizzles of extra virgin olive oil, and lemon juice across the bread.
- ✓ Then sprinkle the dried basil, garlic granules, dried oregano, salt, and pepper.
- ✓ With your hands, coat the cubed bread evenly by tossing it into the spices mixture.
- ✓ For easy coating, ensure that the spices are on the bread instead of being stuck on the sides of the bowl.
- ✓ Transfer the bread into the air fryer, and allow cooking for 5 minutes at 400 F.
- ✓ Shake the basket once or twice within this cooking time. Serve as toppings for your favorite salad.

523) Garlic Bread Recipe

Ingredients:

- 1 small egg
- 1 oz whole milk
- ½ French bread stick
- 2 tsp garlic puree
- 2 tbsp olive oil
- 1 tsp parsley

Direction: Cooking Time: 50 minutes | Servings: 4

- ✓ Get a clean mixing bowl, and in it, combine the milk and egg. Beat until you have a smooth mixture.
- ✓ Chop your French bread into garlic bread pieces. Submerge them in the egg and milk mixture until the pieces are entirely coated with the egg and milk.
- ✓ Shake off any excess coating. Place the bread in the air fryer grill pan, spreading it out to ensure that the bread pieces do not overlap.
- ✓ Get a small bowl, and in it, mix the garlic, olive oil, and parsley. With the aid of your pastry brush, brush the garlic mixture over the top of the bread.
- ✓ Return the grill pan into the air fryer and allow cooking for 2 minutes at 360 F.
- ✓ After two minutes of cooking, turn the sides, and brush the other side too.
- ✓ Cook for an extra 2 minutes. Withdraw and serve immediately.

524) British Fish and Chip Shop Healthy Battered Sausage and Chips

Ingredients:

- 2 large potatoes, peeled
- 1 tbsp olive oil
- 2 slices wholemeal bread Salt and ground black pepper to taste
- 1 medium egg beaten
- 4 oz plain flour
- 4 medium thick sausages

Direction: Cooking Time: 45 minutes | Servings: 2

- ✓ Ensure that your air fryer is preheated to 360 F. Cut your peeled potatoes into chips, transfer them into the air fryer, and add a tablespoon of olive oil. Prepare your breaded crust by transferring the whole wholemeal bread in the air fryer, right on the chips, and harden it for about 5 minutes. Withdraw the bread after 5 minutes and break into bread crumbs.
- ✓ Combine the breadcrumbs with some salt and pepper, in a clean dish. Get another dish and add the egg. And in the third dish, add the flour.
- ✓ Make the breaded sausage by placing each sausage into your hand and rolling it in the flour, and the egg, and finally in the bread crumbs mixture.
- ✓ Repeat for all the sausage pieces or at least four battered sausages.
- ✓ Transfer the battered sausages into the air fryer, on top of the potatoes. Allow cooking for 10 minutes at 360 F.
- ✓ Withdraw the chips after 10 minutes and cook only the sausages for an extra 5 minutes. Serve.

525) Pigs In a Blanket

Ingredients:

- 1 can (8 oz) of crescent rolls
- 1 pack (12 oz) of cocktail franks or mini smoked sausages

Direction: Cooking Time: 25 minutes | Servings: 16

- ✓ Withdraw and drain the cocktail franks from the package.
- ✓ To get rid of any remaining moisture, dry with a paper towel.
- ✓ Remove the crescent rolls dough from the can, and form eight triangles from it. Make two thin triangles from each of the eight triangles.
- ✓ In the end, you will have 16 triangles. Place one frank on the triangle (on the widest part) and roll up.
- ✓ Do the same for the other franks and triangles.
- ✓ Transfer about 8 "Pigs in a Blanket" into the air fryer basket, and air fry for 8 minutes at 330 F.
- ✓ Do the same for the other 8.
- ✓ Serve the fried Pigs in a Blanket alongside hot ketchup, gesso dip, salsa, or mustard.

526) Chicken Breasts in a Bag

Ingredients:

- 1 carrot (thinly sliced)
- Butter Salt and ground black pepper to taste
- 2 chicken breast halves
- 1 lemon (halves)
- Bunch of sage

Direction: Time: 1 hour 10 minutes | Servings: 1-2

- ✓ Ensure that your air fryer is preheated at 375 F.
- ✓ Cut your parchment papers (2 pcs) into a square shape.
- ✓ Divide the sliced carrots equally on each paper.
- ✓ To each portion, add a sufficient lump of butter plus pepper and salt (or other seasonings)
- ✓ Place the chicken breast on the carrot slices.
- ✓ Then add a squeeze of lemon juice, a couple of sage leaves, and finally, a knob of butter again.
- ✓ Fold all the four corners of each parchment paper to make it air tight. Place the first bag on the baking tray, and allow to bake for about 20-25 minutes.
- ✓ Remove once the carrot feels soft.
- ✓ Do the same for the other bag.
- ✓ Open the bag
- ✓ serve.

527) Stuffed Chicken Breasts (Mexican-Style)

Ingredients:

- 4 extra-long toothpicks
- 4 tsp ground cumin, divided
- 4 tsp chili powder, divided 1
- skinless, boneless chicken breast
- 2 tsp chipotle
- flakes Salt and ground black pepper
- 2 tsp Mexican oregano
- ½ red bell pepper, sliced into thin strips
- 1 fresh jalapeno pepper, sliced into thin strips
- ½ onion, sliced into thin strips
- 2 tsp olive oil
- ½ lime, juiced

Direction: Time: 30 minutes | Servings: 2

- ✓ Soak your toothpicks into a small bowl of water.
- ✓ This ensures that they do not burn while cooking.
- ✓ Get a shallow dish and make a mixture of 2 teaspoons cumin and two teaspoons of chili powder.
- ✓ Ensure that your air fryer is preheated at 400 F.
- ✓ While placing on a flat work surface, slice the chicken horizontally through the middle.
- ✓ With the aid of a rolling pin or kitchen mallet, pound each half of the chicken until you have a thickness of about ¼ inch.
- ✓ Mix the remaining chili powder, cumin, chipotle, pepper, salt, and oregano.
- ✓ Sprinkle the mixture on each breast half, equally.
- ✓ Place ½ of the bell pepper, jalapeno, and onion in the center of one breast half.
- ✓ With the aid of two toothpicks, keep the chicken in the position where the tapered end faces upward.
- ✓ Repeat the process for the other breast – add spices, vegetables, and secure with the unused toothpicks.
- ✓ Roll each breast half in the chili-cumin mixture.
- ✓ Then, drizzle olive oil on them until it covers all the surface evenly.
- ✓ Transfer the roll-ups into the air-fryer basket such that the toothpick side faces up.
- ✓ Set your air fryer timer to six minutes.
- ✓ After six minutes, turn the roll-ups over on the other side.
- ✓ Cook again in the air fryer, and continue until the juices run clear and a reading of 165 F is seen on an instant-read thermometer.
- ✓ Cook at this temperature for an additional five minutes.
- ✓ Withdraw the roll-ups from the air fryer, and drizzle lime juice on each evenly.
- ✓ Serve.

528) Chicken Wings in Nandos Marinade

Ingredients:

- 1½ lbs chicken wings
- 10 oz homemade Nandos marinade
- Salt and ground black pepper to taste

Direction: Time: 25 minutes | Servings: 2-4

- ✓ Season the chicken wings by rubbing thoroughly with pepper and salt.
- ✓ Transfer the seasoned chickens in a Ziplock bag or foil.
- ✓ Cover the wings with about 3 oz Nandos marinade and lock the Ziplock bag.
- ✓ Place in the fridge and leave for 10-12 hours.
- ✓ The following day, ensure that your air fryer is preheated to 360 F.
- ✓ Withdraw the chicken from the fridge and place them in the air fryer.
- ✓ Set the timer to 20 minutes and allow cooking.
- ✓ The unused Nandos marinade should be served alongside the cooked wings as the dipping sauce.

529) Herb Seasoned Turkey Breast

Ingredients:

- 2 lbs turkey breast
- 1 tsp fresh sage, chopped
- 1 tsp fresh rosemary, chopped
- 1 tsp fresh thyme, chopped
- Pepper Salt

Direction: Time: 45 minutes - Serve: 4

- ✓ Spray air fryer basket with cooking spray.
- ✓ In a small bowl, mix together sage, rosemary, and thyme.
- ✓ Season turkey breast with pepper and salt and rub with herb mixture.
- ✓ Place turkey breast in air fryer basket and cook at 390 F for 30-35 minutes.
- ✓ Slice and serve.

530) Delicious Rotisserie Chicken

Ingredients:

- 3 lbs chicken, cut into eight pieces
- 1/4 tsp cayenne
- 1 tsp paprika
- 2 tsp onion powder
- 1/2 tsp garlic powder
- 1/2 tsp dried oregano
- 1/2 tbsp dried thyme
- Pepper Salt

Direction: Time: 30 minutes Serve: 6

- ✓ Season chicken with pepper and salt.
- ✓ In a bowl, mix together spices and herbs and rub spice mixture over chicken pieces.
- ✓ Spray air fryer basket with cooking spray.
- ✓ Place chicken in air fryer basket and cook at 350 F for 10 minutes.
- ✓ Turn chicken to another side and cook for 10 minutes more or until the internal temperature of chicken reaches at 165 F.
- ✓ Serve and enjoy.

531) Chicken Wings in Orange Sauce

Ingredients:

- 6 chicken wings
- Orange juice from 1 orange
- 1 tsp orange zest
- 1½ tbsp Worcestershire sauce
- Country herbs (basil, oregano, mint, parsley, thyme, rosemary and sage)
- 1 tbsp sugar Salt and ground black pepper to taste

Direction: Time: 1 hour 5 minutes | Servings: 2

- ✓ Ensure that the Air Fryer is preheated to 360 F.
- ✓ Ensure that the chicken wings are washed well and pat dry.
- ✓ Mix juice and orange zest in a big clean bowl.
- ✓ Place the chicken wings inside the bowl and stir well until the wings are fully coated.
- ✓ Make a mixture of Worcestershire sauce, country herbs, sugar, salt, and black pepper in another bowl.
- ✓ Rub all sides of the wing with this mixture.
- ✓ Wrap the rubbed/coated chicken wings, alongside the sauce, with an aluminum foil.
- ✓ Transfer the wrapped wings into the air fryer and let it cook for 20 minutes.
- ✓ Remove the cooked chicken wings with the sauce and place them in a bowl.
- ✓ Using the sauce, brush the wings before returning them into the air fryer.
- ✓ Do not dispose of the remains of the orange sauce.
- ✓ Let the wings cook for another 15 minutes in the air fryer.
- ✓ Remove and brush again with the remains of the orange source.
- ✓ Cook for an additional ten minutes.
- ✓ Remove from the fryer

532) Spicy Asian Chicken Thighs

Ingredients:

- 4 chicken thighs, skin-on, and bone-in
- 2 tsp ginger, grated
- 1 lime juice
- 2 tbsp chili garlic sauce
- 1/4 cup olive oil
- 1/3 cup soy sauce

Direction: Time: 30 minutes Serve: 4

- ✓ In a large bowl, whisk together ginger, lime juice, chili garlic sauce, oil, and soy sauce.
- ✓ Add chicken in bowl and coat well with marinade and place in the refrigerator for 30 minutes.
- ✓ Place marinated chicken in air fryer basket and cook at 400 F for 15-20 minutes or until the internal temperature of chicken reaches at 165 F.
- ✓ Turn chicken halfway through.
- ✓ Serve and enjoy.

533) Spicy and Crispy Chicken Wing Drumettes

Ingredients:

- 10 large chicken wing drumettes
- Cooking spray
- 1 tbsp soy sauce
- 3/8 tsp red pepper, crushed
- 2 tbsp chicken stock, unsalted
- 1 clove garlic, chopped
- ¼ cup rice vinegar
- 1 tbsp toasted sesame oil
- 3 tbsp honey
- 2 tbsp roasted peanuts, unsalted and chopped
- 1 tbsp fresh chives, chopped

Direction: Time: 40 minutes | Servings: 2

- ✓ Ensure that the Air Fryer is preheated to 400 F.
- ✓ For better space management, arrange the drumettes to the sides of the chicken in the air fryer basket.
- ✓ While in the basket, spray them with the cooking spray. Allow the sprayed chicken to cook for 15 minutes before flipping on the other side and allowing to cook for 15 minutes again.
- ✓ Make a mixture of soy sauce, red pepper, chicken stock, garlic, rice vinegar, sesame oil, and honey in a clean skillet.
- ✓ Using a medium-height heat, stir and bring the honey sauce till it simmers.
- ✓ Then cook for 6 minutes – the sauce will appear slightly thickened.
- ✓ Put the cooked chicken wings into a clean bowl and add the honey sauce, then stir mildly.
- ✓ Once the wings are well coated, sprinkle with peanuts and chopped chives. Serve.

534) Turkey Scotch Eggs

Ingredients:

- 4 hard-boiled eggs, peeled
- 1 cup panko breadcrumbs
- 1 egg, beaten in a bowl
- 1 lb ground turkey
- ½ tsp dried rosemary
- Salt and black pepper to taste

Direction: Time: 20 minutes Servings: 4

- ✓ Preheat the air fryer to 400 F. In a bowl, mix panko breadcrumbs with rosemary.
- ✓ In another bowl, pour the ground turkey and mix it with salt and pepper.
- ✓ Shape into 4 balls.
- ✓ Wrap the balls around the boiled eggs to form a large ball with the egg in the center.
- ✓ Dip in the beaten egg and coat with breadcrumbs.
- ✓ Place in the greased frying basket and Bake for 12-14 minutes, shaking once.
- ✓ Serve and enjoy!

535) Air-Fried Chicken Drumettes

Ingredients:

- ½ lbs chicken wing drumettes
- Olive oil cooking spray
- 1 tbsp lower-sodium soy sauce
- ½ tsp cornstarch
- 1 tsp finely chopped garlic
- ½ tsp finely chopped fresh ginger
- 1 tsp sambal oelek (ground fresh chili paste)
- 1/8 tsp kosher salt
- 1 tsp fresh lime juice
- 2 tsp honey
- 2 tbsp chopped scallions

Direction: Time: 30 minutes | Servings: 2-4

- ✓ Pat the rinsed chicken drumettes dry using the paper towels and then spray with olive oil.
- ✓ Ensure that your air fryer is preheated to 400 F.
- ✓ Transfer the chicken drumettes in the air fryer, maintaining a single layer.
- ✓ Allow cooking in the air fryer for 22 minutes, while shaking twice or thrice.
- ✓ Withdraw the drumettes when crispy.
- ✓ With the drumettes in the air fryer, get a clean saucepan, and combine the soy sauce and cornstarch.
- ✓ Toss in the garlic, ginger, sambal, salt, lime juice, and honey.
- ✓ Stir the mixture thoroughly and transfer to medium-high heat.
- ✓ Cook until the mixture becomes thickened and starts to form bubbles.
- ✓ Remove the chicken drumettes and place them in a big bowl.
- ✓ Pour the sauce mixture over the drumettes and stir mildly.
- ✓ Add chopped scallions and toppings before serving.

536) Wings in a Peach-Bourbon Sauce

Ingredients:

- ½ cup peach preserves
- 1 tbsp brown sugar
- ¼ tsp kosher salt
- 1 garlic cloves, minced
- 2 tbsp white vinegar (or white wine)
- 2 tbsp bourbon
- 1 tsp cornstarch
- 1 tsp water
- Olive oil cooking spray
- 2 lbs chicken wings, without wing tips

Direction: Time: 50 minutes | Servings: 2-4

- ✓ Ensure that your Air Fryer is preheated to 400 F.
- ✓ Clean your blender or food processor.
- ✓ Put the peach preserves, sugar, salt, and garlic in it and blend until the mixture is smooth.
- ✓ Get a clean saucepan and transfer the blended peach mixture into it.
- ✓ On medium-high heat, boil the mixture of vinegar and bourbon.
- ✓ When boiling, reduce the heat and simmer of about four to six minutes, until there is a little thickness.
- ✓ Make a mixture of cornstarch and water in a clean bowl, and stir until you have a smooth mixture.
- ✓ Add the cornstarch mixture to the peach mixture.
- ✓ Boil and allow to cook for one to two minutes with frequent stirring.
- ✓ Keep ¼ of this sauce separately.
- ✓ Brush each wing with the sauce.
- ✓ Each brushed wing should be arranged in a single layer in the basket.
- ✓ Allow to cook for seven minutes before flipping and brushing the other side of the wing with the sauce.
- ✓ Then allow cooking for additional 8 minutes.
- ✓ For best results, you may have to divide the wings into two groups and treat each group separately.
- ✓ Serve the cooked wings with the ¼ sauce reserved.

537) Spicy Drumsticks with Barbecue Marinade

Ingredients:

- 1 tsp chili powder
- 2 tsp brown sugar
- 1 clove garlic, crushed
- ½ tbsp mustard
- salt, Freshly ground black pepper
- 1 tbsp olive oil
- 4 drumsticks

Direction: Time: 45 minutes | Servings: 4

- ✓ Ensure that the Air Fryer is preheated to 390 F.
- ✓ Create a mixture of the chili powder, brown sugar, garlic, mustard, and add a pinch of salt and freshly ground pepper to taste.
- ✓ Add oil to this mixture, stir.
- ✓ Do a thorough rubbing of the drumsticks, using the marinade and allow the rubbed sticks to marinate for 20 minutes.
- ✓ Now, place the drumsticks in the basket, and put the basket into the Air Fryer, allowing to roast for 10 minutes, or until they are brown.
- ✓ Drop the air fryer temperature to 300 F and allow them to roast for additional 10 minutes.
- ✓ Remove the roasted drumsticks.
- ✓ serve with French bread and corn salad.

538) Chicken Quesadillas

Ingredients:

- Cooking spray
- Soft taco shells
- Mexican cheese, shredded
- Chicken fajita strips
- ½ cup onions, sliced
- ½ cup green peppers, sliced
- Sour cream, optional Salsa, (optional)

Direction: Time: 40 minutes | Servings: 4

- ✓ Ensure that your air fryer is preheated to 370 F for 3 minutes and spray the pan with some vegetable oil.
- ✓ Get a pan and place one soft taco shell in it, add the shredded cheese on the shell.
- ✓ Arrange the fajita chicken strips to form a single layer and add the onions and green peppers on the strips.
- ✓ Add extra shredded cheese.
- ✓ Now place another soft taco shell on the top and spray with some vegetable oil.
- ✓ To hold the shell in place, put the rack that came with the air fryer on the top.
- ✓ Set the air fryer timer for 4 minutes, and then change to the other side using a large spatula.
- ✓ Spray again with vegetable oil and place the rack on the top of the shell to hold it in place. Set the timer for four minutes.
- ✓ If you want it to be crispier, let it stay a couple of additional minutes in the air fryer.
- ✓ Withdraw when you are satisfied with the crispiness.
- ✓ Cut into four or six slices.
- ✓ Serve alongside sour cream and Salsa (not compulsory).

539) Coconut and Turmeric Chicken

Ingredients:

- 3 pcs whole chicken leg (de-skin or with skin is totally up to you)
- 4-5 tsp ground turmeric
- ½ tbsp salt
- 2 oz galangal
- 2 oz pure coconut paste (or coconut milk)
- 2 oz old ginger

Direction: Time: 4 hours 40 minutes | Servings: 2-3

- ✓ Do not pound or blend the chicken meat; all other ingredients should be pounded or blended.
- ✓ With a focus on the thick parts, cut a few slits on the leg of the chicken.
- ✓ The cuttings will increase the absorption of the flavor during marinating.
- ✓ Add the blended ingredients to the chicken and allow to marinate for not less than four hours, or if possible, overnight.
- ✓ During the marinating process, the seasoned chicken should be wrapped with a cling film and stored inside the refrigerator.
- ✓ Set the Air Fryer to 375 F and allow to preheat at this temperature, then air-fry the chicken for about 20-25 minutes, frying each side for half of the total time.
- ✓ Once you have a golden brown chicken, you can proceed to serve.

540) Sandwich

Ingredients:

- 3 tbsp half and half ¼ tsp vanilla extract, 1 egg
- 2 slices sourdough, white or multigrain bread
- 2½ oz sliced Swiss cheese
- 2 oz slices deli ham
- 2 oz sliced deli turkey
- 1 tsp butter, melted
- Powdered sugar Raspberry jam

Direction: Time: 25 minutes | Servings: 1

- ✓ Mix the half and half, vanilla extract and the egg in a shallow bowl.
- ✓ Build your sandwich by putting your bread on the counter, and then add a slice of Swiss cheese, the ham, the turkey, and then the second slice of Swiss cheese on one slice of the bread.
- ✓ Finally, top with the other side of the bread.
- ✓ To flatten the combination, simply press down slightly.
- ✓ Ensure that your air fryer is preheated to 350 F.
- ✓ Brush an aluminum foil (almost the same size as the bread) with melted butter.
- ✓ Dip the two sides of the sandwich in the egg batter, one after the other.
- ✓ Allow the batter soak into either side of the bread for 30 seconds each.
- ✓ Transfer the soaked sandwich on the greased aluminum foil and transfer it to the air fryer basket.
- ✓ You can get an extra brown sandwich by brushing the top with melted butter.
- ✓ Set the air fryer temperature to 350 F and timer to 10 minutes.
- ✓ After 10 minutes, flip the sandwich over, and brush again with butter.
- ✓ Now, air-fry for an extra 8 minutes.
- ✓ Place the air-fried sandwich on a serving plate and add sprinkles of powdered sugar.
- ✓ Serve alongside raspberry or blackberry preserves.

541) Chick-fil-A Chicken Sandwich

Ingredients:

- 2 boneless/skinless chicken breasts, pounded
- ½ cup dill pickle juice
- 2 eggs
- ½ cup milk
- ½ tsp garlic powder
- 2 tbsp powdered sugar
- 1 tsp paprika
- ¼ tsp ground celery seed ground
- Salt
- freshly ground black pepper
- 1 tbsp extra virgin olive oil
- 1 cup all purpose flour
- 1 oil mister
- 4 hamburger buns toasted/buttered
- 8 dill pickle chips or more Homemade mayonnaise
- cayenne pepper for spicy sandwiches

Direction: Time: 30 minutes | Servings: 2

- ✓ Put the chicken into a Ziploc Baggie and pound.
- ✓ This is to ensure an even thickness – of about 0.5 inches thick.
- ✓ Depending on how big your chicken is, you may cut into two or three pieces.
- ✓ Transfer the cut chicken back into the Ziploc bag and pour the pickle juice in the bag.
- ✓ Allow resting in the refrigerator for 30 minutes to ensure that it marinates.
- ✓ Get a medium-sized bowl and in it, beat the egg and add milk.
- ✓ Get another bowl, and in it, mix the spices and the flour.
- ✓ With the aid of tongs, coat the chicken generously with the egg mixture; dip it into the flour mixture while also ensuring that it is well coated.
- ✓ Shake off excess flour. Spray the base of the air fryer with the cooking coil.
- ✓ Transfer the coated chicken into the air fryer, and spray again with the cooking oil.
- ✓ Allow the chicken to cook for 6 minutes at 340 F.
- ✓ Use your silicone tongs to flip the chicken gently, then spray with oil and cook for an extra 6 minutes.
- ✓ After this, increase the temperature to 400 F and cook for two minutes extra on each side.
- ✓ Serve on toasted and buttered buns, alongside two pickle chips and possibly a small dollop of mayonnaise.

542) Chicken Popcorn

Ingredients:

- 4 eggs
- 1/2 lbs chicken breasts, cut into small chunks
- 1 tsp paprika
- 1/2 tsp garlic powder
- 1 tsp onion powder
- 2 1/2 cups pork rind, crushed
- 1/4 cup coconut flour
- Pepper, Salt

Direction: Time: 20 minutes Serving: 6

- ✓ In a small bowl, mix together coconut flour, pepper, and salt.
- ✓ In another bowl, whisk eggs until combined.
- ✓ Take one more bowl and mix together pork panko, paprika, garlic powder, and onion powder.
- ✓ Add chicken pieces in a large mixing bowl.
- ✓ Sprinkle coconut flour mixture over chicken and toss well.
- ✓ Dip chicken pieces in the egg mixture and coat with pork panko mixture and place on a plate.
- ✓ Spray air fryer basket with cooking spray.
- ✓ Preheat the air fryer to 400 F. Add half prepared chicken in air fryer basket and cook for 10-12 minutes.
- ✓ Shake basket halfway through.
- ✓ Cook remaining half using the same method.
- ✓ Serve and enjoy.

543) Delicious & Easy Meatballs

Ingredients:

- 1 lb ground chicken
- 1 egg, lightly beaten
- 1/2 cup mozzarella cheese, shredded
- 1/2 tbsp taco seasoning
- 3 garlic cloves, minced
- 3 tbsp fresh parsley, chopped
- 1 small onion, minced
- Pepper Salt

Direction: Time: 20 minutes - Serve: 4

- ✓ Add all ingredients into the large mixing bowl and mix until well combined.
- ✓ Make small balls from mixture and place in the air fryer basket.
- ✓ Cook meatballs for 10 minutes at 400 F.
- ✓ Serve.

544) Garlic Parmesan Breaded Fried Chicken Wings

Ingredients:

- 16 chicken wing drumettes
- Chicken seasoning to taste
- Ground black pepper to taste
- 2 tbsp soy sauce
- ½ cup flour
- 1 tsp garlic powder
- ¼ cup parmesan, grated
- ¼ cup buttermilk, low-fat
- Cooking spray
- 1 tsp parmesan, grated

Direction: Time: 40 minutes | Servings: 4-6

- ✓ With the aid of a paper towel, clean and pat dry the chicken wing drumettes.
- ✓ Add chicken seasoning as well as black pepper, preferably in sprinkles.
- ✓ Put in a Ziploc bag after a quick brush with a soy sauce, and refrigerate the bag for 60 to 120 minutes.
- ✓ Mix flour, garlic powder, and ¼ cup of parmesan in another bowl.
- ✓ Pour the buttermilk in a new bowl.
- ✓ Now, take each of the refrigerated chicken drumettes and dip in the buttermilk, before coating them with the mixture.
- ✓ Ensure that the Air Fryer is preheated to 400 F.
- ✓ Before placing the chicken in the air fryer pan, spray the inside with the cooking spray.
- ✓ Now, sprinkle the cooking spray over the drummettes.
- ✓ Proceed to cook for about 20 minutes.
- ✓ Shake the pot twice or thrice while cooking.
- ✓ After 20 minutes of cooking, let the wings cool down a little before serving with one tablespoon of parmesan.
- ✓ Serve.

545) Quick & Easy Chicken Breast

Ingredients:

- 4 chicken breasts, skinless and boneless
- 1/2 tsp dried oregano
- 1/2 tsp dried basil
- 1/2 tsp dried thyme
- 1/2 tsp garlic powder
- 2 tbsp olive oil
- 1/8 tsp pepper
- 1/2 tsp salt

Direction: Time: 32 minutes Serve: 4

- ✓ In a small bowl, mix together olive oil, oregano, basil, thyme, garlic powder, pepper, and salt.
- ✓ Rub herb oil mixture all over chicken breasts.
- ✓ Spray air fryer basket with cooking spray.
- ✓ Place chicken in air fryer basket and cook at 360 F for 10 minutes.
- ✓ Turn chicken to another side and cook for 8-12 minutes more or until the internal temperature of chicken reaches at 165 F.
- ✓ Serve and enjoy.

546) Spicy Air-Fried Chicken Thighs

Ingredients:

- ½ tsp cayenne pepper
- 1 tsp paprika 2 cups low-fat buttermilk
- 4 (6- to 7-oz.) boneless, skinless chicken thighs
- 1 cup (about 4¼ oz.) all-purpose flour
- 2 large eggs
- 2 tbsp water
- 2 cups whole-wheat panko (Japanese-style breadcrumbs)
- ½ tsp kosher salt Cooking spray
- 2 tsp hot sauce (such as Franks Red-hot)

Direction: Time: 6 hours 30 minutes | Servings: 4

- ✓ Get a large, clean bowl and make a mixture of cayenne pepper, paprika, and buttermilk inside it.
- ✓ Add the chicken thighs, allowing both sides to coat. Then cover and marinate the coated chicken thighs in the refrigerator overnight or for not less than 6 hours. In a shallow dish, add some flour. In another shallow dish, add eggs and water and whisk the mixture mildly.
- ✓ Get a third shallow dish and place the panko in it. Remove the chicken from the marinade and dispose of the remnants. Sprinkle the chicken with salt and then dredge in flour.
- ✓ Shake the chicken to get rid of the excess flour. Dip into the egg mixture, and allowing excess egg to drip off.
- ✓ Dredge the chicken in the panko, while adding a bit of force for adherence, before coating the chicken on either side, using the cooking spray. Spray the air fryer basket mildly with the cooking spray.
- ✓ The chicken is best placed in the basket in a single layer, and start cooking in batches, at 400 F for each batch.
- ✓ Continue this until a thermometer placed in the chicken reads 165 F, with the coating turning golden brown and crispy.
- ✓ Leave for 16 minutes.
- ✓ Ensure that you turn the chicken over midway through cooking. It is best served immediately, with each chicken thigh on a plate, drizzled with ½ teaspoon hot sauce.

547) Simply Fried Chicken Thighs

Ingredients:

- 1 tsp kosher salt
- ½ cup all purpose flour
- 1 egg beaten
- 4 small chicken thighs
- 1½ tbsp Old Bay cajun seasoning

Direction: Cooking Time: 30 minutes | Servings: 4

- ✓ Ensure that your Air Fryer is preheated to 390 F. Combine the salt, flour, and the Old Bay, and mix the mixture.
- ✓ Submerge the chicken in the flour mixture, and into the egg, before taking it back into the flour mixture again.
- ✓ Remove all excess flour by shaking them off.
- ✓ Transfer the four chicken thighs into the cooking compartment of your Air Fryer – preferably at the bottom.
- ✓ Allow to cook for 25 minutes in this position, or until the chicken reaches the temperature of 180 F.
- ✓ Once either of this happens, it means the chicken is ready. Remove and serve.

548) Buttermilk Chicken Thighs

Ingredients:

- 2 lbs chicken thighs (skin on, bone in) Marinade
- 2 tsp black pepper
- 2 tsp kosher salt
- 1 tsp paprika powder
- 2 cups buttermilk Seasoned Flour
- 1 tbsp garlic powder
- 1 tsp kosher salt
- 1 tbsp baking powder
- 2 cups all-purpose flour

Direction: Time: 6 hours 45 minutes | Servings: 3-4

- ✓ Get rid of any visible residue or fat from the chicken thighs by rinsing, then pat dry using paper towels.
- ✓ Get a large, clean bowl, put the chicken pieces in it and add black pepper, salt, and paprika.
- ✓ Pour your buttermilk over the chicken until the entire chicken is coated. Place inside the refrigerator overnight or for not less than 6 hours.
- ✓ Ensure your Air Fryer is preheated at 355 F Get another bowl, and mix garlic powder, salt, paprika, baking powder, and flour.
- ✓ Now, take each piece of the chicken from the buttermilk, dredging them in the flour mixture.
- ✓ To get rid of any excess flour, shake the dredged chicken before transferring to a plate.
- ✓ Place the chicken pieces in one layer of the basket in your fryer, such that the skin side is facing upwards.
- ✓ Now, slide the basket containing the chicken into the air fryer.
- ✓ Let it air fry for 8 minutes – you can set the air fryer's timer.
- ✓ After 8 minutes, remove the tray and change the sides of the chicken such that the skin side is facing downwards.
- ✓ Air fry for another 10 minutes.
- ✓ Withdraw the air-fried chickens on paper towels (to drain)
- ✓ serve.

549) Bacon-Wrapped Chicken Breasts

Ingredients:

- 2 chicken breasts
- 8 oz cream cheese
- 1 tbsp butter
- 6 turkey bacon slices
- Salt to taste
- 1 tbsp fresh parsley, chopped

Direction: Time: 25 minutes – Servings: 4

- ✓ Preheat the air fryer to 390 F.
- ✓ Stretch out the bacon and lay the slices in 2 sets; 3 bacon strips together on each side.
- ✓ Place the chicken on each bacon set.
- ✓ Use a knife to smear the cream cheese on both.
- ✓ Spread the butter on top and sprinkle with salt.
- ✓ Wrap the turkey bacon around the chicken and secure the ends into the wrap.
- ✓ Place the wrapped chicken in the greased frying basket and Air Fry for 16-18 minutes, turning halfway through.
- ✓ Top with fresh parsley and serve with steamed greens.

550) Air-Fried Chicken Popcorn

Ingredients:

- 2 chicken breasts, cut into small cubes
- 2 cups panko breadcrumbs
- Salt and black pepper
- 1 tsp garlic powder

Direction: Time: 30 minutes - Servings: 4

- ✓ Preheat the air fryer to 360 F.
- ✓ Rub the chicken cubes with salt, garlic powder, and black pepper.
- ✓ Coat in the panko breadcrumbs and place them in the greased frying basket.
- ✓ Spray with cooking spray and Air Fry for 16-18 minutes, flipping once until nice and crispy.
- ✓ Serve with tzatziki sauce if desired.

551) Spicy Buffalo Chicken Wings

Ingredients:

- 2 lb chicken wings
- ½ cup cayenne pepper sauce
- 2 tbsp coconut oil
- 2 tbsp Worcestershire sauce
- Salt to taste
- ½ cup sour cream
- ¼ cup mayonnaise
- 1 tbsp scallions, chopped
- 1 tbsp fresh parsley, chopped
- 1 garlic clove, minced

Direction: Time: 25 minutes + marinating time - Servings 4

- ✓ In a mixing bowl, combine cayenne pepper sauce, coconut oil, Worcestershire sauce, and salt.
- ✓ Add in the chicken wings and toss to coat.
- ✓ Cover with a lid and marinate for 1 hour in the fridge.
- ✓ Preheat the air fryer to 400 F.
- ✓ Place the chicken in a greased frying basket and Air Fry for 15-18 minutes or until the marinade becomes sticky and the wings are cooked through.
- ✓ Meanwhile, in a small bowl, mix together sour cream, mayonnaise, garlic, parsley, and salt.
- ✓ Top the wings with scallions and serve with the prepared sauce on the side.
- ✓ Enjoy!

552) Classic Chicken Wings

Ingredients:
- 2 lbs chicken wings
- For sauce:
- 1/4 tsp Tabasco
- 1/4 tsp Worcestershire sauce
- 6 tbsp butter, melted
- 12 oz hot sauce

Direction: Time: 50 minutes Serve: 4

- ✓ Spray air fryer basket with cooking spray.
- ✓ Add chicken wings in air fryer basket and cook for 25 minutes at 380 F.
- ✓ Shake basket after every 5 minutes.
- ✓ After 25 minutes turn temperature to 400 F and cook for 10-15 minutes more.
- ✓ Meanwhile, in a large bowl, mix together all sauce ingredients.
- ✓ Add cooked chicken wings in a sauce bowl and toss well to coat.
- ✓ Serve and enjoy.

553) Sweet Garlicky Chicken Wings

Ingredients:
- 16 chicken wings
- ¼ cup butter
- 1 tsp honey
- ½ tbsp salt
- 4 garlic cloves, minced
- ¾ cup potato starch

Direction: Time: 20 minutes - Servings 4

- ✓ Preheat the air fryer to 370 F.
- ✓ Coat the chicken with potato starch and place in the greased frying basket.
- ✓ Bake for 5 minutes.
- ✓ Whisk the rest of the ingredients in a bowl.
- ✓ Remove the wings from the fryer, pour the sauce over them, and Bake for another 10 minutes, until crispy.
- ✓ Serve.

554) BBQ Chicken Wings

Ingredients:
- 1/2 lbs chicken wings
- 2 tbsp unsweetened BBQ sauce
- 1 tsp paprika
- 1 tbsp olive oil
- 1 tsp garlic powder
- Pepper Salt

Direction: Time: 30 minutes - Serve: 4

- ✓ In a large bowl, toss chicken wings with garlic powder, oil, paprika, pepper, and salt.
- ✓ Preheat the air fryer to 360 F.
- ✓ Add chicken wings in air fryer basket and cook for 12 minutes.
- ✓ Turn chicken wings to another side and cook for 5 minutes more.
- ✓ Remove chicken wings from air fryer and toss with BBQ sauce.
- ✓ Return chicken wings in air fryer basket and cook for 2 minutes more.
- ✓ Serve and enjoy.

555) Flavorful Fried Chicken

Ingredients:
- 5 lbs chicken, about 10 pieces
- 1 tbsp coconut oil
- 1 tsp white pepper
- 1 tsp ground ginger
- 1/2 tsp garlic
- 1 tbsp paprika
- 1 tsp dried mustard
- 1 tsp pepper
- 1 tsp celery salt
- 1/3 tsp oregano
- 1/2 tsp basil
- 1/2 tsp thyme
- 2 cups pork rinds, crushed
- 1 tbsp vinegar
- 1 cup unsweetened almond milk
- 1/2 tsp salt

Direction: Time: 50 minutes Serve: 10

- ✓ Add chicken in a large mixing bowl.
- ✓ Add milk and vinegar over chicken and place in the refrigerator for 2 hours.
- ✓ I a shallow dish, mix together pork rinds, white pepper, ginger, garlic salt, paprika, mustard, pepper, celery salt, oregano, basil, thyme, and salt.
- ✓ Coat air fryer basket with coconut oil.
- ✓ Coat each chicken piece with pork rind mixture and place on a plate.
- ✓ Place half coated chicken in the air fryer basket.
- ✓ Cook chicken at 360 F for 10 minutes then turn chicken to another side and cook for 10 minutes more or until internal temperature reaches at 165 F.
- ✓ Cook remaining chicken using the same method.
- ✓ Serve.

556) Easy Chicken Nuggets

Ingredients:
- 1 lb chicken breast, skinless, boneless and cut into chunks
- 6 tbsp sesame seeds, toasted
- 4 egg whites
- 1/2 tsp ground ginger
- 1/4 cup coconut flour
- 1 tsp sesame oil
- Salt

Direction: Time: 22 minutes Serve: 4

- ✓ Preheat the air fryer to 400 F.
- ✓ Toss chicken with oil and salt in a bowl until well coated.
- ✓ Add coconut flour and ginger in a zip-lock bag and shake to mix.
- ✓ Add chicken to the bag and shake well to coat.
- ✓ In a large bowl, add egg whites.
- ✓ Add chicken in egg whites and toss until well coated.
- ✓ Add sesame seeds in a large zip-lock bag.
- ✓ Shake excess egg off from chicken and add chicken in sesame seed bag.
- ✓ Shake bag until chicken well coated with sesame seeds.
- ✓ Spray air fryer basket with cooking spray.
- ✓ Place chicken in air fryer basket and cook for 6 minutes.
- ✓ Turn chicken to another side and cook for 6 minutes more.
- ✓ Serve and enjoy.

557) Buffalo Style Skinny Chicken Wings

Ingredients:
- ½ cup frank's hot sauce
- 1 lb chicken wings, fresh Blue cheese, crumbled,

Direction: Time: 25 minutes | Servings: 2-4

- ✓ Apply the hot sauce on all sides of the chicken wings.
- ✓ Ensure that your air fryer is preheated to 400 F.
- ✓ Transfer the chicken wings in the air fryer, maintain a single layer of arrangement.
- ✓ Allow to cook for 18 minutes, and shake twice or thrice while cooking.
- ✓ Add blue cheese and celery as toppings on the cooked chicken wings.
- ✓ Serve.

558) Italian Seasoned Chicken Tenders

Ingredients:

- 2 eggs, lightly beaten
- 1/2 lbs chicken tenders
- 1/2 tsp onion powder
- 1/2 tsp garlic powder
- 1 tsp paprika
- 1 tsp Italian seasoning
- 2 tbsp ground flax seed
- 1 cup almond flour
- 1/2 tsp pepper
- 1 tsp salt

Direction: Time: 20 minutes Serve: 2

- ✓ Preheat the air fryer to 400 F.
- ✓ Season chicken with pepper and salt.
- ✓ In a medium bowl, whisk eggs to combine.
- ✓ In a shallow dish, mix together almond flour, all seasonings, and flaxseed.
- ✓ Dip chicken into the egg then coats with almond flour mixture and place on a plate.
- ✓ Spray air fryer basket with cooking spray.
- ✓ Place half chicken tenders in air fryer basket and cook for 10 minutes.
- ✓ Turn halfway through.
- ✓ Cook remaining chicken tenders using same steps.
- ✓ Serve

559) Lemon Pepper Chicken Wings

Ingredients:

- 1 lb chicken wings
- 1 tsp lemon pepper
- 1 tbsp olive oil
- 1 tsp salt

Direction: Time: 26 minutes Serve: 4

- ✓ Add chicken wings into the large mixing bowl.
- ✓ Add remaining ingredients over chicken and toss well to coat.
- ✓ Place chicken wings in the air fryer basket.
- ✓ Cook chicken wings for 8 minutes at 400 F.
- ✓ Turn chicken wings to another side and cook for 8 minutes more.
- ✓ Serve and enjoy.

560) Easy and Delicious Whole Chicken

Ingredients:

- 3 lbs whole chicken, remove giblets and pat dry chicken
- 1 tsp Italian seasoning
- 1/2 tsp garlic powder
- 1/2 tsp onion powder
- 1/4 tsp paprika
- 1/4 tsp pepper
- 1/2 tsp salt

Direction: Time: 60 minutes - Serve: 4

- ✓ In a small bowl, mix together Italian seasoning, garlic powder, onion powder, paprika, pepper, and salt.
- ✓ Rub spice mixture from inside and outside of the chicken.
- ✓ Place chicken breast side down in air fryer basket.
- ✓ Roast chicken for 30 minutes at 360 F.
- ✓ Turn chicken and roast for 20 minutes more or internal temperature of chicken reaches at 165 F.
- ✓ Serve.

561) Barbeque Chicken Wings

Ingredients:

- 2 tbsp honey
- Salt and ground black pepper to taste
- BBQ chicken seasoning
- 1 tbsp olive oil
- 1 lb chicken wings

Direction: Time: 25 minutes | Servings: 2-4

- ✓ Get a clean bowl and in it, mix the honey, salt, pepper, BBQ chicken seasoning, and the olive oil.
- ✓ Using the BBQ mixture, brush the chicken wings generously.
- ✓ Ensure that your air fryer is preheated to 400 F.
- ✓ Transfer the chicken wings into the air fryer, while maintaining a single layer.
- ✓ Allow frying for 18 minutes, while turning the wings after 9 minutes.
- ✓ Withdraw when both sides are fried.
- ✓ Serve.

562) Southern Chicken Drumsticks

Ingredients:

- 2 large slices bread
- Salt and ground black pepper to taste
- 1 tbsp dried garlic and onion
- 1 tsp basil
- ½ tsp cayenne pepper 1 tbsp plain flour
- 2 tbsp paprika 5 oz buttermilk
- 4 chicken drumsticks
- 1 tbsp oregano
- 1 tbsp rosemary
- 1 tbsp thyme
- 1 tsp olive oil

Direction: Cooking Time: 55 minutes | Servings: 4

- ✓ Ensure that the Air Fryer is preheated to about 365 F – it takes about two minutes. In addition to the bread, add the salt, pepper, dried garlic, onion, basil, and a pinch of cayenne. Blend the mixture in the blender until the blend looks like breadcrumbs.
- ✓ Put the blend into a separate bowl and set aside. In a new bowl, add flour and mix with ½ the paprika, while adding pepper and salt to taste. Set aside this bowl also.
- ✓ Get a third bowl and make a mixture of the buttermilk, the chicken drumsticks, and the rest of the seasonings.
- ✓ Stir the mixture well, while the drumsticks are submerged.
- ✓ Take out each chicken drumstick from the bowl and place it in the flour, and after that in the breadcrumbs.
- ✓ Once you are done with the dipping for each, place them into the basket in your air fryer.
- ✓ After coating all the chicken drumsticks, sprinkle a bit of olive oil to ensure that they do not dry while improving their taste.
- ✓ Place all coated and oiled drumsticks in the air fryer and cook for about 30 minutes at 365 F.
- ✓ Reduce the heat to 345 F and cook for an extra two minutes. Remove from the air fryer and serve.

563) Nando's Chicken Drumsticks

Ingredients:

- 2 corn on the cobs
- 1 small fresh red chilli
- ½ bunch of fresh parsley, chopped
- 1 tsp paprika
- 5 garlic cloves, peeled
- 3 bay leaves
- 3 tbsp olive oil
- 8 chicken drumsticks
- Salt and ground black pepper to taste
- ½ tsp Piri Piri seasoning
- 1 tsp butter

Direction: Cooking Time: 35 minutes | Servings: 4

- ✓ Pick each corn on the cob and chop it into three equal pieces, thus giving you six equal small pieces of chopped corn.
- ✓ Put these pieces into the steamer basket of your Instant Pot, which already has 1 cup of water under it.
- ✓ Seal the lid and allow to cook for 15 minutes on the Steamer button.
- ✓ Open the blender and add the red chili, parsley, paprika, garlic, bay leaves, and olive oil.
- ✓ Blend until you have a grainy or almost-smooth blend.
- ✓ On a clean chopping board, arrange the chicken drumsticks and drizzle on them salt and pepper.
- ✓ With the aid of your pastry brush, brush each drumstick with the blended marinade.
- ✓ Proceed by placing the brushed drumsticks into the grill pan of the air fryer. Set the temperature to 355 F and cook for 12 minutes. Once you get a beep tone from the Instant Pot, remove the corn on the cob by using the Quick pressure release.
- ✓ Transfer it to the chopping board, and season with Piri Piri seasoning, alongside salt and pepper to taste. Set the temperature to 390 F and allow this to cook for an extra three minutes on the other side, plus the corn on the cob.
- ✓ This will give them that barbecue well done look.. You can add a little butter to the corn on the cob, before serving with the Peri Peri chicken drumettes.

564) Spicy Air Fryer Chicken Breasts

Ingredients:

- 2 tbsp Dijon mustard
- 2 cups buttermilk
- 1- ½ tsp garlic powder 2 tsp salt
- 2 tsp hot pepper sauce
- 8 bone-in chicken breast halves, skin removed (8 oz each)
- 2 cups soft bread crumbs
- ½ tsp cayenne pepper
- ¼ tsp dried parsley flakes
- ½ tsp poultry seasoning
- ½ tsp paprika
- ½ tsp ground mustard
- ¼ tsp dried oregano
- 1 cup cornmeal
- 2 tbsp canola oil

Direction: Prep + Cook Time: 1 hour 45 minutes | Servings: 8

- ✓ Ensure that your Air Fryer is preheated at 375 F. Get a large bowl and make a mixture of the first five ingredients on the list above. Coat the chicken with this mixture.
- ✓ Keep the coated chicken in the refrigerator, covered, for an hour or overnight.
- ✓ Drain the chicken of excess coatings and dispose of the marinade. In another shallow dish, add all the unused ingredients together and stir to mix.
- ✓ Coat each piece of the chicken with this spice mixture, and transfer them into the basket of the air fryer in a single layer.
- ✓ Ensure that the air fryer basket has already been sprayed. Air fry the chicken until you have a reading of 170 F on the thermometer.
- ✓ This will take about 20 minutes, and you need to turn the chicken halfway. Do the same for the remaining chicken.
- ✓ After all the chicken is cooked, transfer all of them to the basket again. Air fry for about two or three minutes to heat through

565) Balsamic Glazed Chicken Breasts

Ingredients:

- 1 large mango
- 15 tsp olive oil
- 4 garlic cloves
- 5 tbsp balsamic vinegar
- 1 tbsp parsley
- 1 tbsp oregano
- Salt and ground black pepper to taste
- Pinch mustard powder
- 2 chicken breasts
- 1 medium avocado
- 1 red pepper Fresh parsley to garnish

Direction: Cooking Time: 3 hours 20 minutes | Servings: 2

- ✓ After peeling and getting rid of the stone in your mango, set aside about ¾ of it into a separate bowl, and dice the remaining. Place the diced mango, olive oil, garlic, the balsamic vinegar, and all the seasonings into your blender.
- ✓ Blend until you have a smooth mixture. Transfer the blended mixture into a clean bowl, and submerge the whole chicken breasts in it.
- ✓ Refrigerate for about 3 hours to allow it to soak. Separate the chicken and the marinade. Switch your air fryer basket with the grill pan.
- ✓ Coat the top of the chicken with the marinade using a pastry brush.
- ✓ Set your Air Fryer to 355 F and allow the coated chicken breast to cook for 12 minutes.
- ✓ When the coking is halfway, withdraw the pan and turn the chicken to the other side, giving it another balsamic coating.
- ✓ This ensures that the two sides have the coating.
- ✓ Slice the mango, pepper, and avocado thinly.
- ✓ Add some drizzles of some balsamic vinegar. Serve with fresh parsley.

566) Buffalo Chicken Breasts

Ingredients:

- 1 tsp hot sauce (such as Frank's)
- 1 tbsp hot sauce (such as Frank's)
- ¼ cup egg substitute
- ½ cup plain fat-free Greek yogurt
- 1 tbsp cayenne pepper
- 1 tbsp garlic pepper seasoning
- 1 tbsp sweet paprika
- 1 cup panko breadcrumbs
- 1 lb skinless, boneless chicken breasts, cut into 1-inch strips

Direction: Cooking Time: 40 minutes | Servings: 3-4

- ✓ Get a clean bowl and add one teaspoon and one tablespoon hot sauce, egg substitute, and Greek yogurt.
- ✓ Whisk the mixture. In another clean bowl, make a mix of cayenne pepper, garlic pepper, paprika, and breadcrumbs. Set your Air Fryer to 355 F.
- ✓ Dip each chicken strip into the yogurt mixture.
- ✓ Coat the dipped chicken strips with the panko breadcrumb mixture.
- ✓ Place the coated chicken strips in your air fryer, such that they all are in a single layer.
- ✓ Cook in the air fryer for about 8 minutes, turn the chicken to the other side and cook for another eight minutes.
- ✓ It is cooked when the chicken is evenly browned. Serve.

567) Syn Free Slimming World Chicken Tikka

Ingredients:

- 2 large chicken breasts
- Chicken tikka marinade:
- 10 oz Greek yoghurt
- ½ small diced onion 2 tsp garlic puree
- 2 tsp paprika
- 2 tsp cumin
- 2 tsp garam masala
- 2 tsp turmeric
- 1 tsp grated ginger
- Pinch of chilli Juice and rind of 1 lemon

Direction: Cooking Time: 20 minutes | Servings: 4

- ✓ Make a smooth mixture of all the chicken tikka marinade ingredients in a clean mixing bowl.
- ✓ Place the chicken breasts into the bowl and leave overnight to marinade.
- ✓ The next day, separate the chicken breasts from the marinade.
- ✓ Transfer the chicken breasts to a chopping board, and chop the chicken into tikka bite shapes. Switch your air fryer basket with a grill pan.
- ✓ Cook the chopped chicken in the pan at a temperature of 360 F for about 10 minutes.
- ✓ Serve the cooked chicken while warm.

568) Air Fried Chicken Schnitzel

Ingredients:

- 2 chicken breast
- Salt and ground black pepper to taste
- 2 medium eggs
- 12 tbsp gluten free oats
- 2 tbsp mustard powder Fresh parsley, chopped

Direction: 25 minutes | Servings: 3-4

- ✓ Flatten out your chicken breasts on a clean chopping board, such that there are four flat pieces of them.
- ✓ Season the flat pieces with pepper and salt on either side – to ensure thorough seasoning. Get a separate mixing bowl, and beat two eggs in it using a fork. Place the gluten free oats, mustard, the fresh parsley, and another round of salt and pepper in your blender.
- ✓ Blend until you have the appearance of coarse breadcrumbs.
- ✓ Transfer the blend into another separate dish. First roll the chicken in the oats, before transferring it into the egg.
- ✓ Return it to the oats again.
- ✓ Place the rolled chicken in your air fryer's grill pan, and set the temperature to 350 F.
- ✓ Allow cooking for 12 minutes. With the aid of tongs, turn the chicken halfway through.
- ✓ Serve the cooked chicken warm alongside warm potatoes.

569) Thai Mango Chicken

Ingredients:

- Mixed herbs chicken seasoning
- ½ mango peeled and diced
- Salt and ground black pepper to taste
- Spicy chicken seasoning
- 1 tsp red Thai curry paste
- 2 tbsp olive oil
- 1 lime rind and juice
- 2 chicken breasts

Direction: Cooking Time: 20 minutes | Servings: 2

- ✓ Ensure that your Air Fryer is preheated to 355 F. Make a mixture of your mixed herbs seasoning, mango, salt, pepper, spicy chicken seasoning, Red Thai Curry Paste, olive oil, and lime into a clean mixing bowl.
- ✓ Ensure that you mix thoroughly so that the seasoning is evenly distributed in the mixture. With the aid of your vegetable knife, cut slightly into your chicken without the cut reaching the bottom of the breasts.
- ✓ Sprinkle the seasoning mixture in the mixing bowl and ensured that sufficient seasoning gets into the cuts.
- ✓ Transfer the sprinkled chicken into your air fryer, on the baking mat.
- ✓ Set the timer for 15 minutes and allow to cook.
- ✓ Always check well to ensure that the chicken is well-cooked in the center.
- ✓ Garnish some fresh tomatoes and extra lime, and serve with the cooked chicken.

570) Philadelphia Herby Chicken Breasts

Ingredients:

- 2 chicken breasts
- Mixed herbs chicken seasoning
- Salt and ground black pepper to taste
- 2 tbsp soft cheese

Direction: Cooking Time: 20 minutes | Servings: 2

- ✓ Ensure that your Air Fryer is preheated to 355 F.
- ✓ Slice midway into the breasts to create ample space to accommodate the seasoning.
- ✓ Add salt and pepper into the spaces created.
- ✓ Cover the entire chicken with soft cheese; use your hands to ensure a nice creamy layer.
- ✓ Have the seasoned chicken breasts rolled in the mixed herbs. Place them on a reusable baking mat and transfer into the air fryer.
- ✓ Cook until the chicken breasts are cooked in the middle (for about 15 minutes). Serve.

571) Lemon Pepper Chicken Breasts

Ingredients:

- 2 lemons rind and juice
- 1 tbsp chicken seasoning
- Handful black peppercorns
- 1 tsp garlic puree
- 1 chicken breast
- Salt and ground black pepper to taste

Direction: Cooking Time: 20 minutes | Servings: 1-2

- ✓ Ensure that your air fryer is preheated to 360 F. Prepare your workstation by first placing a large silver foil sheet on the worktop and then adding it to the lemon rind and all the seasonings.
- ✓ With your chicken breasts spread on a chopping board, trim off any fatty parts or little bones present.
- ✓ Using pepper and salt, season each side generously until you have a slightly different color.
- ✓ Transfer the seasoned chicken onto the silver foil sheet and rub again to ensure that the seasoning is evenly distributed. Then seal the foil up tightly such that air cannot enter.
- ✓ This is to ensure that the flavor penetrates the chicken well. Slap the sealed chicken with a rolling pin.
- ✓ This flattens it out while ensuring that it releases more flavor.
- ✓ Place the chicken in the air fryer and cook for 15 minutes. Ensure that it is cooked in the middle before taking it off the fryer. Serve."

572) Panko Breaded, Chicken Parmesan, Marinara Sauce

Ingredients:

- Cooking spray
- 16 oz skinless chicken breasts sliced in half to make
- 4 breasts ½ cup parmesan cheese, grated
- 1 cup panko bread crumbs
- 2 tsp Italian Seasoning
- Salt and ground black pepper to taste
- 1/8 cup egg whites
- ¾ cup marinara sauce
- ½ cup mozzarella cheese, shredded

Direction: Cooking Time: 35 minutes | Servings: 4

- ✓ Ensure that the air fryer is preheated at 400 F, with the basket well sprayed with the cooking spray. Create four thinner chicken breasts by cutting the chicken breasts horizontally into half.
- ✓ Pound the chicken breasts on a hard surface to flatten them completely. Grate your parmesan cheese and set it aside.
- ✓ Get a large, clean bowl and mix the grated cheese, panko breadcrumbs, and seasonings. Stir to have a uniform mixture.
- ✓ Get another bowl of similar size and place the egg whites in it. Immerse the chicken into the bowl containing the egg whites, and then the one containing the breadcrumbs mixture.
- ✓ Transfer the immersed chicken into the air fryer, with the top sprayed with the cooking spray. Allow the chicken to cook for 7 minutes in the air fryer.
- ✓ After this, use the marinara sauce and the shredded mozzarella to top the breasts. The topped chicken should be cooked until the cheese melts completely (for about 3 minutes). Serve.

573) Chicken Parmesan and Fries

Ingredients:

- 2 large potatoes
- 2 medium eggs 1 tbsp basil, dried
- 1 tbsp oregano, dried
- Salt and ground black pepper to taste
- 1 tbsp garlic puree Parmesan crisps
- 2 medium chicken breasts
- 1 tbsp olive oil
- 1 oz mozzarella cheese, shredded
- 1 oz parmesan cheese, grated

Direction: Cooking Time: 35 minutes | Servings: 4

- ✓ Without removing the skin, chop the potatoes into French Fries. Create your production line. Get a bowl and beat the eggs in it, adding the basil, oregano, salt, pepper, and some garlic puree.
- ✓ Blend the crisps until you have a fine texture and transfer it into a separate bowl, adding black pepper and a handful of unused breadcrumbs, then mix everything thoroughly. Butterfly the chicken before transferring them onto a clean chopping board.
- ✓ With the French Fries in the air fryer, set it to 360 F, and add a tablespoon of olive oil before cooking for 12 minutes. After withdrawing the basket from the air fryer, insert the grill pan.
- ✓ Dip the butterflied chicken completely in the parmesan coating, then in the egg, and the parmesan coating again.
- ✓ Transfer the dipped chicken to the grill pan. Set the air fryer to 360°F before cooking the chicken for 10 minutes. When the air fryer beeps, place the chicken over the French Fries and decorate the upper part with the cheese.
- ✓ Place in the air fryer again and cook at the same temperature for an additional four minutes. Serve.

574) Crumbed Chicken Tenderloins

Ingredients:

- 1 egg ½ cup dry breadcrumbs
- 2 tbsp vegetable oil
- 8 chicken tenderloins

Direction: Cooking Time: 30 minutes | Servings: 4

- ✓ Ensure that your Air Fryer is preheated to 350°F. Get two clean bowls; in the first bowl, whisk an egg, in the other bowl, make a loose and crumbly mixture of oil and breadcrumbs. Place each chicken tenderloin into the bowl containing whisked egg. Remove any extra egg by shaking.
- ✓ Then immerse in the crumb mixture until the mixture covers the chicken thoroughly and evenly.
- ✓ Place the chicken tenderloins carefully into the air fryer basket.
- ✓ Cook the chicken for about 12 minutes, or until you can no longer see the pink in the middle.
- ✓ Once cooked, measure the temperature with an instant-read thermometer inserted into the center of the chicken. It should read not less than 165 F. Serve.

575) Chicken Tenders

Ingredients:

- 2 large eggs
- 2 small lemons, juice only
- ½ tsp garlic puree
- 8 oz gluten free oats
- Salt and ground black pepper to taste
- 1 tbsp parsley, dried
- 1 tbsp mustard powder
- 2 tbsp basil
- 3 medium chicken breasts
- 1 tbsp mayonnaise, optional

Direction: Cooking Time: 15 minutes | Servings: 6

- ✓ In a clean bowl, make a mixture of egg and half of the lemon juice, alongside the garlic puree. Keep the mix somewhere safe.
- ✓ Blend a combination of ½ of the gluten-free oats until it appears like fine oats.
- ✓ The blended oats should be transferred into a bowl and the non-blended oats into another bowl.
- ✓ Mix both the blended oats and the non-blended oats by adding ¼ of the blended oats into the non-blended, and another ¼ non-blended oat into the blended oats.
- ✓ After the mixing, you should have two bowls – one containing more of blended oats, and the other containing more of unblended oats.
- ✓ Use the unblended oats mixture as your fake breadcrumbs and the blended oats mixture as your fake flour.
- ✓ Add salt, pepper, parsley, and mustard to the fake flour. Add salt, pepper, and basil to the fake breadcrumbs.
- ✓ Cut the chicken breast such that you have tender shapes of medium sizes. Place the chicken tenders into the flour bowl, before soaking it in the egg mixture. Coat the soaked chicken tenders with the breadcrumbs mixture.
- ✓ Transfer the coated tenders into the air fryer basket. Set your Air Fryer to 350 F and cook for about 10 minutes.
- ✓ While the chickens are cooking, prepare your mayonnaise mixture by adding pepper, salt, lemon, and a bit of mustard powder and mixing well. Serve.

576) Spatchcock Chicken

Ingredients:

- 1 tsp mixed herbs
- 1 tbsp garlic puree
- 2 tsp olive oil
- Salt and ground black pepper to taste
- 2 lbs spatchcock chicken

Direction: Cooking Time: 55 minutes | Servings: 4

- ✓ Create a really thick paste by combining all the seasonings, including the garlic puree and the olive oil. While placing the spatchcock chicken on the grill pan of the air fryer, apply the garlic paste on every visible part of the skin to ensure that you have an even and total coating.
- ✓ Set your air fryer to 360°F and cook each side of the chicken for 25 minutes. Serve warm with salad and rice. Notes: The usual practice is to cook the whole chickens in the main basket of the air fryer. However, the chicken was longer than normal this time around.
- ✓ Thus, only the grill pan can accommodate it conveniently. You may reduce the cooking time by five minutes if you are working with a thawed chicken.
- ✓ Air fryers work differently, thus, be sure to check that the chicken is cooked before serving.
- ✓ You can avoid getting burnt while turning the spatchcock chicken over by using kitchen tongs.

577) General Tso's Chicken

Ingredients:

- 1 lb boneless, skinless chicken thighs, patted dry and cut into 1 to 1¼ -inch chunks
- 1 large egg
- 1/3 cup plus
- 2 tsp cornstarch, divided
- ¼ tsp ground white pepper
- ¼ tsp kosher salt
- 2 tbsp ketchup
- 2 tbsp soy sauce
- 2 tsp sugar
- 7 tbsp chicken broth
- 2 tsp unseasoned rice vinegar
- 1½ tbsp canola oil
- 3 to 4 chiles de árbol, chopped and deseeded
- 1 tbsp finely chopped garlic
- 1 tbsp finely chopped fresh ginger
- 1 tsp toasted sesame oil
- 2 tbsp thinly sliced green onion
- ½ tsp toasted sesame seeds

Direction: Cooking Time: 40 minutes | Servings: 4

- ✓ In a large bowl, coat your chicken well in the beaten egg. In another bowl, make a mixture of 1/3 cup cornstarch, pepper, and salt.
- ✓ Using a fork, transfer the chicken into the cornstarch mixture. Ensure that every area is well coated by using a spatula.
- ✓ Divide the chickens into batches, and transfer them into the air-fryer basket. If you are using the air-fryer oven racks instead, you can cook the entire chicken by moving them into the oven racks but leaving little space between the pieces. Set your Air Fryer to 400 F and allow it to preheat for 3 minutes.
- ✓ Place the battered chicken and allow to cook for 12 to 16 minutes, while shaking midway. Allow the cooked chicken to dry for three to five minutes, if a side of the chicken is still damp, cook again for about 1 or 2 minutes.
- ✓ Whisk the remaining two teaspoons of cornstarch alongside ketchup, soy sauce, sugar, broth, and rice vinegar. Get a large, clean skillet and heat canola oil and chiles in it over medium heat.
- ✓ Once the mixture starts to sizzle, add the garlic and ginger, and cook for about 30 seconds until you have a fragrance. Whisk the cornstarch mixture again, and stir into a mixture in the skillet.
- ✓ Set the heat to medium-high, and once you have the sauce bubbling, add the chicken. Stir the chicken to ensure even coating, and continue cooking until you have a thickened sauce that clutches to the chicken tightly.
- ✓ This takes about one and a half minutes. Turn off the heat and stir the chicken in 1 tablespoon sesame oil and 1 tablespoon green onion. Transfer into a serving plate, and add the remaining one tablespoon green onion as well as the sesame seeds.

578) Southern-Style Chicken

Ingredients:

- Ingredients:
- 1 tbsp minced fresh parsley
- 1 tsp paprika
- 1 tsp garlic salt
- 2 cups crushed Ritz crackers (about 50)
- ½ tsp pepper
- ¼ tsp rubbed sage
- ¼ tsp ground cumin
- 1 large egg, beaten
- 1 chicken (3 to 4 lbs), cut up

Direction: Cooking Time: 40 minutes | Servings: 6

- ✓ Ensure that your Air Fryer is preheated to 375 F, and spritz the basket using a cooking spray. Get a clean shallow bowl. In the bowl, make a mixture of the first seven ingredients. Get another clean shallow bowl and place the egg in it.
- ✓ After dipping the chicken in the egg, dip again in the cracker mixture, while patting, to ensure that the coating doesn't remove.
- ✓ Arrange the chickens in a single layer in the air fryer basket and spritz with cooking spray.
- ✓ Allow the chicken to cook for 10 minutes before turning and spraying with additional cooking spray.
- ✓ Cook again (for about 10-20 minutes) until you have a golden brown color and juices running clear. Do the same for the remaining chicken.

579) Rotisserie Chicken

Ingredients:

- 1 whole chicken (3 lbs)

Brine:

- 2 tsp thyme
- 1 tbsp paprika
- Salt and ground black pepper to taste 1 chicken oxo cube Chicken Rub:
- 1 tsp celery salt
- 1 tbsp paprika
- 1 tbsp olive oil
- Salt and ground black pepper to taste

Direction: Cooking Time: 45 minutes | Servings: 4-5

- ✓ Collect all your brine ingredients into a freezing bag. Place the whole chicken inside, and then fill it up with cold water until the chicken is immersed. Zip the freezing bag, and place it in the fridge overnight.
- ✓ When you are ready to cook the next day, withdraw the chicken from the freezing bag and remove the giblets. Separate the brine stock also and dry the entire chicken by patting it dry with a kitchen towel. Get a clean bowl and prepare your chicken rub in it.
- ✓ With the breast facing down, put the entire chicken in the air fryer basket/pan. Rub every visible part of the chicken skin with ½ of the chicken rub and ½ of the olive oil. Set your Air Fryer to 370 F and allow the chicken to cook at this temperature for 20 minutes.
- ✓ Using the kitchen tongs, turn over the chicken to the other side and add the remaining oil and chicken rub, then cook again for another 20 minutes without changing the temperature. Serve warm.

580) Thai Peanut Chicken Egg Rolls

Ingredients:

- 2 cups rotisserie chicken, shredded
- ¼ cup Thai peanut sauce
- 4 egg roll wrappers
- 1 medium carrot, very thinly sliced or ribboned
- ¼ red bell pepper, julienned
- 3 green onions, chopped Non-stick cooking spray or sesame oil

Direction: Cooking Time: 20 minutes | Servings: 3-4

- ✓ Ensure that your air fryer is preheated to 390 F. Get a small bowl and place the chicken in it alongside the Thai peanut sauce. With the egg roll wrappers laid out on a clean, dry surface, arrange ¼ carrot, bell pepper, and onions to accommodate the bottom third of the egg roll wrapper.
- ✓ Spread ½ cup of the chicken mixture over the vegetables. Using water, moisten the outer edges of the wrapper.
- ✓ Roll the wrapper tightly by folding the sides of the wrapper towards the center.
- ✓ Do the same for the other wrappers (pending this time, cover them with a damp paper towel).
- ✓ Using a non-stick cooking spray, spread both sides of the assembled egg rolls well.
- ✓ Transfer the sprayed egg rolls into your air fryer. Bake for 6-8 minutes at 390 F or until you have a crispy and golden brown appearance.
- ✓ Slice the baked chicken into half and serve with extra Thai Peanut Sauce for dipping.

581) Friendly Airfryer Whole Chicken

Ingredients:

- Medium whole chicken (about 3 lbs)
- Salt and ground black pepper to taste
- 1 tbsp mixed herbs
- 1 tbsp olive oil 1 large onion

Direction: Cooking Time: 45 minutes | Servings: 4

- ✓ Ensure that your air fryer is preheated to 340 F. To the skin of your nice and dry chicken, sprinkle salt, pepper, and mixed herbs, before rubbing olive oil.
- ✓ Take away the giblets present in the chicken. Without removing the skin of the onion, chop it into half and place in the chicken's cavity.
- ✓ Transfer the chicken into the air fryer upside down and with the bottom stuck in the air. Allow cooking for 20 minutes before turning it over.
- ✓ This time around, the breast faces up. Cook for another 20 minutes. Remove and serve warm.

582) KFC Chicken in the Air Fryer

Ingredients:

- 1 whole chicken 1 oz KFC spice blend
- 10 oz bread crumbs
- 4 oz plain flour
- 3 small eggs beaten

Direction: Cooking Time: 30 minutes | Servings: 4

- ✓ After chopping your chicken into pieces of desired sizes, set them aside. You may separate the wings, things, drumsticks, and breast, or have the wings and the breast together.
- ✓ Get a clean bowl, and make a mixture of the KFC spice and breadcrumbs.
- ✓ Get another clean bowl and place your flour. In a third clean bowl, place your beaten eggs. After rolling the chicken pieces in the flour, roll it in the egg, and finally in the spicy breadcrumbs.
- ✓ Set your air fryer to 360 F and cook the rolled chicken for 18 minutes. Do not withdraw until it is well cooked in the middle. Serve.

583) KFC Easy Chicken Strips in the Air Fryer

Ingredients:

- 1 chicken breast, chopped into strips
- Salt and ground black pepper to taste
- 3 oz bread crumbs
- ½ oz plain oats
- ½ oz desiccated coconut
- ¼ oz KFC spice blend get our recipe here
- 2 oz plain flour
- 1 small egg, beaten

Direction: Cooking Time: 25 minutes | Servings: 2

- ✓ Make strips out of your chicken breast. Get a clean bowl, and make a mixture of salt, pepper, breadcrumbs, oats, coconut, and the KFC spice blend.
- ✓ Get another clean bowl and place your egg. In the third clean bowl, add your plain flour. Dip the strips in the plain flour first, before the egg, and finally the spicy layer.
- ✓ Set your Air Fryer to 360 F and cook the dipped chicken for eight minutes.
- ✓ Reduce the temperature to 320 F and cook for an extra four minutes to ensure that the chicken cooks well in the middle. Serve.

584) KFC Popcorn Chicken in the Air Fryer

Ingredients:

- 1 chicken breast
- 2 oz plain flour
- 1 small egg, beaten
- Salt and ground black pepper to taste
- 2 oz bread crumbs
- ¼ oz KFC spice blend get the recipe here

Direction: Cooking Time: 25 minutes | Servings: 2

- ✓ Blend your chicken in your food processor until you have something like a minced chicken.
- ✓ Create your factory line – first bowl containing your flour; the second containing your beaten egg; and the third containing a mixture of salt, pepper, bread crumbs, and finally the KFC spice blend.
- ✓ Like another factory line, transform the minced chicken into balls.
- ✓ Roll the balls in the flour first, then in the egg, and finally in the spiced breadcrumbs. Transfer the rolled chicken balls into the air fryer. Set it to 360 F and cook for about 10 to 12 minutes, or until you are sure the chicken is well cooked in the middle.

585) Everything Bagel Chicken Strips

Ingredients:

- 1 day-old everything bagel, torn
- ½ cup panko bread crumbs
- ½ cup grated parmesan cheese
- ¼ tsp red pepper flakes, crushed
- 1 lb chicken tenderloins
- ½ tsp salt
- ¼ cup butter, cubed

Direction: Cooking Time: 25 minutes | Servings: 4

- ✓ Ensure that your Air Fryer is preheated to 400 F. Pulse the torn bagel in a food processor and withdraw only when you have coarse crumbs. Separate ½ of the cup bagel crumbs and transfer it into a shallow bowl, mix it with panko, cheese, and pepper flakes.
- ✓ You may retain or discard the other half of the bagel crumbs. Get a shallow bowl that is safe for use in a microwave, heat microwave butter until it melts. Sprinkle your chicken with salt and dip it in warm butter before coating it with crumb mixture.
- ✓ You may pat the chicken to ensure it retains the crumb. After spraying the air fryer basket with cooking spray, transfer the chicken to form a single layer in the basket. You may divide the chicken into batches.
- ✓ Cook each batch for seven minutes before turning over to the other side.
- ✓ Cook until the pink appearance of the chicken is replaced by the golden brown coating (for about seven to eight minutes). Serve immediately.

586) Buffalo Chicken Strips

Ingredients:

- ¾ cup panko crumbs or bread crumbs ¼ cup flour
- 1 egg, beaten
- Garlic salt and ground black pepper to taste
- Cooking spray
- 12 oz chicken breast strips
- Buffalo sauce (I used about ½ cup)

Direction: Cooking Time: 35 minutes | Servings: 3

- ✓ Get three separate bowls. In each bowl, place the panko crumbs, flour and egg.
- ✓ You may mix the panko alongside some pepper, garlic, and salt.
- ✓ The bottom of the air fryer should be sprayed with a little cooking spray.
- ✓ Place the chicken in the flour, egg, and the panko respectively. Ensure that the chicken is entirely coated.
- ✓ Transfer the coated chicken into the air fryer while spraying the top with a little cooking spray again. Set your Air Fryer to 375 F and fry for 10 minutes. At the same temperature, flip and cook for further 3-5 minutes or until the pink color disappears completely.
- ✓ Transfer the chicken into the cooked chicken into a mixing bowl. Immerse in a buffalo sauce until the whole chicken is well coated. Serve alongside carrots, ranch, and celery.

587) Flourless Cordon Bleu

Ingredients:

- 2 chicken breasts
- 1 tbsp tarragon
- Salt and ground black pepper to taste
- 1 tsp parsley
- 1 tsp garlic puree
- 1 tbsp soft cheese
- 1 slice ham 1 slice cheddar cheese
- 1 small egg, beaten
- 1 oz oats
- 1 tbsp thyme

Direction: Cooking Time: 35 minutes | Servings: 2

- ✓ Ensure that your air fryer is preheated to 365 F. Using a chopping board, chop your chicken breasts at a side angle to the right, near the corner. This is to ensure that they can be folded over easily while adding the ingredients to the middle.
- ✓ Using a mixture of tarragon, pepper, and salt, sprinkle the sides of your chicken very well. Get a clean mixing bowl and make a mixture of parsley, garlic, and soft cheese. Add a layer of the cheese mixture in the middle, plus half a slice each of the ham and cheddar cheese. With the filling inside, press down the chicken till it appears almost sealed.
- ✓ Add your egg and blended oats in another bowl, alongside thyme. Mix well.
- ✓ Roll the chicken in the oats first, and in the egg.
- ✓ Roll in the oats again. Transfer the rolled pieces of chicken on a baking sheet inside your air fryer.
- ✓ Cook for 30 minutes. After the first 20 minutes of cooking, turn the chickens over to ensure that the crispiness is present on both sides. Serve alongside new potatoes.

588) Jamaican Chicken Meatballs

Ingredients:

- 2 chicken breasts
- 1 large onion peeled and diced

Jamaican seasonings:

- 3 tbsp soy sauce
- 2 tbsp honey
- 1 tbsp cumin
- 1 tsp chili powder
- 1 tbsp mustard powder
- 1 tbsp thyme
- 1 tbsp basil
- Salt and ground black pepper to taste
- 2 tsp jerk paste, optional

Direction: Cooking Time: 25 minutes | Servings: 10

- Blend your chicken in the blender until it appears like chicken mince. Blend the onion in the blender as well.
- Place the Jamaican seasonings and blend again for the third time. Make ten medium-sized meatballs from the blended products.
- Transfer the medium-sized meatballs into your Air Fryer and allow them to cook at 360 F for 15 minutes.
- After cooking, place them on sticks before spooning some of the sauce over them.
- You can get the source from the sides of your blender.
- This gives the sticky meatballs a great taste sensation.
- Sprinkle with fresh herbs. Serve.

589) Chicken Fried Rice

Ingredients:

- 3 cups cooked white rice cold
- 6 tbsp soy sauce
- 1 tbsp vegetable oil
- ½ cup onion diced
- 1 cup cooked chicken diced
- 1 cup frozen peas and carrots

Direction: Cooking Time: 35 minutes | Servings: 4-6

- Get a mixing bowl and place the cold cooked white rice into it. Add the soy sauce alongside the vegetable oil and mix thoroughly.
- Add the diced onion, diced chicken, and the frozen carrots and peas before mixing well again.
- Now, transfer the rice mixture into the nonstick pan. In the case of aluminum pan, spray the inside with a non-stick cooking spray before adding the rice.
- Transfer the pan into the air fryer, and with the temperature set at 360 F, cook for 20 minutes.
- Withdraw the pan as soon as the air fryer timer goes off.
- Serve the cooked rice only, or alongside your favorite meat.

590) Crispy Fried Spring Rolls

Ingredients:

- 4 oz cooked chicken breast
- 1 oz carrot
- 1 oz mushrooms 1 celery stalk
- 1 tsp chicken stock powder
- 1 tsp sugar
- ½ tsp finely chopped ginger
- 1 egg, beaten
- 1 tsp corn starch
- 8 spring roll wrappers

Direction: Cooking Time: 30 minutes | Servings: 4

- Cut the breasts into shreds. Cut the carrot, mushroom, and celery into long thin strips. Transfer the shredded chicken into a bowl before mixing it with the mushroom, carrot and celery strips.
- Add the chicken stock powder, sugar, and ginger. Stir the entire contents evenly to make the spring roll filling.
- Add cornstarch to the whisked egg, and stir to create a thick paste.
- Keep the paste separately. Add some filling into each spring roll wrapper and roll them up. Seal the ends of each roll with the egg mixture.
- It is recommended that you brush the spring rolls with oil to achieve a crispy result.
- Ensure your Air Fryer is preheated to 390 F before placing the rolls into its basket. With the timer at 4 minutes, cook the rolls. Serve alongside sweet chili sauce.

591) Turkey Spicy Rolled Meat

Ingredients:

- 1 lb turkey breast fillet
- ½ tsp chili powder
- 1 tsp cinnamon
- 1½ tsp ground cumin
- 1 tsp salt
- 2 tbsp olive oil
- 1 small red onion, finely chopped
- 3 tbsp flat-leafed parsley, finely chopped
- 1 clove garlic, crushed String for rolled meat

Direction: Cooking Time: 60 minutes | Servings: 4

- To create a long piece of meat, ensure that the meat is positioned on the cutting board, such that the short side is facing towards you, then slit it horizontally along the full length, i.e., about a 1/3 of the way from the top and stopping 1-inch from the edge.
- With this part folded open, slit it again from this side and open it. Prepare a mixture of chili powder, pepper, cinnamon, cumin, one teaspoon salt in a big bowl.
- After adding the olive oil, take away one tablespoon of the mixture into a new small bowl. Add onion and parsley in the mixture in the big bowl.
- Ensure that your air fryer is preheated to 360 F.
- Use the onion mixture to coat the meat.
- Coat by rolling the meat firmly and start from the short side. Ensure that the string is tied firmly around the meat, such that each tie is 1-inch away from another.
- Then rub the outside of the rolled meat with the herb mixture.
- Cook for 40 minutes. After the first 25 minutes of cooking, turn the roll over to ensure that the crispiness is present on both sides. Serve.

592) Turkey Breast Glazed with Maple Mustard

Ingredients:

- 2 tsp olive oil
- 5-pound whole turkey breast
- 1 tsp salt
- ½ tsp freshly ground black pepper
- ½ tsp smoked paprika
- 1 tsp dried thyme
- ½ tsp dried sage
- 2 tbsp Dijon mustard
- 1 tbsp butter
- ¼ cup maple syrup

Direction: Cooking Time: 45 minutes | Servings: 6

- ✓ Ensure that your air fryer is preheated to 350 F. Apply the olive oil all over the turkey breast.
- ✓ Prepare a mixture of salt, pepper, paprika, thyme, and sage.
- ✓ Rub the mixture on the outside of the turkey breast.
- ✓ Place the seasoned turkey breast into the basket of your air fryer and air fry for 25 minutes at 350 F. After 25 minutes, change the position of the turkey breast such that the other side is facing up, and then air fry for another 12 minutes.
- ✓ Measure with an instant-read thermometer – once you have about 165 F as the internal temperature of the turkey breast, it means it is fully cooked.
- ✓ While the turkey is still in the air fryer, prepare a mixture of mustard, butter, and maple syrup in a clean saucepan.
- ✓ Once the turkey is done, apply the glaze on every part of the turkey while it stands in an upright position. Air fry again for five minutes, by which the skin will be crispy and nicely browned. Allow the turkey to cool for about five minutes, while covering it slightly with a foil. Slice and serve.

593) Turkey Goujons and Sweet Chilli Dip

Ingredients:

- Turkey goujons:
- 2 oz breadcrumbs
- 1 oz gluten free oats
- 1 oz cheddar cheese
- 1 tsp thyme
- 1 tsp parsley
- Salt and ground black pepper to taste
- 1 large egg beaten
- 2 oz plain flour
- 4 oz leftover turkey breast cut into strips
- Sweet chilli dip:
- 4 oz white sugar
- 1 small red chilli finely chopped and seeds removed
- 2 tbsp garlic puree

Direction: Cooking Time: 25 minutes | Servings: 4

- ✓ Ensure that your air fryer is preheated to 360 F. Prepare a mixture of breadcrumbs, oats, thyme, parsley and cheese in a clean bowl and season to taste. Place your egg in a different bowl, and your flour into another bowl.
- ✓ While laying your turkey on your worktop, cover it in salt and pepper. Be generous with the salt to ensure that the turkey is adequately flavored. Transfer each of the turkey strips into the flour, egg, and the breadcrumbs respectively.
- ✓ The coated turkey strips should be transferred into your air fryer and allowed to cook for 7 minutes (7 turkey goujons).
- ✓ The next seven goujons should be cooked for another 7 minutes and continue like this till all the turkey strips are cooked. While the turkey is in the air fryer, prepare your sweet chili dip.
- ✓ Combine sugar and cold water into a medium pan, and allow to boil on high heat.
- ✓ Add the other ingredients and lower the heat to a simmer for about 10 minutes or until it has reduced.
- ✓ Let the mixture cool and then transfer it into the fridge for another 10 minutes. Serve.

594) Brazilian Mini Turkey Pies

Ingredients:

- 1 oz turkey stock
- 2 oz whole milk
- 2 oz coconut milk
- 8 oz homemade tomato sauce
- 1 tsp oregano
- 1 tbsp coriander
- Salt and ground black pepper to taste
- 2 oz turkey, cooked and shredded Flour
- 8 slices filo pastry
- 1 small egg beaten

Direction: Cooking Time: 15 minutes | Servings: 8

- ✓ Get a clean mixing bowl and put all your wet ingredients, except the egg.
- ✓ Mix well.
- ✓ The result should be a pale-looking sauce – the stock for your pie.
- ✓ Now add the seasoning and turkey before mixing again. Finally, set the mixture aside.
- ✓ To each of your little pie cases, line them with a bit of flour before the filo pastry. This prevents them from sticking.
- ✓ Each pie should use up one sheet of filo, and it should be centrally positioned such that you can easily fold over the extra pastry for the top of the pie.
- ✓ Add the mixture to every mini pie pot until they are ¾ full. Cover the top with the remaining pastry before brushing the egg along the top.
- ✓ Transfer the mini pie pot into the air fryer, set the temperature to 360 F and allow to cook for 10 minutes.
- ✓ Serve Leftover

595) Turkey Spring Rolls

Ingredients:

- 1 oz leftover turkey breast shredded
- 1 tbsp Chinese five spice
- 1 tsp coriander
- Salt and ground black pepper to taste
- 1 tsp Worcester sauce
- 1 tbsp soy sauce
- 1 tbsp honey
- 2 tortilla wraps get our recipe here
- 2 large eggs, beaten

Direction: Cooking Time: 40 minutes | Servings: 1

- ✓ Get a clean mixing bowl and place your leftover turkey plus all the seasonings listed above. Use your hands to ensure that the turkey is coated very well.
- ✓ Your tortilla wraps should be rolled out well to give the best possible thin sheets without breaking.
- ✓ Brush the sheets first with a little water on either side and then with the egg. Transfer the brushed sheet into the fridge for about 30 minutes.
- ✓ This ensures that the egg is adequately absorbed. Withdraw from the fridge after 30 minutes and then cut them into eight different spring roll sheets. Before rolling into a spring roll, put the turkey filling into each sheet.
- ✓ Brush the rolls with another layer of the egg mix before placing them into the air fryer.
- ✓ Set the air fryer to 360 F and allow to cook for 5 minutes. Serve.

596) Sizzling Turkey Fajitas Platter

Ingredients:

- 1 large avocado
- ½ small red onion
- 1 large green pepper
- 1 large yellow pepper
- 1 large red pepper
- 4 oz leftover turkey breast
- 2 tbsp mexican seasoning
- 1 tsp cumin
- 3 tbsp cajun spice
- Fresh coriander
- Salt and ground black pepper to taste
- 5 tbsp soft cheese
- 6 tortilla wraps

Direction: Cooking Time: 30 minutes | Servings: 2-3

- ✓ The first step is to slice up your salad.
- ✓ Cut your avocado into little wedges.
- ✓ Also, dice the red onion and slice the peppers into thin slices. Cut the turkey breast into small little chunks.
- ✓ Transfer the turkey, onions, and peppers into a separate bowl and mix.
- ✓ Then add all seasonings and the soft cheese and mix again.
- ✓ Place all the contents into a silver foil and air fry at 390 F for about 20 minutes. Serve.

597) Turkey Stuffed Bread Recipe

Ingredients:

- 2 oz butter
- 11 oz plain flour
- 1 tsp yeast
- 1 oz shredded turkey wing meat
- 7 oz whole milk
- Salt and ground black pepper to taste
- Handful cooked spinach
- 4 oz soft cheese
- 4 oz white cheddar cheese

Direction: Cooking Time: 45 minutes | Servings: 2

- ✓ Rub the butter into the plain flour so that it appears like breadcrumbs. Then mix in the yeast and the turkey, and finally the warm milk.
- ✓ The next is mixing in pepper and salt. The mixing should be intensive such that the mixture gives a good dough. Then knead the dough for about 10 minutes.
- ✓ Finally, get a clean floury worktop and roll your dough on it. Get a clean mixing bowl and make a mixture of spinach and soft cheese. Layer the top of the bread with the mixture.
- ✓ Then cover it with the cheddar cheese before rolling up the bread. When rolling, the spinach and cheese should form as the center of the bread.
- ✓ Transfer the rolled bread into your Air Fryer, precisely on the baking mat. Set to 360 F and allow to bake for 20 minutes.
- ✓ Reduce the temperature to 320 F and allow to cook for 8 minutes, to ensure that the bread is fully cooked at the center.
- ✓ Serve alongside nice chili dip.

598) Leftover Turkey Muffins

Ingredients:

- Handful spinach
- 2 oz sweet potato
- ½ red onion
- 2 oz brown turkey meat
- 1 large egg
- 1 tbsp soft cheese
- 4 oz cheddar cheese grated
- 1 tsp parsley
- 1 tsp oregano
- 1 tsp garlic puree
- 1 tsp mustard
- Salt and ground black pepper to taste
- 4 oz plain flour

Direction: Cooking Time: 25 minutes | Servings: 8

- ✓ The first step is to gather your vegetables in a bowl. Using your hands, mash up the vegetables.
- ✓ The result should be a few small lumps that can easily form into meatballs if there is the need to.
- ✓ Make a mixture of all the ingredients, except the flour.
- ✓ The mixture should be wet, due to the presence of the egg.
- ✓ Add the flour gradually to the mixture, so that it looks like average meatballs. To ensure that the balls don't stick to your hands, flour your hands. Now, mold the mixture into eight medium-sized balls.
- ✓ Transfer the balls onto a baking mat inside your Air Fryer, set it to 360 F and allow the balls to cook for 15 minutes.
- ✓ Then, turn them over and cook for an additional 5 minutes, but at 320 F. Remove and serve.

599) Turkey Curry Samosas

Ingredients:

- 2 oz shredded turkey wing meat
- 1 tsp coriander
- 1 tsp turmeric
- 1 tsp garam masala
- Salt and ground black pepper to taste
- Coconut milk
- 1 small egg beaten
- 2 pastry sheets

Direction: Cooking Time: 10 minutes | Servings: 2

- ✓ Get a clean mixing bowl and combine the turkey and all the seasonings. Mix well.
- ✓ To get a soft and creamy mixture that would not dry out, put a little coconut milk to the mixture.
- ✓ Transfer the contents onto your pastry sheets. Fold the sheet over to appear like samosa in shape.
- ✓ Beat your eggs into a bowl, and brush the folded sheets until they have a golden glow. Set your Air Fryer to 320 F and allow to cook for 3 minutes. Serve.

600) Leftover Turkey and Cheese Calzone

Ingredients:

- Homemade pizza dough
- 1 tsp basil 1 tsp oregano
- 1 tsp thyme
- Salt and ground black pepper to taste
- 1 tbsp tomato puree
- 4 tbsp homemade tomato sauce
- Leftover turkey brown meat shredded
- 1 oz mozzarella cheese, grated
- 4 oz cheddar cheese, shredded
- 1 oz back bacon, diced
- 1 large egg, beaten

Direction: Cooking Time: 25 minutes | Servings: 4

- ✓ Ensure that your Air Fryer is preheated to 360 F.
- ✓ The first step is to roll out your pizza dough so that they have the size of small pizzas.
- ✓ Get a small mixing bowl, and in it, combine all the seasonings including the puree and the tomato sauce.
- ✓ Add a layer of the tomato to your pizza bases with the aid of a cooking brush.
- ✓ Ensure that the layer doesn't touch the edge. Leave 1/2 - inch space. Now layer up your pizza on one side with the turkey, cheese, and bacon. With ½ - inch gap around your pizza base, use your cooking brush to brush the space with beaten egg.
- ✓ Then fold your pizza base over to look like an uncooked Cornish pasty and brush every area that is visible on the pizza dough with more egg. Transfer to the air fryer and cook for 10 minutes at 360 F. Serve.

601) Thanksgiving Turkey Sandwich Recipe

Ingredients:

- 1 tbsp leftover turkey gravy
- 3 slices wholemeal bread
- Handful fresh lettuce leaves
- 4 slices turkey breast skin still on 1 oz cranberry sauce
- 2 oz leftover turkey stuffing

Direction: Cooking Time: 20 minutes | Servings: 1

- ✓ Use ½ of your leftover gravy in spreading two slices of your bread.
- ✓ The third slice should be transformed into breadcrumbs, and then mixed with the unused gravy.
- ✓ Layer your bread with lettuce, breadcrumbs, turkey, cranberry sauce, and turkey stuffing.
- ✓ While placing the second slice of bread on top, push it down to ensure that it all fits in. Add some small skewers into the sandwich to keep it in place.
- ✓ Transfer into the air fryer and allow to cook at 360 F for 5 minutes, or until nicely warm.
- ✓ Detach the skewers before serving.

602) Airfryer Turkish Cheese and Leek Koftas

Ingredients:

- Leek 1-inch in length
- 1 tsp garlic puree
- 1 tbp parsley
- 1 tbsp mint
- 1 tbsp cumin
- 1 mixed spice
- Salt and ground black pepper to taste
- Feta cheese, broken up
- 11 oz minced beef

Direction: Cooking Time: 30 minutes | Servings: 2

- ✓ After cleaning your leeks, dice them into very thin slices. Get a small ceramic dish that can fit into your air fryer, and in it, add your leeks and the garlic puree.
- ✓ Mix thoroughly. Set your Air Fryer to 360 F and allow the mixture to cook for 10 minutes. Get a mixing bowl and in it, place all your seasonings alongside the cheese.
- ✓ . Add minced beef and mix well. Now add the leeks, and mix well again. Make the mixture into kofta shapes and place them onto sticks.
- ✓ Let the sticks cook in the air fryer for 15 minutes at a temperature of 360 F.
- ✓ Serve alongside ketchup and mayonnaise.

603) Steak in the Air Fryer 1

Ingredients:

- 2 rump steaks
- Salt and ground black pepper to taste

Direction: Cooking Time: 10 minutes | Servings: 2

- ✓ With the aid of a tenderizer, pound your steak so that it appears and feel tenderer.
- ✓ Using salt and pepper, season the grill plan of your air fryer.
- ✓ Transfer the steaks to the top of the seasoning before seasoning the top of the steak in salt and pepper as well.
- ✓ Set your Air Fryer to 400 F.
- ✓ Allow the steaks to cook for 12 minutes, but flip the steak at 6. Withdraw and serve immediately.

604) Steak in the Air Fryer 2

Ingredients:

- Steak with a thickness of 1-inch
- Olive oil Salt and ground black pepper to taste

Direction: Cooking Time: 10 minutes | Servings: 2

- ✓ Withdraw the steak from the fridge. Insert your baking tray into the air fryer, and preheat it for about 5 minutes at 390 F.
- ✓ Use your olive oil to coat the steak at either side generously.
- ✓ Use your salt and pepper to season the steak at either side.
- ✓ Transfer the steak into the air fryer's baking tray.
- ✓ Allow cooking for 3 minutes. Once the timer goes off, flip the steak to the other side and cook for another 3 minutes.
- ✓ Transfer the cooked steak to a plate. Let it cool for 3 minutes more before serving.
- ✓ Note that when the meat is cooling down, the meat fibers are in turn resting. Thus, some of the loose juices are absorbed, and subsequently, the cooled meat is more tender and juicier.

605) Rib Eye Steak

Ingredients:

- 2 lbs rib eye steak
- 1 tbsp steak rub
- 1 tbsp olive oil

Direction: Cooking Time: 20 minutes | Servings: 3-4

- ✓ Ensure that your air fryer is preheated to 400 F and adjust the cooking time to 14 minutes and the mode to
- ✓ French Fries. After seasoning the steak on either side, rub with olive oil too.
- ✓ Transfer the steak into the basket of the air fryer. Allow to cook for the first 7 minutes, then remove and flip the steak.
- ✓ After 14 minutes, withdraw the steak and allow it to rest for 10 minutes. Slice and serve.

606) Herb and Cheese-Stuffed Burgers

Ingredients:

- 2 green onions, thinly sliced
- 2 tbsp minced fresh parsley
- ¼ cup cheddar cheese, cubed
- 3 tsp Dijon mustard, divided
- 2 tbsp ketchup
- ½ tsp salt
- ½ tsp rosemary, dried and crushed
- ¼ tsp sage leaves, dried
- 3 tbsp dry bread crumbs
- 1 lb lean ground beef (90% lean)
- 4 hamburger buns, split Optional toppings: lettuce leaves and tomato slices

Direction: Cooking Time: 45 minutes | Servings: 4

- ✓ Ensure that your air fryer is preheated to 375 F.
- ✓ Get a small bowl, and in it, make a mixture of green onions, parsley, cheddar cheese, and one teaspoon mustard.
- ✓ Get another clean bowl and make a mixture of ketchup, unused mustard, seasonings, and breadcrumbs, and beef.
- ✓ Mix thoroughly but lightly.
- ✓ Portion the mixture into eight thin patties. Using a spoon, add a little out of the cheese mix to the center of the four patties. Top with the remaining patties, while pressing edges together firmly to seal completely.
- ✓ Transfer the burger into the air fryer basket, arranging them in a single layer. If you have several burgers, you may work in batches.
- ✓ Air fry each batch for 10 minutes, then flip and continue cooking for about 8-10 minutes again (until you have a reading of 160 F on your instant-read thermometer).

607) Bunless Burgers

Ingredients:

- Handful lettuce
- Handful fresh basil
- Handful fresh thyme
- 1 medium avocado
- 1 small red onion
- 3 medium tomatoes
- 1 tbsp parsley, dried
- Salt and ground black pepper to taste
- 1 lb minced beef
- 1 tbsp tomato puree
- Handful green beans
- 1 tbsp olive oil
- 4 slices back bacon

Direction: Cooking Time: 35 minutes | Servings: 3-4

- ✓ Ensure that your air fryer is preheated to 360 F.
- ✓ Dice your clean, fresh herbs.
- ✓ Peel and get rid of the stones in the avocado before slicing it.
- ✓ Also, peel and dice the red onion as well as the fresh tomato.
- ✓ Get a clean mixing bowl and make a mixture of all the seasonings, the minced beef, 1/5 of the red onion, and the tomato puree.
- ✓ Then mix well and shape the mixture into four burger shapes. Place the baking mat at the bottom of your air fryer. Transfer the burgers onto your baking mat and cook for 10 minutes.
- ✓ After 10 minutes, place the green beans in the olive oil and place it inside the air fryer alongside the burgers.
- ✓ Cook for extra 5 minutes before adding the slices of bacon. Then cook for an additional 5 minutes. Serve the burgers alongside the avocado, bacon, green beans and salad garnish.

608) Air Fryer Meatloaf

Ingredients:

- 1 pound lean ground beef
- 1 small onion, finely chopped
- 1 tbsp chopped fresh thyme
- 3 tbsp dry bread crumbs
- 1 egg, lightly beaten
- 1 tsp salt
- Ground black pepper to taste
- 2 mushrooms, thickly sliced
- 1 tbsp olive oil, or as needed

Direction: Cooking Time: 45 minutes | Servings: 4

- ✓ Ensure that your air fryer is preheated to 390 F. Get a clean bowl and make a mixture of ground beef, onion, thyme, bread crumbs, egg, salt, and pepper.
- ✓ Knead the mixture and mix thoroughly.
- ✓ Get a clean baking pan and transfer the beef mixture in it and smooth the top, while pressing the mushrooms into the top and coating with olive oil.
- ✓ Transfer the pan into the air fryer basket and slide into the air fryer.
- ✓ Roast the meatloaf inside the air fryer for 25 minutes or until you have a nice brown color.
- ✓ Allow the roasted meatloaf to cool for at least 10 minutes.
- ✓ Slice into wedges and serve.
- ✓ Meatloaf Flavored with Black

609) Peppercorns

Ingredients:

- 4 lbs minced beef
- 3 tbsp tomato ketchup
- 1 tbsp mixed herbs
- 1 tbsp oregano
- 1 tbsp parsley
- 1 tbsp basil
- 1 large onion peeled and diced
- 1 tsp Worcester sauce Breadcrumbs made from one slice of wholemeal bread
- Salt and ground black pepper to taste

Direction: Cooking Time: 40 minutes | Servings: 6

- ✓ Get a large mixing bowl and place the mince in it alongside the tomato ketchup, herbs, onion, and Worchester sauce. Mix all the ingredients well.
- ✓ Massage and mix the ingredients thoroughly for about five minutes to ensure that the slice is evenly distributed in the meatloaf slice.
- ✓ Add the breadcrumbs, salt and pepper to the mixture and mix thoroughly again.
- ✓ Get a small dish and place the mixture in it.
- ✓ Slide the dish into your air fryer and cook for 25 minutes at 360 F. Withdraw and serve.

610) Fried Meatballs in Tomato Sauce

Ingredients:

- 1 small onion
- 1 egg, beaten
- 11 oz minced beef
- 1 tbsp fresh thyme leaves, chopped
- 1 tbsp fresh parsley, chopped
- 3 tbsp bread crumbs
- ¾ cup of your favourite tomato sauce
- Salt and ground black pepper to taste

Direction: Cooking Time: 20 minutes | Servings: 2

- ✓ Ensure that your air fryer is preheated to 390 F.
- ✓ Chop your onion into fine pieces and transfer it, alongside all other ingredients, into a clean mixing bowl.
- ✓ Mix well and shape the mixture into 10 to 12 balls.
- ✓ Separate the balls into two batches and transfer each batch into the air fryer basket. Fry each batch for 7 minutes.
- ✓ Transfer the meatballs into an oven dish, put the tomato sauce and place the oven dish into the air fryer basket.
- ✓ Then set the temperature to 320 F and allow to cook for 5 minutes. This will warm everything through before you finally serve.

611) Roasted Stuffed Peppers

Ingredients:

- 1 tsp olive oil
- ½ medium onion, chopped
- 1 clove garlic, minced
- 1 tsp Worcestershire sauce
- ½ cup tomato sauce
- 8 oz lean ground beef
- ½ tsp salt
- ½ tsp black pepper
- 2 medium green peppers, stems and seeds removed - cooked in boiling salted water for
- 3 minutes
- 4 oz cheddar cheese, shredded

Direction: Cooking Time: 40 minutes | Servings 2

- ✓ Ensure that your air fryer is preheated to 390 F or your convection toaster oven to 400 F. Get a small nonstick skillet and pour some olive oil into it.
- ✓ Then stir-fry your onion and garlic in it until you have a golden appearance. Withdraw from the burner and allow to cool.
- ✓ Combine your Worcestershire, ¼ cup tomato sauce, cooked garlic and onion, beef, salt, and pepper.
- ✓ Blend the mixture alongside half the shredded cheese and transfer the blended mixture into a medium bowl.
- ✓ Divide the peppers into halves and top each with the remaining cheese and tomato sauce.
- ✓ Arrange them into the air fryer basket or in a small baking dish that has been sprayed with cooking oil. Air fry or bake for about 15 to 20 minutes, or until the meat is well cooked. Withdraw and serve.

612) Air Fryer Party Meatballs

Ingredients:

- 2 ½ tbsp Worcester sauce
- ¾ cup tomato ketchup
- 1 tbsp lemon juice
- 1 tbsp Tabasco
- ½ tsp dry mustard
- ¼ cup vinegar
- 3 gingersnaps crushed
- ½ cup brown sugar
- 1 lb mince beef

Direction: Cooking Time: 25 minutes | Servings: 24 meatballs

- ✓ Get a large mixing bowl and mix all your seasonings thoroughly to ensure even coating.
- ✓ Toss the mince into the bowl and mix well again. Create medium sized meatballs from the mixture and transfer them into the air fryer.
- ✓ Set the timer to 15 minutes and temperature to 400 F.
- ✓ Allow to cook, and when done, you will have a nice, crispy, and well-cooked meatballs.
- ✓ If not, cook for a few minutes more.
- ✓ Place the cooked meatballs on sticks. Serve.

613) Mustard Honey Beef Balls

Ingredients:

- 11 oz beef, minced
- 1 tsp garlic, minced
- 2 oz onion, peeled and diced
- 1 tbsp cheddar cheese, grated
- 1 tsp honey
- 1 tsp mustard
- Handful basil, fresh and chopped
- Salt and ground black pepper to taste

Direction: Cooking Time: 35 minutes | Servings: 4

- ✓ Get a large, clean bowl and make a mix of all the ingredients above in it.
- ✓ Form small balls from the mixture.
- ✓ Transfer the balls into the air fryer and cook for 15 minutes at 390 F.
- ✓ Serve hot alongside egg fried rice.

614) Easy Spring Rolls

Ingredients:

- 2 oz rice noodles, dried
- 1 tbsp sesame oil
- 3 cloves garlic, crushed
- 1 small onion, diced
- 1 cup frozen mixed vegetables
- 7 oz ground beef
- 1 tsp soy sauce
- 1 (16 oz) package egg roll wrappers
- 1 tbsp vegetable oil, or to taste

Direction: Cooking Time: 55 minutes | Servings: 3-4

- ✓ Ensure that your air fryer is preheated to 350 F.
- ✓ Get a clean bowl and pour some hot water in it.
- ✓ Then soak your noodles in hot water for about 5 minutes.
- ✓ Cut the soaked noodles into shorter strands.
- ✓ Heat your sesame oil in a suitable cooking pan and over medium-high heat.
- ✓ Add the garlic, onion, mixed vegetables, and ground beef.
- ✓ Cook the mixture until you have a browned beef – this takes about 6 minutes.
- ✓ Withdraw from heat.
- ✓ Stir in the noodles, and allow it to cool for a while so that the juices are well absorbed.
- ✓ Add soy sauce to the filling. Get a flat work surface and lay one egg roll wrapper. Then place a diagonal strip of filling across the wrapper. Fold the top corner over the filling, and fold in the two side corners. Then brush the center with cold water and roll over the spring rolls to seal finally.
- ✓ Do the same for the other wrappers and filling. Brush the tops of the spring rolls using vegetable oil.
- ✓ Arrange the rolls in batches into the air fryer basket. Cook each batch until the rolls are crispy and lightly browned – this takes about 8 minutes. Repeat the process until all the rolls are cooked. Serve.

615) Beef Wellington

Ingredients:

- 2 lb beef fillet
- Salt and ground black pepper to taste
- Homemade short crust pastry
- Homemade chicken liver pate
- 1 medium egg, beaten

Direction: Cooking Time: 55 minutes | Servings: 4

- ✓ Clean out your beef fillet, remove any visible fat, and season with pepper and salt. Then seal it up using cling film and fridge it for an hour.
- ✓ Create your homemade short crust pastry and your chicken liver pate. With your short crust pastry rolled out, use your pastry brush to coat all around the edges with beaten egg.
- ✓ This ensures that it is sticky for sealing. Right inside the outer egg line, place a thin layer of the homemade pate until the white pastry is no longer visible.
- ✓
- ✓ Withdraw the cling film from the meat and put the meat in the middle, on the top, of the pate and apply a little force to push it down a bit.
- ✓ Seal the pastry around the pate and the meat. Ensure that you score the top of the pastry to ensure that the meat is not entirely devoid of air.
- ✓ Transfer into the grill plan of the air fryer. Allow cooking for 35 minutes at 320 F. Remove after 35 minutes and allow to rest for some minutes. Slice and serve alongside roast potatoes.

616) Pork Tenderloin with Bell Pepper

Ingredients:

- 2 tsp Provençal herbs
- 1 red or yellow bell pepper, in thin strips
- 1 red onion, in thin slices
- Salt to taste
- Freshly ground black pepper to taste
- 1 tbsp olive oil
- 1 (15 oz) pork tenderloin
- ½ tbsp mustard Round
- 6-inch oven dish

Direction: Prep + Cook Time: 30 minutes | Servings: 2

- ✓ Ensure that your air fryer is preheated to 390 F.
- ✓ Get a clean dish and make a mixture of the Provencal herbs, bell pepper strips, and onion.
- ✓ Add salt and pepper to taste, and finally a ½ tablespoon olive oil.
- ✓ Cut the pork tenderloin into four pieces. Rub each piece with pepper, mustard, and salt.
- ✓ Coat each piece thinly using olive oil, and transfer them into the dish uprightly, on top of the pepper mixture. Transfer the bowl into the air fryer basket.
- ✓ Allow the meat to roast for 15 minutes, alongside the vegetables. Halfway into roasting, turn the meat and mix the peppers.
- ✓ Withdraw after 15 minutes. Serve with mashed potatoes and a fresh salad for the best taste.

617) Air-Fried Pork Dumplings with Dipping Sauce

Ingredients:

- 1 tsp canola oil
- 4 cups bok choy (about 12 oz), chopped
- 1 tbsp garlic (3 garlic cloves), chopped
- 1 tbsp fresh ginger, chopped
- 4 oz ground pork
- ¼ tsp crushed red pepper
- 18 (3 1/2-inch-square) dumpling wrappers or wonton wrappers
- Cooking spray 2 tbsp rice vinegar
- ½ tsp packed light brown sugar
- 1 tbsp finely chopped scallions 1 tsp toasted sesame oil
- 2 tsp lower-sodium soy sauce

Direction: Cooking Time: 1 hour 10 minutes | Servings: 6

- ✓ Get a clean large nonstick skillet and heat your canola oil in it over medium-high heat. Add bok choy and cook while stirring consistently until the mixture is wilted and almost dry – this takes about 6 to 8 minutes.
- ✓ Toss in garlic and ginger, and cook again for a minute, constantly stirring this time. Remove the bok choy mixture and place in a plate for 5 minutes. Using a paper towel, pat the mixture dry.
- ✓ Get a medium bowl and in it, stir the bok choy mixture, the ground pork, and crushed red pepper together. Lay a dumpling wrapper on your work surface, and using a spoon, place one tablespoon filling into the center of the wrapper.
- ✓ Use your fingers or your pastry brush to moisten the edges of the wrapper lightly with water. Fold the wrapper over to give a shape of a half-moon, and press the edges to seal.
- ✓ Do the same for the other wrappers and filling. Coat the air fryer basket lightly using the cooking spray.
- ✓ Arrange six dumplings in the basket, such that there is a little space between each. Spray the dumplings lightly with the cooking spray.
- ✓ Set your Air Fryer to 375 F and allow to cook for 12 minutes until the dumplings are lightly browned.
- ✓ Turn the dumplings over halfway through cooking (at 6 minutes). Do the same for all the dumplings while keeping the cooked dumplings warm.
- ✓ While cooking the dumplings, create a mixture of rice vinegar, brown sugar, scallions, sesame oil, and soy sauce in a small bowl.
- ✓ Stir together until the sugar is dissolved. Serve by placing three dumplings on each plate alongside two teaspoons sauce.

618) Pork Chops

Ingredients:

- ½ cup Dijon mustard
- 4 pork loin chops (3/4-inch thick)
- ¼ tsp cayenne pepper
- ½ tsp black pepper
- ½ tsp salt
- 1 cup Italian bread crumbs Cooking spray

Direction: Cooking Time: 20 minutes | Servings: 4

- ✓ Ensure that your Air Fryer is preheated to 400 F.
- ✓ Spread the mustard on either side of the pork chops.
- ✓ Ensure it is evenly spread.
- ✓ Get a shallow dish and combine the cayenne, black pepper, salt, and the bread crumbs.
- ✓ Dip the pork chops in the crumbs such that the two sides are well and evenly coated.
- ✓ Arrange the chops in a single layer in the air fryer basket, and spray lightly with the cooking spray.
- ✓ Place the sheet in the oven, leaving a space of about 4 inches between the heating element and the sheet.
- ✓ Cook until you have a golden brown color of the chops, for about 10 minutes.
- ✓ Turn the pork chops to the other side after 5 minutes. Once cooked, serve

619) Crispy Breaded Pork Chops

Ingredients:

- Olive oil spray Kosher salt
- 6 (3/4-inch thick) center cut boneless pork chops, fat trimmed (5 oz each)
- ½ cup panko crumbs (check labels for GF)
- 2 tbsp parmesan cheese, grated
- ½ tsp garlic powder
- 1/3 cup crushed cornflakes crumbs
- ½ tsp onion powder
- 1/8 tsp black pepper
- 1¼ tsp sweet paprika
- ¼ tsp chili powder
- 1 large egg, beaten

Direction: Cooking Time: 25 minutes | Servings: 2

- ✓ Ensure that your Air Fryer is preheated to 400 F for about 2 minutes. Also, spritz the air fryer basket with oil. Use ½ tsp kosher salt to season the pork chops on either side.
- ✓ Place the panko, parmesan cheese, garlic powder, ¾ tsp kosher salt, cornflake crumbs, onion powder, black pepper, paprika and chili powder in a large shallow bowl.
- ✓ Get another large shallow bowl and beat the egg in it.
- ✓ Then dip the pork into the beaten egg and the crumb mixture respectively.
- ✓ Transfer about 3 of the chops into the sprayed air fryer basket and sprinkle the top with cooking oil lightly.
- ✓ Allow cooking for 12 minutes, while turning the chops to the other side after 6 minutes.
- ✓ Spritz either side of the chops with oil. Withdraw the cooked chops after 12 minutes and cook the remaining chops.
- ✓ Serve while warm.

620) Breaded Pork Chops (ver. 2)

Ingredients:

- 4 slices homemade bread
- Salt and ground black pepper to taste
- 5 pork chops bone in
- 2 tbsp olive oil
- 4 oz plain flour
- 1 tbsp pork seasoning 1 large egg
- 3 oz apple juice
- 3 tbsp Parsley

Direction: Cooking Time: 20 minutes | Servings: 5

- ✓ Ensure that your Air Fryer is preheated to 350 F for about 2 minutes. Prepare your breadcrumbs by blending the bread. Using salt and pepper, season your pork chops, and rub little olive oil into the meat.
- ✓ Get a clean mixing bowl and place the plain flour, salt, pork seasoning, and pepper. Get another clean bowl and beat an egg and add the apple juice.
- ✓ Get a third bowl and mix the breadcrumbs with pepper, parsley, and salt.
- ✓ Dredge the pork chops into the flour mixture and egg mixture respectively before coating it generously with the breadcrumbs.
- ✓ Allow the coated pork chops to cook for 10 minutes at 350 F. Serve.

621) Balsamic Smoked Pork Chops

Ingredients:

- Cooking spray 2 large Nellie's Free Range Eggs, beaten
- ¼ cup 2% milk
- 1 cup finely chopped pecans
- 1 cup panko (Japanese) bread crumbs
- 4 smoked bone-in pork chops (7-1/2 ounces each)
- ¼ cup all-purpose flour

For sauce:
- 2 tbsp seedless raspberry jam
- 2 tbsp brown sugar
- 1/3 cup balsamic vinegar
- 1 tbsp thawed frozen orange juice concentrate

Direction: Cooking Time: 35 minutes | Servings: 4

- : Ensure that your Air Fryer is preheated to 400 F.
- Spray the air fryer basket with the cooking spray.
- Get a shallow bowl and whisk the eggs and milk together in it.
- Get another shallow bowl and place the pecans alongside the breadcrumbs.
- Coat the pork chops with flour, and shake to remove the excess flour.
- Dip the coated pork chops into the egg mixture and the crumb mixture respectively.
- Pat occasionally to ensure that the mixtures do not fall off.
- You may work in batches if you have many pork chops. Arrange the chops in a single layer in the air fryer basket, and spray lightly with the cooking spray.
- Allow the pork chops to cook inside the air fryer for 12 to 15 minutes or until they appear golden brown. After 6-7 minutes, turn the chops and spray lightly again. After cooking, withdraw and keep warm.
- Then cook the other chops. While cooking, place the unused ingredients in a small saucepan and boil while stirring until the mixture is slightly thickened.
- This should take about 6 to 8 minutes. Serve the chops alongside the sauce.

623) Turkey and Cheese Calzone

Ingredients:

- Homemade pizza dough
- 1 tsp basil
- 1 tsp oregano
- 1 tsp thyme
- Salt and ground black pepper to taste
- 1 tbsp tomato puree
- 4 tbsp homemade tomato sauce
- Leftover turkey brown meat shredded
- 1 oz mozzarella cheese, grated
- 4 oz cheddar cheese, shredded
- 1 oz back bacon, diced
- 1 large egg, beaten

Direction: Cooking Time: 25 minutes | Servings: 4

- Ensure that your Air Fryer is preheated to 360 F. The first step is to roll out your pizza dough so that they have the size of small pizzas.
- Get a small mixing bowl, and in it, combine all the seasonings including the puree and the tomato sauce.
- Add a layer of the tomato to your pizza bases with the aid of a cooking brush.
- Ensure that the layer doesn't touch the edge.
- Leave 1/2 -inch space. Now layer up your pizza on one side with the turkey, cheese, and bacon. With ½ - inch gap around your pizza base, use your cooking brush to brush the space with beaten egg.
- Then fold your pizza base over to look like an uncooked Cornish pasty and brush every area that is visible on the pizza dough with more egg.
- Transfer to the air fryer and cook for 10 minutes at 360 F. Serve.

622) Garlic Butter Pork Chops

Ingredients:

- 2 tsp parsley, dried
- Salt and ground black pepper to taste
- 2 tsp garlic cloves grated
- 1 tbsp coconut butter
- 1 tbsp coconut oil
- 4 pork chops

Direction: Cooking Time: 1 hour 25 minutes

- Ensure that your air fryer is preheated to 350 F.
- Combine all the seasonings in a clean mixing bowl, alongside the garlic, butter, and the coconut oil.
- Apply the mixture to either side of the pork chops before sealing them in silver foil.
- Fridge the sealed pork chops for an hour. After an hour, withdraw from the fridge and separate the silver foil from the chops.
- Rub the remaining marinade in the silver foil over the chops. Transfer them into the grill pan of the air fryer.
- Allow to cook for 7 minutes, then turn to the other side and allow to cook for another 8 minutes.
- Serve cooked chops alongside the garden salad. You may drizzle with a bit of olive oil.

624) Country Fried Steak

Ingredients:

- 1 tsp garlic powder
- 1 tsp onion powder
- 1 tsp salt
- 1 tsp ground black pepper
- 1 cup Panko bread crumbs
- 6 oz sirloin steak-pounded thin
- 1 cup flour 3 eggs, beaten

Sausage Gravy (optional):
- 6 oz ground sausage meat
- 2 tbsp flour
- 2 cups milk
- 1 tsp ground black pepper

Direction: Cooking Time: 40 minutes | Servings: 1

- Using the spices as seasoning, season the panko. Dip the steak in flour, egg, and seasoned panko respectively.
- Transfer the dredged steak into the air fryer basket and close. Set the temperature to 370 F and allow to cook for 12 minutes.
- Withdraw the steak after 12 minutes and serve alongside sausage gravy or mash potatoes.
- To prepare your sausage gravy, get a clean pan and cook your sausage in it until it is well cooked.
- Then drain the fat and reserve about 2 tbsp in the pan. Add flour to the sausage in the pan, and mix until the flour is well mixed with the sausage.
- Add the milk and mix slowly. Stir the mixture over medium heat until the milk thickens.
- Finally, season with pepper and allow to cook for 3 minutes.

625) Tender Juicy Smoked BBQ Ribs

Ingredients:

- 1 rack ribs (baby back or spare ribs)
- 1 tbsp liquid smoke
- 2-3 tbsp pork rub
- Salt and ground black pepper to taste
- ½ cup BBQ sauce

Direction: Cooking Time: 1 hour 5 minutes | Servings: 1-2

- ✓ There is always a thin layer, usually tough to remove, at the back of the ribs. Remove the membrane by cutting it and pulling it off.
- ✓ Then cut the ribs in half or almost half, such that each half fits conveniently in the air fryer. Drizzle both sides of the ribs with the liquid smoke.
- ✓ Combine the pork rub, pepper, and salt and season both sides of the ribs with the mixture.
- ✓ Cover the ribs and leave it for 30 minutes at room temperature.
- ✓ Transfer the ribs into the air fryer. You may stack the ribs if you want.
- ✓ Allow cooking for 15 minutes at 360 F. Flip the ribs to the other side after 15 minutes and allow to cook for an extra 15 minutes.
- ✓ Withdraw the cooked ribs from the air fryer and drizzle with BBQ sauce. Serve.

626) Chinese Take Out Sweet 'N Sour Pork

Ingredients:

- 1/8 tsp Chinese Five Spice
- ½ tsp sea salt
- ¼ tsp freshly ground black pepper 1 cup potato starch (or cornstarch)
- 2 large eggs
- 1 tsp pure sesame oil, optional
- 2 lbs pork cut into chunks
- 3 tbsp canola oil
- Cooking oil spray
- 1 prepared Simple sweet 'n sour sauce, optional

Direction: Cooking Time: 30 minutes | Servings: 4

- ✓ Get a clean mixing bowl and mix the
- ✓ Chinese Five Spice, pepper, salt, and potato starch in it. Get another clean mixing bowl and beat the eggs in it; add the sesame oil.
- ✓ Dip the pork pieces into the potato starch mixture; shake to remove any excess starch.
- ✓ Then dip into the egg mixture, and shake again to get rid of excess.
- ✓ Finally, dip it into the potato starch mixture again. Place the coated pork pieces into an already-coated air fryer basket (coated with oil).
- ✓ Spray with oil and allow to cook at 340 F for about 8-12 minutes, or until you see that the pork is well cooked. Shake the basket a few times while cooking.
- ✓ Combine the cooked pork with Simple Sweet 'N' Sour Sauce and serve.

627) Bourbon Bacon Cinnamon Rolls

Ingredients:

- 8 bacon strips
- 3/4 cup bourbon
- 1 tube (12.4 oz) refrigerated cinnamon rolls with icing
- 2 tbsp maple syrup
- ½ cup chopped pecans
- 1 tsp minced fresh gingerroot

Direction: Cooking Time: 40 minutes | Servings: 8

- ✓ Get a clean shallow dish. In the dish, place the bacon and add bourbon. Seal the dish containing the mixture and refrigerate.
- ✓ The next day, remove the bacon and pat dry, throw the bourbon away. Get a large skillet and cook the bacon in it over medium heat. Stop cooking when you have nearly crisp but pliable bacon. You can cook in batches. Remove the cooked bacon and drain using paper towels.
- ✓ Discard all but one teaspoon drippings.
- ✓ Preheat your Air Fryer to 350 F Create eight rolls out of the dough, while keeping the icing packet. Unroll each spiral roll into a long strip, and pat the dough to form 6x1-inches strips.
- ✓ Put one bacon strip on each dough strip, while trimming the bacon as required. .
- ✓ Reroll the strip to form a spiral and seal by pinching the ends. Do the same for the remaining dough. Place four rolls into the basket of the air fryer and allow to cook for 5 minutes.
- ✓ After 5 minutes, turn over the rolls and cook the other side until you have a golden brown color (for about 4 minutes). While cooking the rolls, make a mixture of maple syrup and pecans in a bowl. Stir the contents of the icing packet and ginger together in another bowl.
- ✓ Pour the remaining bacon drippings into the same skillet and heat over medium heat. Then add the pecan mixture and allow to cook until lightly toasted while frequently stirring (for about 2-3 minutes).
- ✓ Drizzle half of the icing over warm cinnamon rolls and top them with half of the pecans. Do the same for the second batch. Serve.

628) Rosemary Sausage Meatballs

Ingredients:

- 2 tbsp olive oil
- 1 tsp curry powder
- 4 garlic cloves, minced
- ¼ cup minced fresh parsley
- 1 tbsp minced fresh rosemary
- ¼ cup dry bread crumbs
- 1 jar (4 ounces) diced pimientos, drained
- 1 large egg, lightly beaten
- 2 lbs bulk pork sausage P
- retzel sticks or toothpicks, optional

Direction: Cooking Time: 30 minutes | Servings: 2

- ✓ Ensure that your air fryer is preheated to 400 F. Grab a small skillet and place over medium heat.
- ✓ Heat the oil in the skillet, alongside curry powder and sauté garlic, until the mixture is tender. It takes about 1-2 minutes.
- ✓ Allow the mixture to cool slightly. Get a clean bowl and make a mixture of parsley, rosemary, bread crumbs, pimientos, egg, and the garlic mixture.
- ✓ Add the sausage and mix thoroughly but lightly. Make 1 to ¼ inches balls from the sausage mix.
- ✓ Transfer the balls into the air fryer basket, arranging them in a single layer.
- ✓ Cook for about 7-10 minutes until the balls are lightly browned and cooked through. Withdraw the cooked balls and keep warm.
- ✓ Do the same for the other meatballs. Serve alone or alongside pretzels.

629) Air-Fried Meatloaf

Ingredients:

- ½ lb ground veal
- ½ lb ground pork
- ½ tsp Sriracha salt
- ½ tsp ground black pepper
- 2 medium spring onions, diced
- 1 large egg, beaten
- ¼ cup chopped fresh cilantro
- ¼ cup gluten-free bread crumbs
- 1 tsp blackstrap molasses
- 1 tsp olive oil
- 2 tsp gluten-free chipotle chili sauce
- ½ cup ketchup

Direction: Cooking Time: 1 day 55 minutes | Servings: 4

- ✓ Ensure that your air fryer is preheated to 400 F. Get a nonstick baking dish that can fit into the air fryer basket, then combine veal and pork in the dish.
- ✓ Mix well and add ½ teaspoon of Sriracha salt, black pepper, spring onions, egg, cilantro, and breadcrumbs.
- ✓ Now mix with your hands, and form a loaf inside the sizable baking dish.
- ✓ Make a mixture of molasses, olive oil, chipotle chili sauce, and ketchup in a small bowl. Whisk the mixture well and set aside without refrigerating.
- ✓ Allow the meatloaf to cook for 25 minutes in the air fryer without opening the basket. After 25 minutes, top the meatloaf with the ketchup mixture, ensuring that the top is entirely covered.
- ✓ Now transfer the covered meatloaf into the air fryer and bake until the internal temperature is 160 F – this takes about 7 minutes or more.
- ✓ Turn off the air fryer with the meatloaf still inside. Allow to rest for 5 minutes and withdraw the meatloaf.
- ✓ Let the baked meatloaf rest 5 minutes outside the air fryer. Slice and serve.

630) Chinese Pineapple Pork

Ingredients:

- 1 lb pork loin, cut into cubes
- ½ tsp pepper
- ½ tsp salt
- 1 tsp fresh ginger, minced 1 clove garlic, minced
- 1 green pepper, cut into cubes
- ½ pineapple, cut into cubes
- 1 tbsp brown sugar
- 2 tbsp soy sauce
- 1 tbsp vegetable oil
- Toasted sesame seeds
- 1 small bunch fresh coriander leaves, chopped

Direction: Cooking Time: 45 minutes | Servings: 4

- ✓ Season your pork with pepper and salt. Combine the seasoned pork alongside ginger, garlic, green pepper and pineapple in the air fryer pan.
- ✓ Get a clean bowl and in it, make a mixture of brown sugar and soy sauce as well as the ingredients. Drizzle the vegetable oil over the ingredients.
- ✓ Ensure that your air fryer is preheated to 360 F. Set the cooking time to 17 minutes.
- ✓ After 17 minutes, check and ensure all ingredients are well cooked.
- ✓ Combine the sesame seeds and chopped coriander as a garnish for the pork. Serve alongside white rice.

631) Chinese Kebabs and Rice

Ingredients:

- 4 oz egg fried rice
- 1 tbsp Chinese five spice
- ½ small onion peeled and diced
- 6 oz minced pork
- 1 tsp garlic puree
- 1 tsp tomato puree
- 1 tbsp soy sauce
- Salt and ground black pepper to taste
- 1 slice wholemeal bread made into breadcrumbs

Direction: Cooking Time: 15 minutes | Servings: 20 slices

- ✓ Start by making your egged fried rice: boil the Chinese rice in a pan, add half the Chinese seasoning once it is cooked, then add a hard-boiled egg and mix thoroughly.
- ✓ To make your kebabs, combine the remaining half of the
- ✓ Chinese seasoning, onion, minced pork, garlic and tomato puree, and soy sauce in a mixing bowl.
- ✓ Mix thoroughly and season with salt and pepper.
- ✓ Toss in the breadcrumbs and shape into sausage shapes. A
- ✓ llow the mixture to cook for 20 minutes at 360 F in the air fryer. Serve.

632) Air Fryer Bacon

Ingredients:

11 slices bacon (I am using Trader Joe's, and it is a thick cut)

Direction: Cooking Time: 25 minutes | Servings: 11 slices

- ✓ Divide the bacon into two equal amounts.
- ✓ Transfer a half into the air fryer and cook for 10 minutes at 400 F.
- ✓ For thinner bacon, you may reduce the cooking time.
- ✓ After 5 minutes of cooking, check and rearrange (if there is the need to). Use tongs here.
- ✓ After rearranging, cook for another 5 minutes.
- ✓ Once it is done, withdraw from the air fryer and serve.

633) Drunken Ham with Mustard

Ingredients:

- 1 joint of ham (1½ lbs)
- 8 oz whiskey
- 2 tbsp French mustard
- 2 tbsp honey

Direction: Cooking Time: 45 minutes | Servings: 4

- ✓ Withdraw the ham from the fridge 30 minutes before cooking – this ensures that the ham is at room temperature before cooking.
- ✓ Make your marinade into a casserole dish that fits into your air fryer – mix the whiskey, mustard, and honey to get your marinade mixture.
- ✓ Transfer the ham into the oven dish and turn it in the marinade.
- ✓ Set your air fryer to 320 F and allow the ham cook for 15 minutes.
- ✓ Withdraw the ham, add another shot of whiskey and turn in the marinade again.
- ✓ Allow the ham to cook for 25 minutes at 320 F (or until it is done).
- ✓ Withdraw from the air fryer and serve immediately.
- ✓ You can serve with potatoes and fresh vegetables.

634) Roasted Rack of Lamb with a Macadamia Crust

Ingredients:

- 1 garlic clove
- 1 tbsp olive oil
- 2 lbs rack of lamb
- Salt and ground black pepper to taste
- 3 oz macadamia nuts, unsalted
- 1 tbsp chopped fresh rosemary
- 1 tbsp breadcrumbs (preferably homemade)
- 1 egg, beaten

Direction: Cooking Time: 45 minutes | Servings: 4

- ✓ Ensure that your air fryer is preheated to 210 F.
- ✓ Chop your garlic into fine pieces, and mix them with oil to make the garlic oil.
- ✓ Season the rack of the lamb with salt and pepper alongside the garlic oil.
- ✓ Chop your nuts finely and transfer the pieces into a bowl, add rosemary and breadcrumbs.
- ✓ Get a clean bowl and whisk the egg in it. Dredge the meat in the egg mixture and drain off any excess. Dip it in the macadamia crust again.
- ✓ Transfer the coated lamb rack in the air fryer basket and allow to cook for 25 minutes. Increase the temperature to 390 F after 25 minutes.
- ✓ Cook for 5 minutes at 390 F. Withdraw from the air fryer and allow to rest for another 10 minutes while covering with aluminum foil. Serve.
- ✓ Note: You can use hazelnuts, cashews, pistachios, or almonds instead of the macadamia nuts.

636) Air Fryer Lamb Burgers

Ingredients:

- Lamb burgers:
- 1 tsp harissa paste 2 tsp garlic puree
- 1 tbsp Moroccan spice
- Salt and ground black pepper to taste
- 1¼ lamb, minced

Greek Dip:

- 3 tbsp Greek yoghurt
- 1 small lemon juice only
- ½ tsp oregano
- 1 tsp Moroccan spice

Direction: Cooking Time: 25 minutes | Servings: 4

- ✓ Get a clean mixing bowl and combine your lamb burger ingredients alongside the lamb mince.
- ✓ Mix thoroughly until you are sure the lamb mince is evenly seasoned.
- ✓ Make the mince into lamb burger shapes with the aid of your burger press.
- ✓ Transfer the lamb burgers into your air fryer and set the temperature to 360 F.
- ✓ Allow cooking for 18 minutes. Meanwhile, prepare your Greek Dip by using your fork to mix the
- ✓ Greek dip ingredients.
- ✓ Serve the cooked lamb burgers alongside the Greek dip.

637) Fish and Chips

Ingredients:

- 2 (10 oz) russet potatoes, scrubbed
- Cooking spray
- 1¼ tsp kosher salt, divided
- 1 cup (about 4¼ oz) all-purpose flour
- 2 large eggs 2 tbsp water
- 1 cup whole-wheat panko (Japanese-style breadcrumbs)
- 4 (6 oz) skinless tilapia fillets
- ½ cup malt vinegar

Direction: Cooking Time: 45 minutes | Servings: 4

- ✓ By following the instructions of the manufacturer, use your spiralizer to cut the potatoes into spirals. Place each batch of the spiral potatoes into the air fryer basket.
- ✓ Spray with cooking spray generously such that every piece is well coated. Set your air fryer to 375 F and cook for 10 minutes (or until they are crispy and golden brown). Turn the potatoes halfway through cooking.
- ✓ Once cooked, transfer them into a separate bowl and cover to keep warm. Do the same for the other batches. Sprinkle all the cooked potatoes with ¼ teaspoon salt.
- ✓ While you cook the potatoes, get a shallow dish and place your flour and add ½ teaspoon of the salt.
- ✓ Whisk the eggs and water together lightly in another shallow dish. Get a third shallow dish and stir the panko and the unused ½ teaspoon salt together.
- ✓ Cut each fish fillet lengthwise into two long strips, and dip each strip into the flour mixture, the egg mixture, and the panko mixture respectively. Use the cooking spray to coat the fish pieces on both sides.
- ✓ Transfer the fish into the air fryer basket (in a single layer). Allow each batch to cook for 10 minutes at 375 F (or until golden brown). Remember to turn fish over halfway through cooking. Serve by placing two pieces of fish alongside equal portions of potato spirals on each plate.
- ✓ Include two tablespoons of malt vinegar for dipping.

635) Meatballs with Feta

Ingredients:

- 6 oz lamb mince or lean minced beef
- 1 slice of stale white bread, turned into fine crumbs
- ½ tbsp lemon peel, grated
- 1 tbsp fresh oregano, finely chopped
- 2 oz Greek feta, crumbled
- Freshly ground black pepper Round, shallow oven dish,
- 6 - inch Tapas forks

Direction: Cooking Time: 20 minutes | Servings: 10

- ✓ Ensure that your Air Fryer is preheated to 390 F.
- ✓ Get a bowl and make a mixture of the mince, breadcrumbs, lemon peel, oregano, feta, and black pepper and knead everything together.
- ✓ Create ten equal portions out of the mixture.
- ✓ With your damp hands, create ten smooth balls from the ten portions.
- ✓ Transfer the balls into the oven dish and then into the basket.
- ✓ Place the basket into the air fryer and allow to bake for 8 minutes. The balls are done when they are nicely brown.
- ✓ Serve while hot in a platter alongside tapas forks.

638) Fish Fingers

Ingredients:

- 2 slices wholemeal bread made into breadcrumbs
- Salt and ground black pepper to taste
- 1 tsp parsley
- 2 oz plain flour
- 1 medium egg, beaten
- 2 white fish fillets skinned and boned
- 1 tsp mixed herbs
- 1 small lemon juice only
- 1 tsp thyme

Direction: Cooking Time: 25 minutes | Servings: 2

- ✓ Ensure that your air fryer is preheated to 360 F.
- ✓ To prepare your breadcrumbs, place it in a clean dish and mix it thoroughly with pepper, parsley, and salt.
- ✓ Transfer your beaten egg in a separate dish and the plain flour in another. Place the fish in a food processor alongside mixed herbs, salt and pepper, lemon juice, and thyme.
- ✓ When the mixture is all mashed up like uncooked fishcakes, start making your fish fingers.
- ✓ Bread your fish – roll it in the flour, the egg, and then in the breadcrumbs. Transfer the rolled fish into the air fryer and allow to cook at 360 F for 8 minutes.
- ✓ Serve the cooked rolled fish alongside potatoes and mayonnaise. You may also serve in a sandwich.

639) Fish and Fries

Ingredients:

- 1 lb potatoes (about 2 medium)
- 2 tbsp olive oil
- ¼ tsp pepper
- ¼ tsp salt Fish:
- ¼ tsp pepper
- 1/3 cup all-purpose flour
- 1 large egg 2 tbsp water
- 1/8 tsp cayenne pepper
- 1 tbsp Parmesan cheese, grated
- 1 lb haddock or cod fillets
- ¼ tsp salt
- 2/3 cup crushed cornflakes Tartar sauce

Direction: Cooking Time: 40 minutes | Servings: 4

- ✓ Ensure that your air fryer is preheated to 400 F. Cut the peeled potatoes lengthwise into thick slices (of 0.5-inch thickness), and then cut the slices into thick sticks (of 0.5-inch thickness). Get a large bowl, and combine the potatoes, oil, pepper, and salt in it.
- ✓ You may work in batches if required. Arrange the potatoes in the air fryer basket to form a single layer.
- ✓ Allow cooking until just tender (for about 5-10 minutes).
- ✓ Transfer the cooked potatoes into the basket to redistribute and continue cooking until they are crisp and lightly browned (for about 5-10 minutes longer).
- ✓ While cooking the potatoes, get a shallow bowl and mix the pepper and flour in it. Mix the whisked egg and water in a separate shallow bowl.
- ✓ Combine the cayenne and cheese in a third bowl. Sprinkle your fish with salt, and dip it into the flour mixture ensuring that the two sides are well coated while shaking off the excess.
- ✓ Dredge in the egg mixture too, and finally in the cornflake mixture. Withdraw the fries from the basket, and allow it to cool. Transfer the fish into the air fryer basket, forming a single layer.
- ✓ Allow the fish to cook until it is lightly browned and flakes easily with a fork. Turn halfway through cooking (say after 8-10 minutes).
- ✓ Endeavor not to overcook the fish. Replace the cooked fish with the fries and heat through. Serve immediately alone, or alongside tartar sauce.

640) Fish and Chips

Ingredients:

- 8 oz white fish filet (tilapia, cod, pollack)
- Salt and ground black pepper to taste
- ½ tbsp lemon juice
- 1 oz tortilla chips
- 1 egg
- 10 oz (red) potatoes
- 1 tbsp vegetable oil

Direction: Cooking Time: 30 minutes | Servings: 2

- ✓ Ensure that your air fryer is preheated to 360 F. Cut the fish into four equal pieces.
- ✓ Rub each piece with pepper, salt, and the lemon juice and allow to rest for 5 minutes. While the fish is resting, grind the tortilla chips in your food processor. Place the ground tortilla chips in a plate.
- ✓ Get a clean deep dish and beat the egg in it.
- ✓ Dredge each fish piece into the egg and roll it through the ground tortilla chips until it is entirely covered.
- ✓ Do the same for the other pieces of fish. Cut the cleaned potatoes lengthwise into thin strips and soak them in water for not less than 30 minutes.
- ✓ After draining the water, pat them dry using your kitchen paper. Finally, coat them with oil in a boil. Fix your separator in the air fryer basket.
- ✓ Arrange the potato strips and fish pieces on either side.
- ✓ Place the basket into the air fryer and allow the potatoes and fish to try for 12 minutes (or until they have a crispy brown appearance).

641) Slimming World Beer Battered Fish and Chips Recipe

Ingredients:

- 5 oz beer 1 tsp turmeric
- 1 tsp paprika
- 1 tsp cayenne pepper
- 1 tsp lemon juice
- 1 tsp garlic puree
- 4 oz plain flour
- 2 large potatoes, peeled
- 1 lb cod fillet
- Salt and ground black pepper to taste
- 1 tbsp olive oil

Direction: Cooking Time: 25 minutes | Servings: 4

- ✓ The first step is to make the batter: combine the beer, seasoning and the plain flour. Mix thoroughly until you have a smooth mixture without any flour lumps.
- ✓ Fridge the batter for about an hour. Slice the peeled potatoes into chip shapes. Remove any excess moisture from the fish by squeezing, then season with pepper and salt. Chop the fish into pieces and immerse in the batter until each piece is well coated.
- ✓ Transfer the chips into the air fryer and drizzle olive oil over them.
- ✓ Allow cooking for 6 minutes at 360 F.
- ✓ Place the potatoes in the baking pan and cook alongside the fish for 7 minutes at the same temperature.
- ✓ Serve alongside the dipping sauce.

642) Chili Lime Tilapia Healthy

Ingredients:

- 1 lb tilapia
- Ground black pepper and salt to taste
- 1 cup panko crumbs
- 1 tbs chili powder (less if you're not into spice)
-) ½ cup flour (I used trader Joe's gluten free flour)
- 1 -2 eggs, beaten
- Juice of 1 lime

Direction: Cooking Time: 30 minutes | Servings: 3-4

- ✓ Grab a plate wide enough to lay tilapia flat. In the plate, mix the pepper, panko, chili powder, and salt.
- ✓ Place the flour in a bowl and the scrambled egg in another. Spray the bottom of the air fryer using a little cooking spray.
- ✓ Dredge both sides of the tilapia in the flour, then the egg, and finally press well into the panko mixture until the tilapia is evenly coated.
- ✓ Transfer the coated tilapia into the air fryer and spray the top with a little cooking spray.
- ✓ You may work in batches if necessary. Fry the fish for 7-8 minutes at 375 F, then flip to the other side and cook for an extra 7-8 minutes or until the fish has cooked through.
- ✓ Withdraw the tilapia and squeeze lime juice over the top. Serve alongside some pico de gallo, avocado, and lime wedges. Otherwise, you can serve with your favorite veggie.

643) Fried Catfish 3 Ingredient

Ingredients:

- 4 catfish fillets
- ¼ cup seasoned fish fry I used Louisiana
- 1 tbsp olive oil
- 1 tbsp chopped parsley optional

Direction: Cooking Time: 1 hour 5 minutes | Servings: 4

- ✓ Ensure that your air fryer is preheated to 400 F. Pat the catfish dry after rinsing well. In a large Ziploc bag, pour the fish fry seasoning, and add the catfish to the bag one after the other.
- ✓ Seal the bag and shake well to ensure that all parts of the fillet are well coated with the seasoning.
- ✓ Spray olive oil on the top of each fillet and transfer them into the air fryer basket. Cook for about 10 minutes before flipping the fish.
- ✓ After flipping, cook for an extra 10 minutes. Flip the fish again, and cook for about 2-3 minutes more (or until as crisp as desired). Top with parsley and serve.

644) Air-Fried Crumbed Fish

Ingredients:

- 1 cup dry bread crumbs
- 4 flounder fillets
- 1 egg, beaten
- ¼ cup vegetable oil 1 lemon, sliced

Direction: Cooking Time: 25 minutes | Servings: 4

- ✓ Ensure that your air fryer is preheated to 355 F. Grab a clean bowl and mix the breadcrumbs and the oil in it. Stir until you have a crumbly and loose mixture.
- ✓ Dip the fish fillets into the egg, and then into the bread crumb mixture. In either case, coat thoroughly and evenly.
- ✓ Place the coated fillets gently in the preheated air fryer.
- ✓ Allow cooking until the fish flakes easily with a fork (it takes about 12 minutes).
- ✓ Garnish with lemon slices and serve.

645) Five Ingredient Super Simple Fisherman's Fishcakes

Ingredients:

- 3 cups white fish boned and cooked
- 1 cup mashed potatoes
- 1 tsp parsley 1 tsp sage
- Salt and ground black pepper
- 3 tbsp butter
- 3 tbsp milk
- 3 tsp flour

Direction: Cooking Time: 60 minutes | Servings: 4

- ✓ Grab a large mixing bowl, and in it, combine fish, potatoes, and the seasoning.
- ✓ Mix very well and add the butter and milk.
- ✓ Mix again until you have a uniform mixture. You may need to add more milk to ensure a nice consistency.
- ✓ Add a little flour to the mixture and make patty cakes from it. Transfer the cakes into the fridge and leave for three hours.
- ✓ This solidifies the cakes.
- ✓ Cook the cakes in the air fryer for 15 minutes at 390 F. Serve.

646) Grilled Fish Fillet with Pesto Sauce

Ingredients:

- 2 white fish fillets (8 oz each)
- 1 tbsp olive oil
- Ground black pepper and salt to taste

Pesto sauce:

- 1 bunch fresh basil
- 1 tbsp pine nuts
- 2 garlic cloves
- 1 cup extra-virgin olive oil
- 1 tbsp grated Parmesan cheese

Direction: Cooking Time: 20 minutes | Servings: 2

- ✓ Ensure that your air fryer is preheated to 360 F. Grab each fish fillet and brush with the oil and season with salt and pepper. Transfer the coated fillet into the air fryer cooking basket and allow to cook for 8 minutes.
- ✓ While cooking the fish fillet, pick the basil leaves and combine them with pine nuts, garlic, olive oil, and the Parmesan cheese.
- ✓ Transfer the mixture into a food processor or mortar and pestle.
- ✓ Pulse or grind the mixture until you have a sauce. Salt to taste.
- ✓ Serve the cooked fish fillets drizzled with pesto sauce on a serving plate.

647) Sesame Seeds Fish Fillet

Ingredients:

- 5 frozen fish fillets (if it's not frozen, just cut the cooking time by roughly 3 minutes)
- 3 tbsp plain flour
- 1 egg, beaten

Coating:

- Handful of sesame seeds
- 3 tbsp oil
- Pinch of ground black pepper Pinch of sea salt
- 5-6 soda biscuit crumbs (or any plain biscuits you have or breadcrumbs)
- Pinch of rosemary herbs, optional

Direction: Cooking Time: 40 minutes | Servings: 3-5

- ✓ Coating Without adding oil to the pan, fry the sesame seed in it for 2 minutes while stirring consistently.
- ✓ Once they become brown, remove them from pan. Get a large plate and make a mixture of all the coating ingredients. Fish Fillet
- ✓ Ensure that your Air Fryer is preheated to 360 F and lined with aluminum foil.
- ✓ Proceed to arrange your ingredients to ensure efficiency following the order below. Dip the fish in the flour, then the egg, and finally in the coating mixture.
- ✓ Place the coated fish inside the air fryer. Cook for 10 minutes if it's frozen fillet, flip the fish and cook for extra 4 minutes. If the fillet is not frozen, cook the first side for 8 minutes and the second for 2 minutes Serve!

648) Thai Fish Cakes with Mango Salsa

Ingredients:

- 1 ripe mango, peeled
- 3 tbsp fresh coriander or flat leaf parsley
- 1½ tsp red chili paste Juice and zest of 1 lime
- 1 lb white fish fillet (pollack, cod, pangasius, tilapia)
- 1 egg, beaten 1 green onion, finely chopped
- 2 oz ground coconut

Direction: Cooking Time: 35 minutes | Servings: 4

- ✓ Ensure that your Air Fryer is preheated to 375 F. Cut the peeled mangoes into small cubes, and mix them in a bowl alongside one tablespoon coriander, ½ teaspoon red chili paste, the juice, and zest of half a lime. In the food processor, puree the fish and add one egg, one teaspoon salt, and the remaining lime zest, red chili paste, and the lime juice.
- ✓ Mix these with the remaining coriander, the green onion, and two tablespoons coconut. Get a clean soup plate and transfer the remainder of the coconut in it.
- ✓ Make 12 portions out of the fish mixture, with each portion shaped into round cakes.
- ✓ Finally, coat each cake with the coconut, Arrange six fish cakes into your air fryer basket and air fry the fish cakes for about 7 minutes, or until the golden brown color is visible.
- ✓ Do the same for the other fish cakes. Withdraw the cooked fish cakes and serve alongside mango salsa.
- ✓ You may also combine with pandan rice and stir-fried pak choi.

649) Air Fryer Salmon

Ingredients:

- : 2 wild caught salmon fillets with comparable thickness (1-1/12-inches thick)
- 2 tsp avocado oil or olive oil
- Salt and ground black pepper to taste
- 2 tsp paprika Lemon wedges, to serve

Direction: Cooking Time: 30 minutes | Servings: 4

- ✓ Ensure that your salmon has no bone, and set it aside for about an hour. Grab each fillet and rub with olive oil, and seasoning with pepper, paprika, and salt.
- ✓ Transfer the rubbed fillets into the air fryer basket. Set the temperature to 390 F and allow the fillet to cook for 7 minutes (for 1 – 1½ inch fillets).
- ✓ After 7 minutes, check the fillets with a fork to ensure they are well cooked according to your taste.

Notes:

- ✓ You can also check if the fillets are done while cooking without necessarily withdrawing the basket from the air fryer. This helps you monitor the fillets better to ensure they are not overdone. Another helpful tip is to set your timer for a little less to enable you regularly check to avoid overcooking any item.

650) Salmon and Fennel Salad

Ingredients:

- 2 tsp fresh flat-leaf parsley, finely chopped
- 1 tsp fresh thyme, finely chopped
- 1 tsp kosher salt, divided
- 4 (6 oz) skinless center-cut salmon fillets
- 2 tbsp olive oil
- 1 garlic clove, grated
- 4 cups thinly sliced fennel (from 2 [15 oz] heads fennel)
- 2 tbsp fresh orange juice (from 1 orange)
- 2/3 cup 2% reduced-fat Greek yogurt
- 2 tbsp chopped fresh dill
- 1 tsp fresh lemon juice (from 1 lemon)

Direction: Cooking Time: 30 minutes | Servings: 4

- ✓ Ensure that your air fryer is preheated to 350 F.
- ✓ Get a small bowl and mix the parsley, thyme, and a ½ teaspoon of the salt in it.
- ✓ Grab the salmon and brush with oil, while sprinkling the herb mixture evenly all over the fish.
- ✓ Transfer two salmon fillets into the air fryer basket and allow them to cook at 350 F. Withdraw the fillets when you are satisfied that they are well cooked (it takes about 10 minutes).
- ✓ Transfer the cooked fillets to the preheated oven to keep them warm. Do the same for other fillets.
- ✓ While you are cooking the salmon, prepare your fennel salad.
- ✓ Get a medium bowl and in it, mix the garlic, fennel, orange juice, yogurt, dill, lemon juice, and the other ½ teaspoon salt.
- ✓ Serve the salmon fillets over the fennel salad.

651) Tandoori Salmon with Refreshing Raita

Ingredients:

- 11 oz grams salmon
- ½ tbsp tandoori spice powder
- 3 cups plain yoghurt, divided, or to taste
- Salt and ground black pepper to taste
- ½ tsp ground cumin
- 1 tbsp minced green chilli, or to taste
- 30 leaves fresh mint, chopped
- 1 small tomato
- ½ red onion
- ½ cucumber

Direction: Cooking Time: 30 minutes | Servings: 4

- ✓ Shape the salmon into 12 cubes. Coat each cube with tandoori spice powder.
- ✓ Place in the fridge and allow to marinate. Separate ¼ of the yogurt, and blend it with the pepper, cumin, chili, mint, and salt. Place in the fridge and allow to steep.
- ✓ After peeling and removing the seeds, dice the tomato into small pieces.
- ✓ Chop the peeled onion into fine pieces. Peel the cucumber also, and cut lengthwise and use a small spoon to get rid of the seeds.
- ✓ Finally, dice the seedless cucumber. Before you serve, cook the salmon in your air fryer at 350 F for about 6 minutes, alongside seasoning. Avoid fat. While cooking the salmon, combine the remaining yogurt and the flavored yogurt, diced onion, cucumber, and tomato.
- ✓ Transfer the sauce into small soup plates or glasses and add the salmon on top. If you want your salmon to be more cooked, you may have to cook for another 4-5 minutes.
- ✓ But you may serve like that if you prefer it half-cooked.

652) Salmon Patties

Ingredients:

- 3 large russet potatoes (15 oz) Breadcrumbs to coat
- Fresh parsley, chopped
- 1 salmon (8 oz) portion
- A handful of frozen vegetables (parboiled and drained)
- Salt and ground black pepper to taste
- 2 sprinkles of dill
- 1 egg, beaten
- Olive oil spray

Direction: Cooking Time: 40 minutes | Servings: 8

- ✓ Chop the peeled potatoes into small pieces. Boil enough water in a pot, transfer the chopped potatoes and allow to cook for 10 minutes (or till the potatoes are tender).
- ✓ Drain the water and let the potatoes continue cooking on low flame. Once the water in the potatoes has evaporated (it takes about 2-3 minutes), mash the cooked potatoes with a whisk.
- ✓ Transfer the mashed potatoes into a large mixing bowl. Place in the fridge and withdraw only when it is no longer hot.
- ✓ While cooling your potatoes, prepare your breadcrumbs (not necessary if you are using packaged panko).
- ✓ Blend 4 pieces of breadcrumbs till you have a fine blend and set aside.
- ✓ Withdraw the mashed potatoes from the fridge, and combine them with chopped parsley, flaked salmon, parboiled vegetables, salt, and dill. You may taste and if the seasonings are not enough, add more. Add the egg to the mixture and stir together.
- ✓ Using your dry hands, make 6-8 patties or smaller balls from the mixture and coat them with breadcrumbs. Spray some oil to ensure the color of the balls come out nice. Air fry the coated balls for about 10-12 minutes (or until golden) at 360 F.
- ✓ You may not line with an aluminum foil if you are working with the grill pan. If you are lining with foil, ensure that you flip halfway once the top of the balls are golden. Serve alongside lemon, mayo, and salad on the side.

653) Air-Grilled Honey-Glazed Salmon

Ingredients:

- 1 tsp water
- 6 tsp soy sauce
- 6 tbsp honey
- 3 tsp hon mirin (alternatively you can use rice wine vinegar)
- 2 pcs salmon fillets (about 4 oz each)

Direction: Cooking Time: 25 minutes | Servings: 2

- ✓ Directions: Combine water, soy sauce, honey and Hon-Mirin (sweet rice wine) in a mixing bowl. Divide the mixture into two.
- ✓ Transfer half or some of the mixture into another bowl and set aside (to be served alongside the salmon).
- ✓ Combine the marinade mixture and the salmon. Allow the mixture to marinate for at least 2 hours. Ensure that your air fryer is preheated to 360 F.
- ✓ Air-grill the salmon for about 8 minutes.
- ✓ Turn the other side up after four minutes, and cook for an extra 5 minutes.
- ✓ Drizzle the salmon with the marinade mixture at intervals of 3 minutes.
- ✓ Prepare the sauce by transferring the remaining sauce into a pan and allow it to boil for a minute. Serve the sauce alongside the salmon.

654) Grilled Cajun Salmon

Ingredients:

- 2 salmon steak
- 2 tbsp cajun seasoning

Direction: Cooking Time: 25 minutes | Servings: 2

- ✓ Start by cleaning and patting the salmon steak dry.
- ✓ Then rub every part of the salmon with Cajun seasoning.
- ✓ Allow it to marinate for about 10 minutes. Ensure that your air fryer is preheated to 390 F.
- ✓ Transfer the salmon steaks to the grill pan and allow it to grill for 8 minutes.
- ✓ After 4 minutes, flip the steaks over.
- ✓ Grill for another four minutes. Serve the grilled salmon.

655) Chili Tuna Puff

Ingredients:

- ½ cup chili tuna
- 1 sheet puff pastry (thawed)

Direction: Cooking Time: 25 minutes | Servings: 2

- ✓ Ensure that your Air Fryer is preheated to 375 F.
- ✓ Make four equal squares out of the pastry.
- ✓ Spread the Chili Tuna on each square pastry, right at the center.
- ✓ Fold the square pastry into a triangle or a rectangle, and press the edges with a fork to seal them off.
- ✓ Transfer the pastry in the baking tray and allow to air bake for 10-12 minutes, or until you have the golden brown color.

656) Tuna Patties

Ingredients:

- 2 cans tuna packed in water
- 1½ tbsp almond flour
- 1 tsp garlic powder
- ½ tsp onion powder
- 1 tsp dried dill
- 1½ tbsp mayo Juice of
- ½ lemon
- Pinch of salt and ground black pepper

Direction: Cooking Time: 20 minutes | Servings: 2

- ✓ Mix all the ingredients thoroughly in a bowl. The tuna should be wet such that it can form into patties.
- ✓ If the dryness is not enough to form patties, add an extra tablespoon of almond flour.
- ✓ Make four patties out of the tuna. Ensure that your air fryer is preheated to 400 F.
- ✓ Transfer the patties into the basket, in a single layer, and allow to cook for 10 minutes.
- ✓ If your preference is the crispier patties, then cook for an extra 3 minutes.

657) Shrimp Spring Rolls and Sweet Chili Sauce

Ingredients:

- 2 ½ tbsp sesame oil, divided
- 1 cup julienne-cut red bell pepper
- 1 cup matchstick carrots
- 2 cups pre-shredded cabbage
- ¼ cup chopped fresh cilantro
- 2 tsp fish sauce
- ¼ tsp crushed red pepper
- 1 tbsp fresh lime juice
- ¾ cup julienne-cut snow peas
- 4 oz peeled, deveined raw shrimp, chopped 8 (8-inch-square) spring roll wrappers
- ½ cup sweet chili sauce

Direction: Cooking Time: 40 minutes | Servings: 4

- ✓ Get a large skillet, pour in 1.5 teaspoons of the oil and let it heat over high heat until it smokes slightly.
- ✓ Now toss in the bell pepper, carrots, and cabbage. Allow it to cook while continually stirring until the mixture is lightly wilted (this takes 1 or 1.5 minutes).
- ✓ Spread on a rimmed baking sheet and allow to cool for 5 minutes. Get a large bowl and combine cilantro, fish sauce, crushed red pepper, lime juice, snow peas, shrimps, and the cabbage mixture. Stir slightly.
- ✓ Place the spring roll wrappers on the work surface such that one corner is facing you. Using your spoon, transfer ¼ cup filling into the center of each spring roll wrapper, while spreading it from left to right and into a 3-inch long strip.
- ✓ Fold the bottom corner of each wrapper over the filling, while tucking the tip of the corner under the filling.
- ✓ Fold right and left corners over filling. Brush the remaining corner lightly using water, and roll the filled end of the wrapper towards the remaining corner.
- ✓ Finally, press gently to seal.
- ✓ Brush the spring rolls with the unused two teaspoons oil. Transfer the first four spring rolls in the air fryer basket and allow them to cook for about 7 minutes at 390°F.
- ✓ After the first five minutes, turn the spring rolls.
- ✓ Do the same for the other spring rolls. Serve the cooked spring rolls alongside sweet chili sauce.

658) Coconut Shrimp and Apricot

Ingredients:

- 1-1/2 lbs large shrimp, uncooked
- 1-1/2 cups sweetened shredded coconut
- ½ cup panko bread crumbs
- 4 large egg whites
- ¼ tsp salt
- ¼ tsp ground black pepper
- 3 dashes Louisiana-style hot sauce
- ½ cup all-purpose flour
- Cooking spray

Sauce:

- 1 cup apricot preserves
- ¼ tsp crushed red pepper flakes
- 1 tsp cider vinegar

Direction: Cooking Time: 40 minutes | Servings: 6

- ✓ Ensure that your air fryer is preheated to 375 F. Peel the shrimp, get rid of the veins, but retain the tails.
- ✓ Get a shallow bowl, and combine coconut and breadcrumbs in it.
- ✓ Get another shallow bowl and whisk your egg whites, salt, pepper, and hot sauce.
- ✓ Get a third shallow bowl and place your flour in it. Dip the shrimp into the flour to coat lightly.
- ✓ Remove any excess flour by shaking. Dip the flour-coated shrimp into the egg white mixture and finally in the coconut mixture.
- ✓ Pat to ensure the coating adheres. Spray the basket in your air fryer with cooking spray. You may work in batches if required. Arrange the shrimps in the air fryer basket such that they form a single layer.
- ✓ Allow cooking for 4 minutes. Turn the shrimps to the other side and cook until the coconut is lightly browned and the shrimp turned pink (this takes about 4 minutes).
- ✓ While cooking the shrimps, get a small saucepan and mix the sauce ingredients in it.
- ✓ Then cook and stir the mixture over medium-low heat until the preserves are melted. Serve the sauce alongside the freshly cooked shrimps.

659) Coconut Shrimp and Lime Juice

Ingredients:

- 1½ tsp black pepper
- ½ cup all-purpose flour
- 2 large eggs
- 2/3 cup unsweetened flaked coconut
- 1/3 cup panko (Japanese-style breadcrumbs)
- 12 oz medium peeled, deveined raw shrimp, tail-on (about 24 shrimp)
- Cooking spray ½ tsp kosher salt

Sauce:

- ¼ cup lime juice
- 1 serrano chile, thinly sliced
- ¼ cup honey
- 2 tsp chopped fresh cilantro (optional)

Direction: Cooking Time: 35 minutes | Servings: 4

- ✓ Get a shallow dish – and make a mixture of the pepper and the flour. In a second shallow dish, beat the eggs. Get a third shallow dish and mix the coconut and panko in it.
- ✓ Hold each shrimp by the tail and dip into the flour mixture without coating the tail. Shake to get rid of the excess flour.
- ✓ Dip in the egg mixture and allow any excess to drip off. Finally, dip in the coconut mixture and press to ensure adherence.
- ✓ Coat the shrimp generously with the cooking spray. Transfer half of the shrimp in the air fryer basket and allow to cook for 6 to 8 minutes at 400 F.
- ✓ Halfway into cooking, turn the shrimp to the other side and season with ¼ teaspoon of the salt.
- ✓ Do the same for the other shrimps and salt also. In the meantime, get a small bowl and whisk the lime juice, Serrano chile, and the honey together. Sprinkle the cooked shrimp with cilantro, and serve alongside the sauce (if desired).

660) Lemon Pepper Shrimp

Ingredients:

- 1 lemon, juiced
- ¼ tsp paprika
- ¼ tsp garlic powder
- 1 tsp lemon pepper
- 1 tbsp olive oil
- 12 oz uncooked medium shrimp, peeled and deveined
- 1 lemon, sliced

Direction: Cooking Time: 20 minutes | Servings: 2

- ✓ Ensure that your air fryer is preheated to 400 F.
- ✓ Make a mixture of lemon juice, paprika, garlic powder, lemon pepper, and olive oil in a bowl.
- ✓ Toss in the shrimp and coat it with the mixture.
- ✓ Transfer the shrimp into the air fryer and cook for about 8 minutes (until the shrimp is firm and pink).
- ✓ Serve alongside lemon slices.

661) Bang Bang Air Fryer Shrimp

Ingredients:

- ¼ cup sweet chili sauce
- 1 tbsp sriracha sauce
- ½ cup mayonnaise
- ¼ cup all-purpose flour
- 1 cup panko bread crumbs
- 1 lb raw shrimp, peeled and deveined
- 1 head loose leaf lettuce
- 2 green onions, chopped, or to taste (optional)

Direction: Cooking Time: 40 minutes | Servings: 4

- ✓ Ensure your Air Fryer is set to 400 F.
- ✓ Make a mixture of chili sauce, sriracha sauce, and mayonnaise in a bowl.
- ✓ Mix until smooth.
- ✓ Keep some bang source aside in a separate bowl for dipping, if you want.
- ✓ Place the flour on a plate, and the panko on another plate.
- ✓ Dip the shrimp into the flour first, and then the mayonnaise mixture. Finally, dip it into the panko.
- ✓ Transfer the coated shrimp on a baking sheet, then into the air fryer basket without overcrowding the basket.
- ✓ Allow cooking for 12 minutes. Do the same for the remaining shrimp.
- ✓ Serve the cooked shrimp in lettuce wraps with green onions as garnish.

662) Crispy Nachos Prawns

Ingredients:

- 18 large prawns, peeled and deveined, tails left on
- 1 egg, beaten
- 1 (10 oz) bag nacho-cheese flavored corn chips, finely crushed

Direction: Cooking Time: 25 minutes | Servings: 6

- ✓ Rinse the prawns and dry by patting them. Get a small bowl and whisk the egg in it. Transfer the crushed chips in a separate bowl.
- ✓ Dip a prawn in the whisked egg and the crushed chips respectively.
- ✓ Transfer the coated prawn into a plate and do the same for the remaining prawns.
- ✓ Ensure that your Air Fryer is preheated to 350 F.
- ✓ Transfer the coated prawns into the air fryer and allow to cook for 8 minutes.
- ✓ Opaque prawns mean they are well cooked.
- ✓ Withdraw from the air fryer and serve.

663) Scampi Shrimp and Chips

Ingredients:

- 2 medium potatoes Salt and ground black pepper to taste
- 1 tbsp olive oil
- 1 lb King prawns
- 1 small egg 5 oz gluten free oats
- 1 large lemon 1
- tsp thyme 1 tbsp parsley

Direction: Cooking Time: 25 minutes | Servings: 4

- ✓ After peeling the potatoes, cut them into chunky chips and season with pepper and salt. Drizzle little olive oil on the chips. Finally, cook for 5 minutes in the air fryer at 360 F. Rinse the prawns and dry by patting them with a kitchen towel.
- ✓ Transfer them to the chopping board and season with pepper and salt. Transfer the egg into a small bowl and mix using a fork until you have a beaten egg. Place 80% of the gluten-free oats into the blender alongside the thyme and parsley.
- ✓ Blend until you have a mixture that appears like coarse breadcrumbs. Transfer the blend into a medium sized mixing bowl.
- ✓ Add the unused 20% gluten-free oats into another separate bowl.
- ✓ Place the prawns into the blended oats, the egg, and the blended oats respectively. Finally, place the prawns in the non-blended oats.
- ✓ Withdraw the chips from the air fryer and place them on the grill pan.
- ✓ Place the prawns rest in the grill pan of the air fryer and allow them to cook at 360 F.
- ✓ Season the cooked prawns and chips with fresh lemon juice. Serve.

664) Gambas 'Pil Pil' with Sweet Potato

Ingredients:

- 12 King prawns
- 4 garlic cloves
- 1 red chili pepper, de-seeded
- 1 shallot
- 4 tbsp olive oil
- Smoked paprika powder
- 5 large sweet potatoes
- 2 tbsp olive oil
- 1 tbsp honey
- 2 tbsp fresh rosemary, finely chopped
- 4 stalks lemongrass
- 2 limes

Direction: Cooking Time: 35 minutes | Servings: 3-4

- ✓ Clean and gut the prawns. Gut the garlic and red chili pepper finely, and chop the shallots.
- ✓ Combine the red chili pepper, garlic, and olive oil alongside the paprika to form a marinade.
- ✓ Let the prawns marinate for about 2 hours in the marinade. Make fine slices by cutting the sweet potato.
- ✓ Mix the potato slices with 2 tablespoons of olive oil, honey, and the chopped rosemary. Bake the potatoes in the air fryer at 360 F for 15 minutes.
- ✓ While baking the potatoes, thread the prawns on the lemongrass stalks.
- ✓ Increase the temperature to 390 F and include the prawn skewers. Allow the combination to cook for 5 minutes. Serve alongside lime wedges.

665) Fried Hot Prawns with Cocktail Sauce

Ingredients:

- 1 tsp chilli powder
- 1 tsp chilli flakes
- ½ tsp freshly ground black pepper
- ½ tsp sea salt
- 8-12 fresh king prawns

For sauce:
- 1 tbsp cider or wine vinegar
- 1 tbsp ketchup
- 3 tbsp mayonnaise

Direction: Cooking Time: 20 minutes | Servings: 4

- Ensure that your Air Fryer is set to 360 F. Get a clean bowl and combine the spices in it.
- Coat the prawns by tossing them in the spices mixture.
- Transfer the spicy prawns into the air fryer basket and place the basket in the air fryer.
- Allow the prawns to cook for 6 to 8 minutes (how long depends on the size of the prawns).
- Get another clean bowl and make a mixture of the sauce ingredients.
- Serve the prawns while hot alongside the cocktail sauce.

666) Crispy Airfryer Coconut Prawns

Ingredients:

- 1 lb fresh prawns 3 oz granola
- 1 tbsp Chinese five spice
- 1 tbsp mixed spice
- 1 tbsp coriander
- Salt and ground black pepper to taste
- 1 lime rind and juice
- 2 tbsp light coconut milk
- 3 tbsp desiccated coconut
- 1 small egg

Direction: Cooking Time: 25 minutes | Servings: 2

- After cleaning your prawns, lay them out on a chopping board.
- Blend the granola in a blender until it appears like fine breadcrumbs.
- Before removing the granola blend from the blender, add all the seasonings, lime, and the coconut mix. Whizz the blender around again.
- Get a clean bowl and beat your egg in it, using a fork. While holding each prawn by the tail, dip it into the egg and the batter one after another. After dipping all the prawns, line the baking sheet at the bottom of the air fryer with your prawns.
- Allow cooking at 360 F for 18 minutes. Serve the cooked prawns.

667) King Prawns in Ham with Red Pepper Dip

Ingredients:

- 1 large red bell pepper, halved
- 10 (frozen) king prawns, defrosted
- 5 slices of raw ham
- 1 tbsp olive oil ½ tbsp paprika 1 large clove garlic, crushed Salt to taste Freshly ground black pepper to taste Tapas forks

Direction: Cooking Time: 30 minutes | Servings: 10

- Ensure that the air fryer is preheated to 390 F. Place the bell pepper in the air fryer basket and allow to roast for 10 minutes; withdraw when the skin is slightly charred. Transfer the roasted bell pepper in a bowl, while covering it with a cling film or lid.
- Allow it to rest for about 15 minutes. Peel your prawns and make a deep incision in the back to allow you to take out the black vein.
- Cut the ham into slices lengthwise, and wrap each prawn in each ham slice. Coat each parcel using a thin film of olive oil and transfer into the basket.
- Return the basket into the air fryer and allow to fry for 3 minutes.
- Withdraw once the prawns appear crispy and just right. While frying the prawns, peel off the skin of the bell pepper halves, and get rid of the seeds too.
- Then cut the pepper into pieces and puree the pieces in the blender alongside olive oil, paprika, and garlic.
- Transfer the sauce into a dish and add pepper and salt to taste. Serve the prawns in harm in a platter alongside tapas forks. Include a small dish of red pepper dip.

668) Crispy Crabstick Crackers

Ingredients:

- 1 packet Crabstick Filament, thawed
- Cooking Spray

Direction: Cooking Time: 25 minutes | Servings: 2-3

- Ensure that your Air Fryer is set at 360 F. After detaching the plastic wrapper on each crabstick filament, peel and unroll them.
- Finally, separate them into little pieces, ½ - inch wide is good for thicker crackers.
- Before transferring them into the frying basket, spray them with some cooking spray.
- Transfer the crab sticks in batches into the air fryer.
- Air fry each batch for 8-10 minutes. In the 4th minute, remove the tray and stir the crabstick crackers with your kitchen tongs – this ensures that they do not stick together.
- When air frying is completed, withdraw and allow to cool before storing them in an airtight container.

669) Wasabi Crab Cakes

Ingredients:

- 2 large egg whites
- 1 celery rib, finely chopped
- 1 medium sweet red pepper, finely chopped
- 3 green onions, finely chopped
- ¼ tsp prepared wasabi
- 3 tbsp reduced-fat mayonnaise
- ¼ tsp salt
- 1/3 cup plus
- ½ cup dry bread crumbs, divided
- 1-1/2 cups lump crabmeat, drained
- Cooking spray Sauce:
- ½ tsp prepared wasabi 1 green onion, chopped
- 1 celery rib, chopped
- 1 tbsp sweet pickle relish
- ¼ tsp celery salt
- 1/3 cup reduced-fat mayonnaise

Direction: Cooking Time: 35 minutes | Servings: 2

- ✓ Ensure that your Air Fryer is preheated to 375 F, and the air fryer basket spritzed with cooking spray. Get a mixing bowl and make a mixture of the first seven ingredients, alongside 1/3 cup breadcrumbs. Fold gently in crab.
- ✓ Get a shallow bowl and transfer the remaining bread crumbs in it.
- ✓ Then add heaping tablespoonfuls of crab mixture into the bowl. Coat and shape the crumbs into patties of ¾-inches thick.
- ✓ You may work in batches if required – each batch of crab cakes should be arranged in the air fryer basket to form a single layer.
- ✓ Only cook after spritzing the crab cakes with cooking spray.
- ✓ The cooking should last for 8 to 12 minutes, or until the cakes turn golden brown.
- ✓ Halfway through cooking, turn the cakes, and spritz again with extra cooking spray.
- ✓ Once cooked, withdraw and keep warm.
- ✓ Do the same for the other batches.
- ✓ While cooking the cakes, place the sauce ingredients in your food processor and blend to the preferred consistency. Serve cooked crabs while hot, alongside the dipping sauce.

670) Flourless Truly Crispy Calamari Rings

Ingredients:

- 1 oz calamari
- 1 cup gluten free oats
- 1 large egg, beaten
- 1 tbsp paprika
- 1 tsp parsley
- 1 small lemon juice and rind
- Salt and ground black pepper to taste

Direction: Cooking Time: 15 minutes | Servings: 2

- ✓ Ensure that your Air Fryer is preheated to 360 F.
- ✓ Slice your calamari thinly to produce small rings of calamari.
- ✓ Using a food processor or a blender, blend your oats until you have a consistency that looks like that of fine breadcrumbs.
- ✓ Transfer the beaten egg in a separate bowl and the oats in another bowl.
- ✓ Mix the oats with the paprika and parsley.
- ✓ Get a chopping board, and coat your calamari rings on it using salt, lemon, and pepper. Your hands may be sticky, thus, ensure you rub them in the oats.
- ✓ Transfer the calamari rings into the oats first, then into the egg, then the oats, why ensuring that they are thoroughly coated at each stage.
- ✓ Get rid of any excess oats and transfer the rings into the baking mat of your air fryer. Allow cooking for 8 minutes at 360 F. Serve!

671) Scallops Wrapped In Bacon

Ingredients:

- 8 scallops
- 8 bacon slices Toothpicks

Direction: Cooking Time: 25 minutes | Servings: 4

- ✓ Wrap the bacon over the scallop. Hold it in place with a toothpick. Set your air fryer to 360 F and air fry the bacon.
- ✓ Withdraw after 18 minutes or when a beautiful golden brown color is observed.

672) Air Fryer Egg in a Hole

Ingredients:

- 1 slice whole wheat bread
- 1 large egg
- Salt and ground black pepper to taste
- 2 oz avocado, optional

Direction: Cooking Time: 10 minutes | Servings: 1

- ✓ With the aid of a cookie cutter, make a hole at the center of your slice of bread.
- ✓ Transfer the slice of bread into the baking pan of the air fryer, and crack the egg into the hole.
- ✓ Allow cooking for 7 minutes at 320 F. Season the top of the cooked egg with pepper and salt. Get a small bowl and make a mixture of avocado.
- ✓ Use a fork to mix well to get rid of lumps. Spread the avocado around the bread edges. Serve.

673) Traditional Welsh Rarebit

Ingredients:

- 3 slices bread
- 2 large eggs separated
- 1 tsp paprika
- 4 oz cheddar cheese
- 1 tsp mustard

Direction: Cooking Time: 30 minutes | Servings: 2

- ✓ Heat the bread in the air fryer at a very light heat so that it is almost like toast – leave for about 5 minutes at 360 F.
- ✓ Get a clean bowl, and in it, whisk the egg whites until you have soft peaks.
- ✓ Combine the egg yolks, paprika, cheddar cheese and mustard in a separate bowl. Fold in the egg whites, and spoon it onto the partly toasted bread.
- ✓ Return the bread into the air fryer and allow to cook for 10 minutes at 360 F. Serve.

674) French Toast Soldiers

Ingredients:

- 4 slices wholemeal bread
- 2 large eggs, beaten
- 1 tsp cinnamon
- ¼ cup brown sugar
- ¼ cup whole milk
- 1 tbsp honey
- Pinch of nutmeg Pinch of icing sugar

Direction: 20 minutes | Servings: 2

- ✓ Make soldiers out of your slices of bread by chopping them – 4 soldiers from a slice.
- ✓ Get a clean mixing bowl and combine all ingredients, except the icing sugar.
- ✓ Mix thoroughly.
- ✓ Dip each soldier into the mixture, ensuring that it is well coated.
- ✓ Transfer the coated soldiers into the air fryer while wet and allow the 16 soldiers to cook at 320 F for 10 minutes. Withdraw when they are crispy, nice, and dry like toast.
- ✓ Turn the soldiers over halfway during cooking to ensure that either side is well cooked.
- ✓ Serve alongside a sprinkle of icing sugar and some fresh berries.

675) Cheese Toastie

Ingredients:

- 8 slices wholemeal bread
- 6 oz cheddar cheese

Direction: Cooking Time: 10 minutes | Servings: 4

- ✓ Fill up the sandwiches with your bread and cheese.
- ✓ Cook each batch of two sandwiches in the air fryer at 360 F, allowing each side to cook for 4 minutes.
- ✓ Serve while warm.

676) Breakfast Potatoes

Ingredients:

- 3 large white potatoes
- 1 medium white onion
- Salt and ground black pepper
- 2 tsp parsley, dried
- 6 slices back bacon
- ½ tsp olive oil

Direction: Cooking Time: 25 minutes | Servings: 4

- ✓ Shape the peeled potatoes into cubes and transfer the cubes into a large mixing bowl.
- ✓ Dice the peeled onions, alongside the bacon.
- ✓ Get a mixing bowl and in it, combine onion, seasoning and the bacon.
- ✓ Mix well. Add the olive oil and mix thoroughly.
- ✓ Transfer the mixture into the air fryer basket and allow to cook at 360 F for 15 minutes.
- ✓ Shake halfway through cooking so that the potatoes will not stick. Serve warm.

677) Breakfast Toad-in-the-Hole Tarts

Ingredients:

- 1 sheet frozen puff pastry, thawed
- 4 tbsp shredded Cheddar cheese
- 4 tbsp diced cooked ham
- 4 eggs, beaten
- Chopped fresh chives, optional

Direction: Cooking Time: 35 minutes | Servings: 4

- ✓ Ensure that your Air Fryer is preheated to 390 F.
- ✓ Having unfolded the pastry sheet on a flat surface, make four squared pieces out of the sheet.
- ✓ Cook 2 pastry squares for 6-8 minutes in the air fryer.
- ✓ Withdraw, and with the aid of a metal tablespoon, press the cooked square gently to form an indentation.
- ✓ Fill the hole made with one tablespoon Cheddar cheese and one tablespoon ham. Finally, pour one egg on the top of each square.
- ✓ Allow the filled square to cook again in the air fryer for about 6 minutes or more. Remove from the basket once it is done and allow to cool for about 5 minutes.
- ✓ Do the same for the other pastry squares, cheese, ham, and eggs. Garnish the tarts with chives and serve.

678) Green Tomato BLT

Ingredients:

- 2 medium green tomatoes (about 10 oz)
- ¼ tsp pepper
- ½ tsp salt 1 cup panko (Japanese) bread crumbs
- ¼ cup all-purpose flour
- 1 large egg, beaten
- 2 green onions, finely chopped
- 1 tsp snipped fresh dill or
- ¼ tsp dill weed
- ½ cup reduced-fat mayonnaise
- 8 slices whole wheat bread, toasted
- 8 cooked center-cut bacon strips
- 4 Bibb or Boston lettuce leaves

Direction: cooking Time: 35 minutes | Servings: 4

- ✓ : Ensure that your air fryer is preheated to 350 F and spray the basket with some cooking spray. Make eight slices out of your tomato, each slice with a thickness of ¼ inch. Finally, sprinkle salt and pepper on the tomato slices.
- ✓ Get three separate shallow bowls and place the bread, flour, and egg in each. Dip the tomato slices in the flour, and shake to remove excess, then into the egg, and finally the crumb mixture.
- ✓ You may divide the slices into batches. Place the tomato slices in the air fryer basket to form a single layer, then spray with cooking spray.
- ✓ Allow to cook for about 8-12 minutes, turning halfway, and spritzing with additional cooking spray. Remove when the golden brown color is consistent, and keep warm.
- ✓ Do the same for the other tomato slices. While cooking the tomato slices, make a mixture of green onions, dill, and mayonnaise.
- ✓ On each of the four slices of bread, lay two bacon strips, one lettuce, and two tomato slices in it. Then spread the mayonnaise mixture over the remaining slices of bread, and place over the top. Serve immediately.

679) Home Bakery Cornish Pasty Recipe

Ingredients:

- 1 large carrot, peeled and sliced into small cubes
- 1 medium potato, peeled and sliced into small cubes 0.
- 5 lb plain flour
- 4 oz butter
- 2 to 3 tbsp water (cold)
- 4 oz minced pork
- 1 tbsp olive oil
- 1 tsp mixed herbs
- Salt and ground black pepper to taste
- 1 tsp thyme
- 1 small egg, beaten

Direction: Cooking Time: 45 minutes | Servings: 4

- ✓ Allow the carrot and potato to cook for 20 minutes or until soft in a food steamer. Set aside the cooked vegetables.
- ✓ Make your pastry by rubbing the butter into the flour until you have an appearance of breadcrumbs.
- ✓ To achieve a nice soft dough, add little cold water intermittently.
- ✓ Roll out your pastry ready for the Cornish pasties. Get a large pan, and in it, mix your mince alongside a little olive oil.
- ✓ Cook the mixture until it has browned through. Then add the seasoning, steamed potato, and carrot.
- ✓ Mix thoroughly again and keep separately. Fill half of a side of the
- ✓ Cornish pastry with the cold filling, generously.
- ✓ Brush the pastry with egg. Transfer the pastry into your air fryer. Allow to cook at 400 F for 25 minutes, or until the pastry is cooked to your satisfaction. Remove and serve.

680) Flaky Buttermilk Biscuits

Ingredients:

- 4 oz butter
- 1.1 lb self raising flour
- 20 oz buttermilk
- ½ small egg, beaten, optional

Direction: Cooking Time: 20 minutes | Servings: 14

- ✓ Get a clean mixing bowl and transfer the butter and flour. Rub the fat into the flour until you have the appearance of coarse breadcrumbs.
- ✓ Pour the buttermilk into the mixture and mix thoroughly with a fork.
- ✓ -Rub your hands with flour, and mold the mixture into a dough ball with your hands.
- ✓ Roll out the dough. Make 16 medium-sized flaky biscuits from the dough by using the biscuit cutters.
- ✓ Arrange the flaky biscuits in batches of four inside the air fryer grill pan, leaving a little space between them.
- ✓ Cook each batch at 360 F for 4-8 minutes. Withdraw and serve while warm.

681) Easy Pull Apart Bread

Ingredients:

- 1 lb plain flour
- 3 oz butter
- 10 oz whole milk
- 1/3 tbsp yeast
- 1 tbsp coconut oil
- 1 tbsp olive oil
- Salt and ground black pepper to taste

Direction: Cooking Time: 2 hours 10 minutes | Servings: 6

- ✓ To prepare the bread, rub the butter into the flour until the butter is well mixed in. Get a pan and pour in the milk and oils – warm until they are lukewarm.
- ✓ Transfer the pan mixture into the bowl, add yeast, and form a dough by mixing with your hands. Knead the bread for 5 minutes, and place a damp tea towel over the bowl while the bread dough is still in it.
- ✓ Place the bowl in a hot place. Wait for an hour and repeat the kneading and proving process, this time for 30 minutes.
- ✓ Make the proved dough into bread roll shapes.
- ✓ For the bread roll to become the "Easy Pull Apart" type, make them into medium-sized bread burns while leaving enough space to avoid contact and allow breathing.
- ✓ And ensure that you transfer the bread rolls straight into the air fryer. If you follow all this, you will have the pull apart appearance in the end.
- ✓ Lastly, allow cooking for 15 minutes at 365 F.

682) Pumpkin Bread

Ingredients:

- 6 tbsp banana flour
- 2 large eggs
- 8 tbsp pumpkin puree
- 2 tbsp vanilla essence
- Pinch of nutmeg
- 4 tbsp Greek yoghurt
- 4 tbsp honey
- 6 tbsp gluten free oats

Direction: Cooking Time: 25 minutes | Servings: 4

- ✓ : In a clean mixing bowl; combine all the ingredients, except the oats, and mix with a hand mixer to form a creamy and smooth mix. Mix in the oats using a fork.
- ✓ Apply some extra banana flour to the sides and base of the baking pan before pouring in the pumpkin-bread mixture. Use your spatula to smoothen the sides to ensure that lumps do not form.
- ✓ Allow the mixture to cook for 15 minutes in the air fryer at 360 F.
- ✓ Use your spatula to smoothen the sides to ensure that lumps do not form.
- ✓ Allow the mixture to cook for 15 minutes in the air fryer at 360 F.
- ✓ To remove the baking pan, cut around the sides and edges of the pan. Leave the cake to cool for about 2-3 minutes before slicing it.
- ✓ Serve the slices alongside some butter.

683) Rock Buns

Ingredients:

- 4 oz butter
- 2 oz caster sugar
- 0.5 lb self raising flour
- 1 tbsp honey
- 3 oz mixed raisins
- 1 medium orange
- 1 medium lemon
- 1 medium egg Milk

Direction: 15 minutes | **Servings:** 8

- ✓ Get a mixing bowl and make a mixture of butter, sugar, and flour in it, while rubbing the fat into the flour.
- ✓ Include the honey and the raisins also.
- ✓ With the aid of a good grater add the orange rind and the lemon as well.
- ✓ Squeeze the juice from the chopped lemon and orange into the mixing bowl.
- ✓ Mix thoroughly with a fork. Crack the egg in and mix thoroughly again.
- ✓ Add little milk intermittently until the dough is soft enough.
- ✓ Shape the dough into small to medium sized scones.
- ✓ Transfer the shaped dough into the air fryer's grill pan.
- ✓ Allow cooking for 10 minutes at 360 F. Serve warm.

684) Buttery Dinner Rolls

Ingredients:

- 1 cup fresh milk (room temperature)
- 4 oz butter, softened
- 2 oz sugar 2 eggs, beaten
- 1½ tsp salt 1 lb bread flour
- 2¼ tsp instant yeast Glaze: Some melted butter

Direction: Cooking Time: 1 hour 15 minutes | **Servings:** 10

- ✓ : Get a clean bread maker pan and add all the ingredients following the order listed above. Select Dough setting, and at the end of the cycle, turn the dough onto a lightly floured surface and punch out the air.
- ✓ Make 22 portions out of the dough, and shape each portion into a round ball.
- ✓ Line your air fryer basket with baking sheet and oil the edges slightly. Then, transfer the shaped dough into the basket.
- ✓ Cover with a damp cloth and allow to proof for until the dough is twice the original size – this takes about 30 minutes.
- ✓ Ensure that your Air Fryer is preheated to 320 F. Air bake the burns for 13-15 minutes at this temperature and withdraw when there is a visible golden brown color.
- ✓ Do the same for the other batches. After baking, brush some melted butter on the buns. Serve.

685) Hot Cross Buns

Ingredients:

- : 6 oz whole milk
- 1 tbsp olive oil
- 2/3 lb strong white bread flour
- ½ tbsp yeast
- 1 tsp mixed spice
- 1 tsp cinnamon
- 2 oz caster sugar
- 3 handfuls raisins
- 1 tsp nutmeg
- 2 oz butter
- 2 tbsp icing sugar
- 4 tbsp plain flour

Direction: Cooking Time: 50 minutes | **Servings:** 6

- ✓ : Ensure that your Air Fryer is preheated to 175 F or the lowest temperature possible.
- ✓ Get a clean saucepan and place the milk and the olive oil.
- ✓ Warm the mixture until the milk is lukewarm. While warming the milk, get a clean bowl and place the bread flour and yeast, alongside the seasonings.
- ✓ Rub the butter into the flour using the rubbing-in method.
- ✓ Add the raisins and thoroughly mix until you have the appearance of a breadcrumb.
- ✓ Put the saucepan ingredients, little at a time, until you have a soft bread dough. Break the bread dough up into hot cross bun sizes and transfer them on the air fryer's baking mat. Allow cooking for 12 minutes at 360 F.
- ✓ Withdraw from the air fryer and allow it cool for 5 minutes before serving. In the meantime, you can create the icing topping by mixing the icing sugar, plain flour, with a little water to form a thick paste.
- ✓ Use a spoon or piping bag to make a cross on each of the tops of the buns. Serve the buns with butter.

686) Rich Fruit Scones

Ingredients:

- : 0.5 lbself raising flour
- 2 oz butter 2 oz sultanas
- 1 oz caster sugar
- 1 medium egg Milk

Direction: Cooking Time: 15 minutes | **Servings:** 4

- ✓ Get a clean mixing bowl and place the flour and butter and rub the fat into the flour.
- ✓ Add the sultanas, followed by the caster sugar, and finally crack the egg into the mixture.
- ✓ Mix thoroughly with a fork until you have a uniform mixture.
- ✓ Add little milk intermittently until you have a smooth scone dough.
- ✓ Shape the dough into scones.
- ✓ Transfer the scones into the grill pan of the air fryer. Allow cooking at 360 F for 8 minutes. Withdraw and serve warm.

687) Strawberry Scones

Ingredients:

- 0.5 lb self raising flour
- 2 oz butter
- 2 oz caster sugar
- Vanilla essence
- 2 oz milk
- 4 tbsp whipped cream
- 1 tbsp homemade strawberry jam
- 2 oz fresh strawberries

Direction: Cooking Time: 20 minutes | Servings: 4

- ✓ Get a clean mixing bowl and place the flour, butter, and sugar. Rub the butter into the sugar and flour until you have the appearance of breadcrumbs.
- ✓ Finally, add the vanilla essence and milk generously until you have a soft dough. Shape the dough into four equal balls that look like scone shapes.
- ✓ Transfer the shaped balls into the baking pan of your air fryer. Allow cooking at 360 F for 10 minutes.
- ✓ Withdraw cooked balls, place them on a cooling rack and allow to cool for some minutes.
- ✓ Then cut in half, and fill the inside with whipped cream, strawberry jam, and fresh strawberries. Serve.

688) Three Ingredient Shortbread Fingers

Ingredients:

- 0.5 lb plain flour
- 3 oz caster sugar
- 6 oz butter

Direction: Cooking Time: 20 minutes | Servings: 10

- ✓ Ensure that your Air Fryer is preheated to 360 F. Get a bowl and make a mixture of the flour and sugar and add the butter. Rub the butter into the flour and sugar.
- ✓ Knead the mixture to give a lovely and smooth mixture.
- ✓ Shape the mixture into finger shapes and decorate with fork markings.
- ✓ Allow cooking on the baking sheet of the air fryer for 12 minutes.
- ✓ Serve.

689) Yorkshire Pudding Recipe

Ingredients:

- 2 oz plain flour
- Salt and ground black pepper to taste
- 1 small egg, beaten
- 5 oz whole milk Olive oil

Direction: Cooking Time: 25 minutes | Servings: 6

- ✓ Ensure that your Air Fryer is preheated to 390 F.
- ✓ Get a bowl and make a mixture of the plain flour and seasoning. Pour in the egg gradually, and stir continuously until you have all the egg in the mixture.
- ✓ Add the milk gradually too, and stir consistently to get a mixture as thick as a batter.
- ✓ Beat well until you have bubbles forming on the top. Add a little olive oil in your Yorkshire pudding dish, and place it in the air fryer for about 5 minutes until it is smoking.
- ✓ Now pour your mixture until it is halfway up the container, and place in the air fryer again.
- ✓ Allow cooking for 15 minutes this time, at 390 F.

690) Crispy Risotto Balls

Ingredients:

For risotto:

- 1 tbsp olive oil
- 1 cup onions, diced
- 1 cup arborio rice, dry
- 4 cups vegetable broth
- 1 cup parmesan cheese, grated
- 1 bunch of parsley, chopped
- Salt and ground black pepper to taste

Breading:

- 1.5 cups Bread Crumbs
- 2 eggs

Direction: Cooking Time: 3 hours 20 minutes | Servings: 4

- ✓ Place your frying or saute pan on the stove top and preheat it over medium heat. Then pour the olive oil and allow to heat.
- ✓ Toss in the diced onions and saute, and stir regularly until the onions are soft.
- ✓ Pour in the rice and allow to cook for an additional minute.
- ✓ Add 2 cups of vegetable broth and allow to cook, while stirring regularly for 5 minutes. Pour in the remaining 2 cups of broth.
- ✓ Leave the rice to cook until the rice is soft and the broth is entirely absorbed – this takes about 15 minutes.
- ✓ Combine the cheese and parsley using the risotto, adding season, pepper, and salt to taste.
- ✓ Pour the risotto in a casserole dish, and leave in the fridge for 2 hours. While the risotto is cooling, get a clean bowl and toss in the breadcrumbs.
- ✓ Find another clean bowl, and beat the eggs in it. Withdraw the rice mixture from the fridge and make it into 1-inch rice balls by rolling.
- ✓ Dip the rice balls into the egg mixture before the breadcrumbs. Transfer the coated rice balls back to the fridge, allow to cool for another 50 minutes.
- ✓ Ensure that your air fryer is preheated to 400 F. With the rice balls in the air fryer, set the timer to 8-10 minutes and allow to cook until golden brown. Withdraw and serve.

691) Sticky Mushroom Rice

Ingredients:

- 16 oz jasmine rice, uncooked
- 4 tbsp maple syrup
- 2 tsp Chinese 5 Spice
- 4 tbsp rice vinegar or white wine
- ½ cup soy sauce, you can use gluten free tamari
- ½ tsp ground ginger
- 4 cloves garlic, finely chopped
- 16 oz cremini mushrooms wiped clean, (any other mushrooms cut in half)
- ½ cup peas, frozen

Direction: Cooking Time: 25 minutes | Servings: 6

- ✓ Keep the cooked rice separately. Get a clean bowl and in it, mix the maple syrup, rice vinegar, soy sauce, ground ginger, garlic, and Chinese 5 spice.
- ✓ Ensure that your air fryer is preheated to 350 F. Allow the mushrooms to cook for 10 minutes in the air fryer.
- ✓ After 10 minutes, open the air fryer and shake or stir the mushrooms. Pour the liquid mixture over the cooked mushrooms, followed by the peas.
- ✓ Stir and allow to cook for extra 5 minutes. Finally, add the mushroom sauce to the cooked hot rice and stir well. Serve.

692) Cool Green Beans

Ingredients:

- 1 lb green beans Oil
- Cooking spray
- Salt and ground black pepper to taste
- Ranch seasoning to taste
- Lemon juice to taste

Direction: Cooking Time: 15 minutes | Servings: 2

- ✓ : Ensure that your air fryer is preheated to 400 F.
- ✓ After spraying the green beans with the olive oil, add salt and pepper to taste.
- ✓ Proceed to fry the seasoned green beans for about 9-10 minutes or until crisp.
- ✓ Add sprinkles of ranch seasoning plus lemon juice to taste. Serve.

693) Spicy Green Beans

Ingredients:

- 12 oz fresh green beans, trimmed
- 1 tsp rice wine vinegar
- 1 tsp soy sauce
- 1 clove garlic, minced
- 1 tbsp sesame oil
- ½ tsp red pepper flakes

Direction: Cooking Time: 45 minutes | Servings: 4

- ✓ Ensure that your air fryer is preheated to 400 F. Keep your green beans in a bowl.
- ✓ Get a separate bowl and in it, combine the rice wine vinegar, soy sauce, sesame oil, red pepper flakes and garlic.
- ✓ Whisk the mixture and pour it over the green beans. Toss to coat and allow marinating for 5 minutes. Divide the green beans into two halves, and place the first batch in the air fryer basket.
- ✓ Allow cooking for 12 minutes, while shaking the basket 6 minutes after cooking. Do the same for the other half of the green beans.

694) Falafel

Ingredients:

- 1 cup dry garbanzo beans
- 1 clove garlic
- 1 small red onion, quartered
- 3/4 cup fresh flat-leafed parsley, stems removed
- 1 ½ cups fresh cilantro, stems removed 1 tbsp ground cumin
- 1 tbsp sriracha sauce 2 tbsp chickpea flour
- 1 tbsp ground coriander
- Salt and ground black pepper to taste ¼ tsp baking soda
- ½ tsp baking powder Cooking spray

Direction: Cooking Time: 1 d 1 h 45 m | Servings: 15

- ✓ : After soaking your chickpeas in water for 24 hours, loosen and remove the skins by rubbing them with your fingers.
- ✓ Rinse and drain the skin-less chickpeas, and spread them on a large, clean dish towel.
- ✓ This will enable them to get dry.
- ✓ Combine the garlic, onion, parsley, cilantro and the chickpeas into a food processor and blend until you have a rough paste.
- ✓ Pour the mixture into a large bowl. Into the bowl containing the blended mixture, toss in cumin, sriracha salt, chickpea flour, coriander, salt and pepper.
- ✓ . Mix thoroughly before covering the bowl. Let the mixture rest for 1 hour. Ensure that your air fryer is preheated at 375 F. Add baking soda and baking powder to the chickpea mixture, before mixing thoroughly with your hands to ensure even combination.
- ✓ Mold the mixture into 15 balls of equal sizes, pressing each ball mildly to form patties. Spray the patties with cooking spray.
- ✓ Arrange seven falafel patties in the air fryer basket, and allow cooking for 10 minutes. Remove the cooked falafel and place them on a plate. Do the same for the other eight falafels, cooking for 10-12 minutes.

695) Macaroni and Cheese Toasties in the Air fryer

Ingredients:

- 2 slices white bread
- 4 tbsp macaroni cheese
- 1 oz cheddar cheese
- 1 small egg, beaten
- Salt and ground black pepper to taste

Direction: Cooking Time: 15 minutes | Servings: 1

- ✓ Make a sandwich by layering the bread alongside the macaroni cheese and the cheddar cheese. With the second slice of bread on the top, slice the sandwich diagonally.
- ✓ Apply the beaten egg to either side of the bread, followed by sprinkles of pepper and salt.
- ✓ Ensure that your air fryer is preheated to 355 F.
- ✓ Transfer the sandwich in the air fryer and allow to cook for 5 minutes.
- ✓ Withdraw when the bread is crunchy, and the cheese melted. Serve.

696) Macaroni and Cheese Mini Quiche Recipe

Ingredients:

- Shortcrust pastry
- 1 tsp garlic puree
- 2 tbsp Greek yoghurt
- 8 tbsp leftover macaroni and cheese
- 2 large eggs, beaten
- 12 oz whole milk
- Grated cheese, optional

Direction: Cooking Time: 30 minutes | Servings: 4

- ✓ After preparing your ramekins, rub the bottom with some flour.
- ✓ Transfer the short crust pastry on the bottom of the ramekins.
- ✓ Get a clean small bowl, and in it, mix garlic, Greek yogurt and the unused macaroni.
- ✓ Fill the ramekins with the yogurt and garlic mixture (up to ¾ full).
- ✓ Get a separate bowl and mix the eggs and milk.
- ✓ Pour the mixture over the macaroni cheese. Ensure that your air fryer is preheated to 355 F.
- ✓ Pour the cheese as toppings on the ramekins and transfer them into the air fryer.
- ✓ Allow cooking for 20 minutes. Withdraw and serve.

697) Patatas Bravas

Ingredients:

- 10 oz red potato, cut into
- 1-inch chunks
- 1 tbsp avocado oil (peanut oil; safflower oil; coconut oil)
- 1 tsp garlic powder
- Pinch of sea salt and ground black pepper Seasoning
- 1 tbsp smoked paprika
- Sea salt and ground black pepper to taste
- ½ tsp cayenne, optional
- Garnish: Garlic aioli Dried chives

Direction: Cooking Time: 27 minutes | Servings: 4

- ✓ Boil enough water in a pot. Place the cut red potatoes into the water, and allow to cook for about 6 minutes.
- ✓ With the aid of a filter, remove the potatoes instantly and transfer them to a kitchen towel to cool and pat dry.
- ✓ Leave the potatoes for about 15 minutes, so that it cools to room temperature.
- ✓ Once they are dry, transfer them to a large bowl, and add avocado oil, garlic powder, pepper, and sea salt.
- ✓ Coat the potatoes in the mixture and place them into the basket of your air-fryer. You may work in batches to avoid overcrowding and ensure proper frying.
- ✓ Set your air fryer to 390 F and allow the potatoes air-fry for about 15 minutes. Withdraw the basket after 7 minutes and shake. You may spray the potatoes with the avocado oil one more time before frying. Once you have a golden brown layer on the outside, and crispy flakes, stop the frying.
- ✓ Place the "fried" potatoes in a bowl. Spray again with avocado oil (lightly), and add the seasonings. Coat the potatoes generously with the seasoned oil and serve immediately with your preferred condiment

698) Rosemary Potato Wedges

Ingredients:

- 2 russet potatoes, sliced into 12 wedges each with skin on
- 1 tbsp extra-virgin olive oil
- 2 tsp seasoned salt
- 1 tbsp finely chopped fresh rosemary

Direction: Cooking Time: 35 minutes | Servings: 4

- ✓ Ensure that your air fryer is preheated to 380 F. Combine the potatoes in a large bowl add the olive oil.
- ✓ Add sprinkles of seasoned salt and rosemary. Mix to coat the potatoes very well. Transfer the coated potatoes into the air fryer basket, maintaining an even layer arrangement.
- ✓ You may work in batches to ensure that all the potatoes are well fried. Each batch should be air-fried for about 10 minutes at first, and then flip using tongs.
- ✓ The frying should resume after flipping and continue until done as desired – perhaps for an additional 10 minutes.

699) Baked Potatoes

Ingredients:

- 2 large russet potatoes, scrubbed
- 1 tbsp peanut oil
- ½ tsp coarse sea salt

Direction: Cooking Time: 1 hour 5 minutes | Servings: 2

- ✓ : Ensure that your air fryer is preheated to 400 F. Coat the potatoes with peanut oil, and sprinkle with salt.
- ✓ Transfer the coated potatoes into the basket of the air fryer.
- ✓ Allow cooking until the potatoes are done – perhaps for 1 hour.
- ✓ Pierce the cooked potatoes to check if they are done.

700) Garlic and Parsley Baby Potatoes

Ingredients:

- 1 pound baby potatoes, cut into quarters
- 1 tbsp avocado oil
- ¼ tsp salt
- ½ tsp granulated garlic
- ½ tsp dried parsley

Direction: Cooking Time: 30 minutes | Servings: 4

- ✓ Ensure that your air fryer is pre-heated to 350 F. In a clean bowl, add the potatoes and oil. Toss the potatoes to coat, and add ¼ teaspoon granulated garlic and ¼ teaspoon parsley.
- ✓ Toss the potatoes again to coat. Add the remaining garlic, parsley, and salt and toss for the last time.
- ✓ Transfer the potatoes into the air fryer basket and allow to cook, while tossing sometime, until you have a golden brown color.
- ✓ This may take about 20 or 25 minutes.

701) Airfryer Crispy Roasted Onion Potatoes

Ingredients:

- 2 lb baby red potatoes
- 2 tbsp olive oil
- 1 envelope Lipton onion soup mix

Direction: Cooking Time: 25 minutes | Servings: 4-6

- ✓ Split the potatoes, and place the pieces into the olive oil placed in a medium bowl.
- ✓ In the same bowl, add the onion soup mix and stir coat all the potatoes very well.
- ✓ Transfer the coated potatoes into the air fryer basket and cook for 17 to 20 minutes at 390 F.
- ✓ Withdraw until the potatoes are tender and golden brown. You may stir the potatoes halfway through. Serve.

702) Rosemary Roast Potatoes

Ingredients:

- : 2 large potatoes 1 tsp rosemary
- 1 tbsp olive oil Salt and ground black pepper to taste

Direction: Cooking Time: 15 minutes | Servings: 4

- ✓ : After peeling the potatoes, quarter them into the shapes suitable for roasting.
- ✓ Transfer the cut potatoes into the air fryer and add a tablespoon of olive oil.
- ✓ Then allow cooking for about 10 minutes at 360 F.
- ✓ After cooking, place them in a mixing bowl.
- ✓ Sprinkle the cooked potatoes with salt, pepper, and rosemary. Mix well and then serve.

703) Potato Hay

Ingredients:

- 2 russet potatoes
- 1 tbsp canola oil Kosher
- salt and ground black pepper to taste

Direction: Cooking Time: 1 hour 10 minutes | Servings: 4

- ✓ Make the potatoes into spiral shapes with the aid of the medium grating attachment on a spiralizer. Then cut the spirals after four or five rotations using kitchen shears.
- ✓ Transfer the potato spirals into a bowl of water, and allow to soak for about 20 minutes. Remove the water and rinse thoroughly. Using paper towels, pat the potatoes dry, getting out as much moisture as possible.
- ✓ Move the dried potato spirals into a large resealable plastic bag. Add salt, pepper, and oil into the bag and toss the spirals to coat them properly. Ensure that your air fryer is preheated to 360 F.
- ✓ Divide the potato spirals into two – transfer one half to the air fryer basket and cook for 5 minutes – until you have a golden color.
- ✓ Then increase the temperature to 390 F. Remove the basket and toss the potato spirals with the aid of tongs, and return them into the fryer.
- ✓ Resume cooking, while sometimes stirring, for the next 10 – 12 minutes or until you have a golden brown color.
- ✓ Reduce the temperature to 360 F and do the same for the other half of the spirals.

704) Easy Potato Gratin

Ingredients:

- 2 large potatoes
- 1 tbsp plain flour
- 4 oz coconut cream
- 2 eggs beaten
- 2 oz cheddar cheese

Direction: Cooking Time: 35 minutes | Servings: 4

- ✓ Cut the potatoes into very thin slices while retaining the skin. Transfer the potato slices into the air fryer – allow to cook for 10 minutes at 360 F.
- ✓ While cooking the potatoes, prepare the sauce by combining flour, coconut cream, and two eggs and mixing till there is a consistent thickness.
- ✓ . Withdraw the potatoes from the air fryer, and line the bottom of four ramekins.
- ✓ Cover with the cream mixture and some sprinkles of cheese.
- ✓ Allow cooking for an extra 10 minutes on 390 F. Serve.

705) Make Loaded Potatoes

Ingredients:

- : 11 oz baby Yukon Gold potatoes (about 8 [2-inch] potatoes)
- 1 tsp olive oil
- 2 center-cut bacon slices
- 1/8 tsp kosher salt
- 2 tbsp reduced-fat sour cream
- ½ oz finely shredded reduced-fat
- Cheddar cheese (about 2 tbsp)
- 1½ tbsp chopped fresh chives

Direction: Cooking Time: 30 minutes | Servings: 2

- ✓ Coat the potatoes in oil and transfer them into the air fryer basket. Allow to cook at 350 F or until they are tender (check with a fork) while stirring sometimes.
- ✓ While cooking the potatoes, get a medium skillet and cook the bacon in it over medium heat for about 7 minutes or until crispy.
- ✓ Remove the bacon and crumble. Transfer the potatoes on a serving platter and split them by crushing them lightly.
- ✓ Drizzle with bacon drippings. Combine crumbled bacon, salt, sour cream, cheese, and chives and top the potatoes with the mixture. Serve.

706) Small Jacket Potatoes with Rosemary

Ingredients:

- 1 lb small new potatoes, unpeeled
- ½ tbsp olive oil
- 1 tbsp fresh rosemary
- 2 cloves garlic, sliced
- Coarse sea salt
- Freshly ground black pepper to taste

Direction: Cooking Time: 30 minutes | Servings: 4

- ✓ Ensure that the air fryer is preheated to 360 F. Wash the small new potatoes thoroughly under running water. When clean, pat-dry using a kitchen paper.
- ✓ Get a clean bowl, and in it, combine olive oil, rosemary, and garlic. Coat the small new potatoes with this mixture. Transfer the coated potatoes into the air fryer and allow to air-fry for 24 minutes or until they are crispy and done.
- ✓ Withdraw the fried potatoes and place them in a serving dish. Add sprinkles of salt and pepper.
- ✓ Serve alongside grilled fish or meat. Another way to go about the potatoes is to slice them into blocks and submerge them under water for about 30 minutes.
- ✓ Then drain them thoroughly and dry them by patting with kitchen paper.

707) Stuffed Potatoes

Ingredients:

- 4 baking potatoes, peeled and halved
- 3 tsp olive oil, divided
- ½ cup Cheddar cheese, divided
- ½ yellow onion, diced fine
- 2 slices bacon

Direction: Cooking Time: 1 hour | Servings: 4

- ✓ Ensure that your air fryer is preheated to 350 F.
- ✓ Using a teaspoon of oil, brush the potatoes gently.
- ✓ Transfer the brushed potatoes into the air fryer basket and allow cooking for 10 minutes.
- ✓ Remove after 10 minutes and brush again with an extra teaspoon oil. Resume cooking in the air fryer, for another 10 minutes.
- ✓ Remove again and coat with the remaining oil. Now cook until tender – for an additional 10 minutes.
- ✓ Cut the cooked potatoes in half and spoon the insides into a bowl. Add ¼ cup Cheddar cheese and mix well.
- ✓ Combine the bacon and onion in a skillet and cook over medium-high heat.
- ✓ Turn sometimes and withdraw once the bacon is evenly browned. This takes about 10 minutes. Combine the potato-Cheddar cheese mixture with bacon and onion. Stuff the skins with the mix, and sprinkle the remaining cheese on top. Put back the stuffed
- ✓ potatoes into the air fryer and allow to cook for about 6 minutes or until you have the cheese melted.

708) Potato-Skin Wedges

Ingredients:

- 4 medium russet potatoes
- 1 cup water
- ¼ tsp ground black pepper
- 1 tsp paprika
- ¼ tsp salt
- 3 tbsp canola oil

Direction: Cooking Time: 55 minutes | Servings: 4

- ✓ : In a large, clean pot, put the potatoes and cover them with salt water.
- ✓ Bring the water to a boil. Once boiling, reduce the heat to medium-low and allow to simmer until the potatoes are tender – it takes about 20 minutes.
- ✓ Remove the water and transfer the potatoes into a bowl, and then into a refrigerator. Leave in the refrigerator for about 30 minutes or until completely cool.
- ✓ Get a clean mixing bowl and make a mixture of black pepper, paprika, salt, and oil. Quarter the cooled potatoes and submerge them in the mixture made in the mixing bowl. Ensure that the air fryer is preheated to 400 F.
- ✓ Divide the potato wedges into two. Place one half into the air fryer basket gently, skin-side down.
- ✓ Avoid overcrowding. Allow cooking for 13-15 minutes or until golden brown. Do the same for the other half of the wedges.

709) Restaurant Style Garlic Potatoes

Ingredients:

- 6 small potatoes
- 3 rashers unsmoked bacon
- 1 tsp garlic puree
- 2 tsp olive oil
- Salt and ground black pepper to taste

Direction: Cooking Time: 25 minutes | Servings: 2

- ✓ Chop the peeled potatoes into medium-sized cubes.
- ✓ Transfer them into the air fryer and add a teaspoon of olive oil.
- ✓ Allow cooking for 10 minutes in the air fryer at 360 F.
- ✓ Meanwhile, dice the bacon and combine the bacon, garlic, extra teaspoon of olive oil, pepper and salt into a separate bowl.
- ✓ Remove the cooked potatoes and toss them into the bowl containing the mixture. Mix thoroughly.
- ✓ Get a big piece of silver foil. On the foil, place the potato and the bacon mixture.
- ✓ Make a small cut in the silver foil to create an avenue for breathing.
- ✓ Return into the air fryer and allow to cook at the same temperature for an extra 10 minutes. Withdraw and serve.

710) Roasted Paprika Potatoes with Greek Yoghurt

Ingredients:

- 1 and 2/3 lbs waxy potatoes
- 1 tbsp spicy paprika
- 2 tbsp olive oil Freshly ground black pepper to taste
- 5 oz Greek yoghurt

Direction: Cooking Time: 55 minutes | Servings: 4

- ✓ Ensure that the air fryer is preheated to 360 F. Chop the peeled potatoes into 1 - inch cubes, and allow them to soak in water for about 30 minutes. Drain the water and pat the cubes dry using kitchen paper.
- ✓ Get a medium-sized bowl, and combine paprika, one tablespoon olive oil, and pepper.
- ✓ Coat the potato cubes in the mixture of spices and oil. Transfer the coated potato cubes into the air fryer basket and allow to fry for 19 minutes or until the cubes are golden brown.
- ✓ Ensure that you turn them regularly during frying.
- ✓ Combine the Greek yogurt with the remaining spoonful of olive oil, salt, and pepper in a small bowl.
- ✓ Add sprinkles of paprika. Serve the potato cubes in a platter and sprinkle with salt, alongside the yogurt mixture as a dip.
- ✓ You may add kebabs or a rib eye.

711) Potato Latkes Bites

Ingredients:

- 4 large potatoes 1 large onion
- 4 large eggs, beaten
- 2 tsp kosher salt
- ½ tsp freshly ground black pepper
- 1/3 cup matzo meal
- 1 tbsp potato starch
- ½ tsp baking powder, optional Grape seed oil Tools:
- 1 (1.5 oz) silicone cheesecake bites mold
- 1 oil mister 1 air fryer

Direction: Cooking Time: 35 minutes | Servings: 14 pieces

- ✓ Peel the washed potatoes, and grate them using the food processor. Transfer the grated potatoes into a bowl containing cold water.
- ✓ Keep the bowl somewhere safe. Rinse the food processor and add onions. Grate. Transfer the grated onions in a tea towel or paper towel to squeeze out all the liquid.
- ✓ Get a medium mixing bowl and in it, combine the eggs, salt, pepper, matzo meal, potato starch, baking powder (optional) and finally, the grated onions.
- ✓ Remove the potatoes from the water and save the starch left in the bowl.
- ✓ Squeeze all the water from the potatoes and transfer them into the onion mixture.
- ✓ Scoop out the starch from the potato bowl into the Latkes mixture. Spray the silicone trays generously with oil. Fill each tray well with the latkes mixture and spray again with enough oil.
- ✓ Transfer into the air fryer basket and allow to cook for 6 minutes at 350 F. Withdraw the air fryer basket and pop out bites into the air fryer.
- ✓ Spray generously and resume cooking for an extra 4 minutes but at 400°F. Serve alongside sour cream and applesauce.

712) Hassleback Potatoes

Ingredients:

- 4 large potatoes
- Salt and ground black pepper to taste
- 1 tbsp parsley
- 1 tbsp fresh rosemary
- 1 tbsp olive oil
- 1 tbsp garlic puree
- 1 oz cheddar cheese, shredded

Direction: Cooking Time: 35 minutes | Servings: 4

- ✓ On a clean chopping board, slice the four potatoes using the Hasselback potatoes method. Add sprinkles of salt, parsley, and pepper on top of the potatoes, with some entering the gaps.
- ✓ Transfer the sprinkled potatoes into the air fryer's grill pan.
- ✓ Allow cooking for 15 minutes at 360 F. Wear an oven glove and withdraw the potatoes from the air fryer.
- ✓ Transfer them onto the chopping board. Get a clean mixing bowl and combine fresh rosemary, olive oil, and garlic. Spread the mixture down the bottom, sides, and top of the potatoes with the fingers and thumbs.
- ✓ This ensures that the mixture goes down the slits while the potatoes cook. Lastly, add sprinkles on top of cheddar cheese. Allow cooking for an additional 10 minutes at 360 F.

713) Homemade Fries

Ingredients:

- 1 and 2/3 lbs waxy potatoes, peeled
- 1 tbsp olive oil
- Salt to taste

Direction: Cooking Time: 1 hour 25 minutes | Servings: 4

- ✓ Slice the potatoes into long French fries – 8 mm thick each. You may use a French fry cutter too. Soak the fries in water for not less than 30 minutes.
- ✓ Drain and pat dry with kitchen paper. Ensure that your air fryer is preheated to 320 F.
- ✓ Transfer the fries into a large bowl and add the oil. Toss the fries to coat them well and place the coated fries into the air fryer basket.
- ✓ Allow cooking for 18 minutes. Withdraw the basket after 18 minutes and shake the fries. Return and allow to cook for an additional 12 minutes at 360 F.
- ✓ Halfway during cooking, remove the basket and shake the fries again.
- ✓ Resume cooking for the remaining 6 minutes or until the fries are golden brown.
- ✓ Sprinkle the fries with salt to taste. Serve on a platter.

714) The Best Ever Air Fryer Fries

Ingredients:

- 4 medium potatoes
- 4 tbsp olive oil
- Salt and ground black pepper to taste

Direction: Cooking Time: 35 minutes | Servings: 2

- ✓ Cut the peeled potatoes into fries. Ensure that your air fryer is preheated to 360 F.
- ✓ Transfer the fries into the air fryer basket and add the olive oil.
- ✓ Allow cooking for 2 minutes and shake.
- ✓ Cook again for 8 minutes before shaking again. Resume cooking and continue for another 15 minutes.
- ✓ If you want the fries to appear golden, cook for 20 minutes at 390 F instead.
- ✓ Add salt and pepper. Serve.

715) Parmesan Truffle Oil Fries

Ingredients:

- 3 large russet potatoes peeled and cut lengthwise
- 1 tbsp olive oil
- 1 tbsp canola oil
- 2 tbsp white truffle oil
- Salt and ground black pepper to taste
- 1 tbsp parsley chopped
- 1 tsp paprika
- 2 tbsp parmesan shredded

Direction: Cooking Time: 55 minutes | Servings: 6

- ✓ Pour cold water into a large bowl and soak the sliced potatoes in it for 30 minutes or an hour.
- ✓ On a flat surface, coat the fries with olive oil, canola oil, one tablespoon of white truffle oil, alongside seasonings.
- ✓ Divide the fries into two, transfer half into the air fryer basket. Set the temperature to 380 F and allow to cook for 15-20 minutes.
- ✓ Pause cooking after 10 minutes and shake the basket once. If you want crispier fries, you may have to cook for more time, depending on your preference.
- ✓ And if the crispiness is obvious before 15 minutes, remove the fries.
- ✓ Do the same for the other half. Once you remove the fries from the air fryer, add the remaining parmesan and truffle oil. Add shredded parsley as toppings. Serve.

716) Five Guys Cajun Fries

Ingredients:

- .5 lbs white potatoes, peeled into chips
- 2 tsp mexican seasoning
- 1 tbsp cajun spice
- Salt and ground black pepper to taste
- 1 tsp coriander 1 tsp mixed spice
- ½ tsp olive oil

Direction: Cooking Time: 35 minutes | Servings: 2

- ✓ Transfer the peeled potatoes into a medium-sized bowl. Pour enough water until the potatoes are submerged.
- ✓ Leave in the fridge for 15 minutes. Drain after 15 minutes and get rid of excess water. Pat the potatoes dry.
- ✓ After seasoning the potatoes thoroughly, add olive oil and mix well using your hands.
- ✓ Ensure that the fries are well and evenly coated.
- ✓ Transfer the French fries into the air fryer basket, and allow cooking for 10 minutes at 320 F.
- ✓ Withdraw the basket and shake after 10 minutes.
- ✓ Resume cooking for another 5 minutes, this time at 390 F to ensure crispiness of the fries.
- ✓ Remove and serve.

717) Skin on French Fries

Ingredients:

- 2 large white potatoes
- 1 tsp olive oil
- 2 tsp chives, dried
- Salt and ground black pepper to taste

Direction: Cooking Time: 20 minutes | Servings: 2

- ✓ While scrubbing the potatoes, get rid of any eyes.
- ✓ Slice the washed potatoes into French fries and transfer the same into a bowl.
- ✓ Add the olive oil and the entire seasoning in the bowl and mix well with your hands.
- ✓ Transfer the coated slices into the air fryer basket, and allow cooking for 15 minutes at 360 F. Shake after 7 or 8 minutes.
- ✓ After 15 minutes, withdraw the fries and serve alongside mayonnaise or ketchup.

718) Garlic Sweet Potato Fries

Ingredients:

- 2 small sweet potatoes, peeled
- ½ tsp garlic powder
- 2 tbsp olive oil
- ¼ tsp salt

Direction: Cooking Time: 20 minutes | Servings: 2

- ✓ Cut your potatoes into fries of desired thickness and transfer them into a food-safe plastic bag.
- ✓ Add the other ingredients and toss to coat thoroughly. Place the coated fries into the air fryer basket, while leveling them as much as you can.
- ✓ Allow cooking for about 7 minutes at 350 F. In the case of thicker fries, stir them after 7 minutes, and cook for an additional 7 minutes.
- ✓ Do the same for all the fries until they are cooked to your taste. Optionally, sprinkle extra salt when serving.

719) Flourless Mashed Potato Cakes

Ingredients:

- 4 lbs white potatoes, peeled and diced
- 9 oz vegetable stock
- 4 tbsp whole milk
- Salt and ground black pepper to taste
- 1 tbsp chives
- 4 oz cheddar cheese

Direction: Cooking Time: 30 minutes | Servings: 4

- ✓ The first step is to prepare the mashed potatoes. Place the peeled and diced white potatoes into the Instant Pot. Pour in the vegetable stock too and place the lid on the Instant Pot. With the valve set to sealing, allow cooking for 25 minutes on manual.
- ✓ After cooking, use the quick pressure release and drain the potatoes, but retain them in the Instant Pot. Use a masher or blender to mash the potatoes, while adding a little milk sometimes.
- ✓ Add salt and pepper to season to taste. Transfer the mashed potato in the freezer until it becomes very cold and a bit hard – this is the perfect texture for making mashed potato cakes.
- ✓ You may decide to leave in the fridge overnight – it offers the same results.
- ✓ Now you can prepare the mashed potato cakes by adding the seasoning and the cheese in the Instant Pot while mixing thoroughly with your hands.
- ✓ Mold the mixture into mashed potato cake shapes.
- ✓ Inside the air fryer grill pan, arrange four mashed potato cakes – the first batch. Allow cooking for 12 minutes at 360 F.
- ✓ Do the same for other batches. Serve the cooked mashed potato cakes while warm.

720) Hash Brown Recipe

Ingredients:

- 4 large potatoes, peeled and finely grated
- 2 tsp vegetable oil
- 2 tsp chili flakes
- 1 tsp onion powder, optional
- 1 tsp garlic powder, optional
- Ground black pepper to taste Salt to taste
- 2 tbsp corn flour

Direction: Cooking Time: 35 minutes | Servings: 8

- ✓ After the shredded potatoes have been soaked in cold water, drain the water and repeat the step to get rid of excess starch from the potatoes. Get a non-stick pan, and in it, heat one teaspoon of vegetable oil.
- ✓ Saute the shredded potatoes until they are cooked slightly – it takes about 3 or 4 minutes.
- ✓ Allow the potatoes to cool down before transferring into a plate. Combine chili flakes, onion powder, garlic, pepper, salt, and corn flour and mix thoroughly.
- ✓ Spread the mixture over the potatoes plate and pat firmly using the fingers. Keep in the fridge for 20 minutes.
- ✓ Ensure that your air fryer is preheated to 360 F.
- ✓ Remove the refrigerated potato and halve it into pieces using a knife.
- ✓ Using some oil, brush the wire basket of the air fryer gently.
- ✓ Transfer the hash brown pieces of potatoes into the basket and allow to air-fry for 15 minutes at 360 F.
- ✓ Withdraw the basket and turn the hash browns to the other side after 6 minutes.
- ✓ This ensures even frying. Serve while hot alongside ketchup.

721) Tex-Mex Hash Browns

Ingredients:

- 1 ½ lbs potatoes, peeled and cut into
- 1-inch cubes
- 1 tbsp olive oil
- 1 red bell pepper, seeded and cut into
- 1-inch pieces
- 1 jalapeno, seeded and cut into 1-inch rings
- 1 small onion, cut into 1-inch pieces
- ½ tsp olive oil
- 1 pinch salt and ground black pepper to taste
- ½ tsp ground cumin
- ½ tsp taco seasoning mix

Direction: Cooking Time: 1 hour 10 minutes | Servings: 4

- ✓ After soaking the potatoes for 20 minutes in cold water, drain and dry with a clean towel, before placing them in a large bowl.
- ✓ Ensure that your air fryer is preheated to 320 F. Spread one tablespoon of olive oil over the potatoes and toss to ensure even coating. Transfer the coated potatoes into the air fryer basket and set the timer for 18 minutes.
- ✓ Meanwhile, combine bell pepper, the jalapeno, and onion in the bowl where the potatoes were initially kept. Add the ½ teaspoon olive oil, salt, pepper, ground cumin, and taco seasoning.
- ✓ Withdraw the potatoes from the air fryer and transfer into the bowl containing the vegetable mixture.
- ✓ With the empty basket back into the air fryer, set the temperature to 365 F. Toss the contents of the bowl to ensure that the potatoes are well mixed with the seasoning and vegetables.
- ✓ Return the mixture into the air fryer basket. Allow cooking for 6 minutes, after which you withdraw and shake the basket.
- ✓ Resume cooking until you have crispy and brown potatoes – this takes about 5 minutes or more. Withdraw the crispy brown potatoes and serve immediately.

722) Poutine

Ingredients:

- 1 ¾ lbs russet potatoes
- 4 tbsp vegetable oil, divided
- ½ tsp salt
- ½ tsp pepper
- 1 tbs all-purpose flour
- 1½ cups beef broth
- 1 dash Worcestershire sauce
- 1 cup part-skim mozzarella cheese, cubed

Direction: Cooking Time: 1 hour | Servings: 4

- ✓ Cut the scrubbed potatoes into fries of the same size – about 0.5-inch thick on all sides. Rinsed the fries in water and drain. Remove the remaining water with a clean kitchen towel.
- ✓ Transfer the fries into the air fryer's pan. Spray half of the oil and cook at 360 F for 25 minutes or until you have golden, crisp, and cooked through fries.
- ✓ Add half of the salt and pepper to season fries. While cooking the fries, heat the remaining oil in a small saucepan over medium heat.
- ✓ Pour in the flour and cook, while stirring. Stop frying after a minute or until the flour is lightly browned.
- ✓ Whisk in broth and Worcestershire sauce and allow the mixture to boil. Cook the mixture, while often stirring, until it is thick enough – this may take about 5 minutes.
- ✓ Add the remaining salt and pepper to taste. Place the fries evenly in four serving plates, while topping each plate with an equal amount of cheese.
- ✓ Melt the cheese by drizzling with hot gravy.

723) Sweet Potato Fries

Ingredients:

- ¼ tsp garlic powder
- ¼ tsp fine sea salt
- 1 tsp chopped fresh thyme
- 1 tbsp olive oil
- 2 (6-oz) sweet potatoes, peeled and cut into
- 1/4-inch sticks
- Cooking spray

Direction: Cooking Time: 1 hour | Servings: 4

- ✓ In a clean medium bowl, combine the garlic powder, salt, thyme, and olive oil.
- ✓ Place the sweet potato in the mixture and toss well to coat thoroughly.
- ✓ Apply some cooking spray as a coating for the air fryer basket. Transfer the sweet potatoes into the basket, ensuring they are arranged in a single layer.
- ✓ If necessary, work in batches. Cook each batch at 400 F until the sweet potatoes are tender on the inside and lightly browned on the outside.
- ✓ This takes about 14 minutes. After the first seven minutes, turn the fries.
- ✓ Do the same for the other batches. Serve the cooked sweet potatoes.

724) Spicy Sweet Potato Wedges

Ingredients:

- 2 large sweet potatoes, peeled
- 1 tsp chilli powder
- 1 tsp cumin
- 1 tsp mustard powder
- 1 tbsp mexican seasoning S
- alt and ground black pepper to taste
- 1 tbsp olive oil

Direction: Cooking Time: 30 minutes | Servings: 2

- ✓ Chop the peeled sweet potatoes into the shape of wedges. Ensure that your air fryer is preheated to 360 F for 5 minutes.
- ✓ Get a clean mixing bowl and in it, combine your seasonings and mix thoroughly. Toss in the potato wedges until they are evenly coated.
- ✓ Transfer the coated wedges into the air fryer, add some olive oil and allow cooking for 20 minutes. Shake the basket at 5 minutes' intervals until the cooking is complete.
- ✓ Serve the cooked sweet potatoes alongside a thousand island dip and sprinkles of a little extra chili powder.

725) Crispy Crunchy Sweet Potato Fries

Ingredients:

- 2 large sweet potatoes peeled and cut lengthwise
- 1 tbsp olive oil
- 1 tbsp canola oil 2 tsp garlic powder
- 2 tsp paprika
- 1 ½ tbsp corn starch
- Salt and ground black pepper to taste

Direction: Cooking Time: 30 minutes | Servings: 6

- ✓ Soak the sliced sweet potatoes in a large bowl containing cold water for an hour. After an hour, transfer them into a Ziploc bag alongside the cornstarch.
- ✓ Seal the bag and shake to ensure that the fries are thoroughly coated.
- ✓ On a clean flat surface, spread the fries and coat them with the olive oil, canola, and seasonings.
- ✓ Transfer the coated fries into the basket of the air fryer. With the temperature set to 380 F, allow cooking for about 25 minutes.
- ✓ Stop the cooking after every 10 minutes to shake the basket. If your preference is the crispy type of fries, allow them to cook for more time while checking to ensure that they do not get burnt.
- ✓ Serve when cool.

726) Sweet Potato Chips

Ingredients:

- 1 medium sweet potato, peeled and sliced crossways into 1/8-inch slices
- 1 tsp avocado oil
- ½ tsp Creole seasoning, or to taste

Direction: Cooking Time: 25 minutes | Servings: 2

- ✓ Ensure that your air fryer is preheated to 400 F.
- ✓ Get a large bowl, and place the sweet potato slices in it, add the avocado oil and stir well to ensure that each piece is well coated.
- ✓ Pour the creole seasoning and stir to make it mix with the potato.
- ✓ Transfer the coated slices into a thin layer on the air fryer basket's base. Allow cooking for 7 minutes, after which you turn and shake the fries to ensure even cooking.
- ✓ Resume cooking until the fries are crisp according to your taste – this may take 6 minutes or more. Place the cooked potato slices on a rack and allow to cool. Serve.

727) Sweet Potato Hash

Ingredients:

- 2 slices bacon, cut into small pieces
- 2 tbsp olive oil
- 1 tbsp smoked paprika
- 1 tsp sea salt
- 1 tsp dried dill weed
- 1 tsp ground black pepper
- 2 large sweet potato, cut into small cubes

Direction: Cooking Time: 30 minutes | Servings: 6

- ✓ Ensure that your air fryer is preheated to 400 F. In a large bowl, combine the bacon, olive oil, paprika, salt, dill, and pepper.
- ✓ Toss the sweet potato in the mixture and then place it in the preheated air fryer.
- ✓ Allow cooking for about 12 or 16 minutes.
- ✓ Check and stir after the first 10 minutes, and then at intervals of 3 minutes until you have browned and crispy potatoes

728) Sweet Potato Tots

Ingredients:

- 2 sweet potatoes, peeled
- ½ tsp Cajun seasoning
- Olive oil cooking spray
- Sea salt to taste

Direction: Cooking Time: 1 hour 10 minutes | Servings: 24

- ✓ Toss sweet potatoes into a pot of boiling water and allow the potatoes to boil until they can be pierced with a fork without losing firmness.
- ✓ This should take about 15 minutes.
- ✓ Avoid excessive boiling as this may lead to messy potatoes. Drain the cooked potatoes and leave to cool.
- ✓ Grate the cool potatoes using a box grater and transfer into a bowl. Combine the grated potatoes alongside Cajun seasoning.
- ✓ Shape the mixture into tot-shaped cylinders. After spraying the olive oil spray in the air fryer basket, transfer the tots in it – forming a single row while leaving space between the tots and the sides of the basket.
- ✓ Spray the arranged tots with olive oil spray and add sprinkles of sea salt. Allow the tots to cook for 8 minutes at 400 F.
- ✓ Withdraw the basket and turn the tots, then spray with more olive oil spray and add more sprinkles of sea salt. Cook for an extra 8 minutes.
- ✓ Allow to cool and serve.

729) Big Fat Veggie Fritters

Ingredients:

- 3 large carrots
- 1 small onion
- 1 large sweet potato
- 4 oz courgette
- 3 oz turmeric granola
- Salt and ground black pepper to taste
- 1 lime rind and juice

Direction: Cooking Time: 35 minutes | Servings: 2

- ✓ Dice the peeled carrots, onion, and sweet potato alongside the courgette too. Transfer everything into the Instant Pot and allow to steam for 5 minutes using the steam option.
- ✓ After cooking for 5 minutes, remove the pressure and drain the vegetables. Squeeze any excess moisture out of the vegetables using a tea towel. When completely drained, transfer into a mixing bowl.
- ✓ Blend the turmeric granola in a blender. Pour the blend into the mixing bowl containing the drained vegetables, and add salt, pepper, as well as the juice and rind of one lime.
- ✓ Mix thoroughly and mold the mixture into fritter-like shapes. Fridge the shapes for about an hour, to harden them a bit.
- ✓ Remove from the fridge after an hour and allow to cook for 15 minutes at 390 F. Serve.

730) Carrot and Pumpkin Recipes

Ingredients:

- 6 large carrots, peeled
- 2 tbsp olive oil
- 1 tbsp oregano
- Salt and ground black pepper to taste
- Fresh parsley

Direction: Cooking Time: 20 minutes | Servings: 4

- ✓ Make your peeled carrots into thick chips by slicing lengthways.
- ✓ Sprinkle your air fryer basket with olive oil and arrange the sliced carrots in it. Allow cooking at 360 F for 12 minutes.
- ✓ Shake thoroughly and add the seasonings after 12 minutes.
- ✓ Return the basket into the air fryer and allow to cook for an extra 2 minutes but at 400 F.
- ✓ Withdraw and serve alongside extra fresh parsley.

731) Honey Roasted Carrots

Ingredients:

- 3 cups of baby carrots or carrots cut into large chunks
- 1 tbsp olive oil
- 1 tbsp honey
- Salt and ground black pepper to taste

Direction: Cooking Time: 17 minutes | Servings: 2-3

- ✓ Get a clean bowl and combine the carrots alongside the olive oil and honey.
- ✓ Immerse the carrots in the mixture.
- ✓ Add salt and pepper to taste. Allow cooking in the air fryer at 395 F for 12 minutes.
- ✓ Serve while hot.

732) Shoestring Carrots

Ingredients:

- 1 bag (10 oz) of julienned carrots (sold for cole-slaw)
- 1 tbsp olive oil
- Salt and ground black pepper to taste
- 1 tsp orange zest
- Apple cider vinegar in a spray bottle

Direction: Cooking Time: 25 minutes | Servings: 1-2

- ✓ Get a clean medium bowl and combine the carrots and the olive oil, while coating the carrots lightly. Ensure that all the pieces of carrots are well coated, and then season with salt and pepper.
- ✓ Transfer the coated carrots in the air-fryer preheated at 390 F. Set the timer to 13 or 16 minutes, and allow the carrots to cook, while mixing them around after every few minutes.
- ✓ Withdraw the carrots from the air fryer when they are becoming nicely brown. Be observant so that the pieces will not get too dark very quickly.
- ✓ Transfer the cooked carrots into a serving bowl. Add some orange zest, little apple cider vinegar sprays, and season to taste with more pepper and salt. Serve while hot.

733) Slimming World Carrot Fritters

Ingredients:

- 6 large carrots peeled and diced
- 1¼ oz gluten free oats
- 1 tbsp thyme 1 tbsp parsley
- 1 tsp mustard powder
- Salt and ground black pepper to taste
- 1 large egg

Direction: Cooking Time: 25 minutes | Servings: 8

- ✓ Put your carrots into your food processor and blitz them until they appear like grated carrots. Season the oats and mix until the oats become blended.
- ✓ After removing the lid of your food processor, withdraw the blade as well and crack your egg into the mixture.
- ✓ After mixing with a fork, make the mixture into shapes of small cakes. Open your air fryer and place the baking mat in the bottom, before layering the fritters on top of it. You may have to work in batches if your air fryer is small.
- ✓ Allow cooking for 15 minutes at 360 F, while turning at the halfway point. Serve the cooked carrots warm.

734) Oil Free Pumpkin French Fries

Ingredients:

- 10 oz pumpkin
- Salt and ground black pepper to taste
- 1 tbsp mustard
- 1 tsp thyme Tomato ketchup, optional

Direction: Cooking Time: 25 minutes | Servings: 2

- ✓ Remove the seeds from the peeled pumpkin before slicing into French fries.
- ✓ Transfer them into the air fryer; set to 395 F and allow cooking for 15 minutes.
- ✓ After 7 minutes, shake and season with salt, pepper, mustard, and thyme.
- ✓ Serve hot alongside tomato ketchup.

735) Oil Free Sticky Pumpkin Wedges

Ingredients:

- ½ medium pumpkin
- Salt and ground black pepper to taste
- 1 tbsp paprika
- 1 tsp turmeric
- 1 tbsp balsamic vinegar
- 1 lime juice only
- 1 cup Paleo ranch dressing, optional

Direction: Cooking Time: 30 minutes | Servings: 2

- ✓ With half of the pumpkin sliced into wedges of medium sizes, transfer them into the grill pan of your air fryer.
- ✓ Set the timer to 20 minutes and allow cooking at 360 F. After 20 minutes, open the air fryer.
- ✓ Sprinkle the sliced pumpkins with the half of the seasonings, plus vinegar and lime. Turn them over with thongs, and sprinkle the other half of the seasonings.
- ✓ Then cook for an extra 5 minutes on either side at 390 F. Serve with ranch dressing.

736) Spiced Pumpkin

Ingredients:

- 1½ lbs pumpkin (about 3 slices) 1 tbsp olive oil
- 3 cloves garlic, unpeeled
- Ground nutmeg
- Ground cinnamon
- Brown sugar Sea salt

Direction: Cooking Time: 25 minutes | Servings: 2-3

- ✓ Using a brush, clean the pumpkin thoroughly, especially the skin, since we will be roasting with it. Remove the seeds and discard them.
- ✓ Ensure that your air fryer is preheated to 360 F. Cut the pumpkin into cubes and slices, and transfer them into a clean bowl.
- ✓ Spray some olive oil on the pumpkin, and rub on all surfaces.
- ✓ Add the unpeeled garlic and season with ground nutmeg, ground cinnamon, sugar, and salt.
- ✓ Transfer the pumpkin cubes/slices onto the baking sheet.
- ✓ Move the baking sheet into the basket of the air fryer. Allow air-roasting for 10-12 minutes, based on how thick the pumpkin slices or cubes are.

737) Pumpkin Tortilla Chips

Ingredients:

- 2 tbsp olive oil
- 1 tbsp nutmeg
- Salt and ground black pepper to taste

Make the pumpkin tortillas:

- 10 oz plain flour
- 2 oz whole milk
- 1 oz butter
- 1 oz pumpkin pie puree
- 1 tbsp olive oil
- 1 tbsp mixed spice
- 1 tbsp nutmeg
- Salt and ground black pepper to taste

Direction: Cooking Time: 1 hour 10 minutes | Servings: 4

- ✓ Following the same way of making regular wraps, make the pumpkin tortillas as well. However, substitute less butter and less milk in the case of the pumpkin puree. Cook the wraps in a frying pan, as usual.
- ✓ To prepare the chips, brush one side of each of the six tortilla wraps with oil before stacking and cutting them into tortilla chip shapes.
- ✓ Place them in the grill pan of the air fryer basket gently, and add sprinkles of salt, pepper, and nutmeg.
- ✓ Set your air fryer to 400 F and allow cooking for 18 minutes or until they become golden brown.
- ✓ Withdraw and serve alongside the pumpkin puree dipping sauce.

738) Butternut Squash Roasties

Ingredients:

- 1 small butternut squash
- 2 tbsp olive oil
- Mixed herbs chicken seasoning
- Salt and ground black pepper to taste

Direction: Cooking Time: 15 minutes | Servings: 2

- ✓ Ensure that your air fryer is preheated to 360 F. Peel the butternut squash and dice it.
- ✓ With the butternut squash drizzled in olive oil, toss it in the unused mixed herb seasoning.
- ✓ Then transfer it in the air fryer.
- ✓ Set the timer to 10 minutes and allow cooking until you have a golden color appearance.
- ✓ Serve alongside fresh herbs.

739) Avocado Fries

Ingredients:

- 1½ tsp ground black pepper
- ½ cup (about 2 1/8 oz) all-purpose flour
- 2 large eggs
- 1 tbsp water
- ½ cup panko (Japanese-style breadcrumbs)
- 2 avocados, cut into
- 8 wedges each
- Cooking spray
- ¼ cup no-salt-added ketchup
- 2 tbsp canola mayonnaise
- 1 tbsp apple cider vinegar
- 1 tbsp Sriracha chili sauce
- ¼ tsp kosher salt

Direction: Cooking Time: 35 minutes | Servings: 4

- ✓ In a clean shallow dish, combine the pepper and flour and stir thoroughly.
- ✓ Get another shallow dish and beat eggs lightly while adding some water. In the third shallow dish, put the panko and set aside.
- ✓ Dip the avocado wedges into flour and shake off excess, then into the egg mixture, allowing any excess to drip off, and finally, dredge in the panko while pressing to adhere.
- ✓ Make a generous coating of the avocado wedges using the cooking spray. In the air fryer basket, arrange the avocado wedges and allow to cook for 7-8 minutes at 400 F.
- ✓ Turn them halfway into cooking. Meanwhile, combine the ketchup, mayonnaise, vinegar, and Sriracha in a separate small bowl to produce the sauce.
- ✓ Withdraw the cooked wedges from the air fryer and sprinkle with salt. Serve four avocado fries on each plate alongside two tablespoons of the sauce.

740) Avocado Slices Recipe

Ingredients:

- 2 large avocados
- 3 limes juice and rind
- Salt and ground black pepper to taste
- 4 tbsp coriander
- 2 tbsp mexican seasoning
- 8 oz gluten free oats
- 3 tbsp Thousand Island
- 1 tbsp basil

Direction: Cooking Time: 20 minutes | Servings: 2

- ✓ Remove the avocados' skin and chop them on the cutting board into shapes similar to the potato wedges. Squeeze the juice in one of the limes over the chopped avocados. Using pepper, salt, and a sprinkling of coriander, season the avocados to taste.
- ✓ Blend the combination of the lime rind, seasoning, and the oats in a blender to produce a coarse mixture – just like the breadcrumbs. Transfer the blended mixture into a shallow mixing bowl. Immerse the avocados into the blended mixture.
- ✓ Withdraw and place them on the grill pan of the air fryer. Set the timer to 6 minutes and allow cooking at 360 F.
- ✓ Increase the heat to 400 F and allow to cook for another 3 minutes.
- ✓ Turn the avocados and let the other side to cook for another 3 minutes at the same heat. Squeeze the remaining juice out of the lime and on to the air-fried avocado slices. Serve alongside a preferred dipping sauce or a Thousand Island.

741) Avocado On Toast

Ingredients:

- 4 slices whole wheat bread
- 4 oz mashed avocado

Direction: Cooking Time: 10 minutes | Servings: 4

- ✓ Allow a slice of toast to cook in the air fryer at 400 F for 4 minutes.
- ✓ Turn it over and allow the other side to cook for an additional 4 minutes.
- ✓ Spread the top of it with mashed avocado and serve.

742) Avocado Egg Boat

Ingredients:

- 2 medium avocados
- Salt and ground black pepper to taste
- Fresh chives Fresh parsley
- 4 small eggs

Direction: Cooking Time: 10 minutes | Servings: 2

- ✓ Cut the avocados in half, thus giving you access to eject the stones and about 20% of the flesh. This makes the avocado wholes bigger.
- ✓ Add salt, pepper, chives, and fresh parsley as seasonings.
- ✓ Into each of the four halves, crack one egg and transfer them into the air fryer. Allow cooking for 8 minutes at 360 F.
- ✓ Add sprinkles of extra fresh parsley plus additional salt and pepper. Serve.

743) Air Fried Guacamole

Ingredients:

- 1 egg 1 egg white
- 1/3 cup almond flour (coconut flour; tapioca or arrowroot powder)
- 3 oz gluten free panko (regular panko; wheat breadcrumbs) Cooking spray olive oil

Guacamole:

- 3 medium ripe avocados
- 1/3 cup chopped onion Juice from 1 lime
- 2 tsp cumin Fresh finely chopped cilantro to taste (about 1/3 cup)
- Sea salt and ground black pepper to taste
- 8 tbsp fine almond flour

Direction: Cooking Time: 5 hours 25 minutes | Servings: 10

- ✓ Get a clean bowl and in it, mix and mash all the guacamole ingredients, except the almond flour. When the taste is what you desire, add the almond flour until the guacamole becomes as thick as the brownie batter. You may need to add extra tablespoons of almond flour to achieve the desired thickness. Add moderate lime juice, as excess will only make the guacamole loosen and wet. Place the bowl in the freezer and allow to harden for about 1-2 hours.
- ✓ Withdraw when the guacamole has hardened. Use a non-stick foil or a parchment paper to line a baking sheet. Scoop out the hardened guacamole and shape it into a ball of a size of a ping pong ball. Transfer the ball-shaped guacamole on the baking tray. Do the same for the remaining guacamole. Cover the tray with the non-stick foil and return to the freezer. Leave overnight or for 4 hours at least. Ensure that your air fryer is preheated to 390 F.
- ✓ Get a clean bowl and in it, beat the eggs together. You may have to work in batches here, but at top speed. Spray a guacamole ball lightly with olive oil, and once sticky, dip it in the almond flour, then the egg mixture, and finally the panko crumbs.
- ✓ Do the same for the remaining guacamole balls, until the air fryer basket is filled. Make sure to leave a breathing space between the balls in the basket. All uncoated balls should be returned to the freezer. Place the basket in the air fryer, and spray with a little olive oil. Set the timer to 6-8 minutes and allow cooking until the outside appears golden brown.
- ✓ If the balls start cracking, remove them from the air fryer. Return them only when they are cold and firmer.
- ✓ Now coat the uncoated balls and air-bake them.
- ✓ Serve and enjoy.

744) Zucchini Chips

Ingredients:

- 1 cup panko bread crumbs
- 3/4 cup grated Parmesan cheese
- 1 medium zucchini, thinly sliced
- 1 large egg, beaten
- Cooking spray

Direction: Cooking Time: 35 minutes | Servings: 3-4

- ✓ Preheat an air fryer to 350 F before you begin preparing the zucchini. Combine panko and Parmesan cheese on a plate.
- ✓ Dip 1 zucchini slice into beaten egg then into panko mixture, pressing to coat.
- ✓ Place zucchini slice on a wire baking rack and repeat with remaining slices.
- ✓ Lightly spray zucchini slices with cooking spray.
- ✓ Place as many zucchini slices in the air fryer basket as you can without overlapping them. Cook for 10 minutes. Flip with tongs. Cook for 2 minutes more.
- ✓ Remove from air fryer and repeat with remaining zucchini slices.

745) Flourless Mini Zucchini Fritter Bites

Ingredients:

- 4 oz zucchini
- 2 large eggs beaten
- 1 tsp mixed herbs
- 1 tsp oregano
- Salt and ground black pepper to taste
- 2 oz cheese
- 2 cups gluten free oats

Direction: Cooking Time: 25 minutes | Servings: 10

- ✓ Preheat your air fryer to 360 F. Start by grating your zucchini and removing any excess water from it by squeezing it out with your hands into a bowl.
- ✓ Place your squeezed out zucchini and your beaten egg into a mixing bowl. Along with seasonings and cheese
- ✓ . In a blender place your oats on the high setting and blend until they resemble fine bread crumbs. Place the oats into the bowl a little at a time as it will go thick rather quickly.
- ✓ Mix together and create bite sized balls. Place in the air fryer for 12 minutes on 360 F. Serve.

746) Guilt-Free Ranch Zucchini Chips

Ingredients:

- 1/8 tsp salt
- 1 pinch ground black pepper
- ¼ cup all-purpose flour
- ½ cup ranch dressing
- ¼ tsp garlic powder
- ½ cup whole wheat bread crumbs
- ¼ cup grated
- Parmesan cheese
- 2 zucchini, thinly sliced
- Cooking spray

Direction: Cooking Time: 25 minutes | Servings: 4

- ✓ Ensure that your air fryer is preheated to 400 F. Get a clean bowl and mix the salt, pepper, and flour.
- ✓ Get another clean bowl and pour in the ranch dressing. In a third bowl, mix the garlic powder, bread crumbs, and Parmesan cheese.
- ✓ Dredge each piece of the zucchini in the flour mixture first, followed by the ranch dressing, and then coat either side while removing the excess dressing by shaking.
- ✓ Finally, dip into the breadcrumb mixture, while pressing the bread mixture lightly to adhere to the zucchini chip. After adding some cooking spray, transfer the breaded zucchini chips in the air fryer basket.
- ✓ Maintain a single layer and leave breathing space. Allow to cook for about 5-6 minutes or until the chips are browned. Do the same for the other zucchini chips.
- ✓ Serve.

747) Baked Zucchini Fries

Ingredients:

- Cooking spray
- 2 large egg whites
- Salt and ground black pepper to taste
- 2 tbsp grated
- Parmesan cheese
- ¼ tsp garlic powder
- ½ cup seasoned bread crumbs
- 3 medium zucchini sliced into sticks

Direction: Cooking Time: 35 minutes | Servings: 1

- ✓ Ensure that your oven is preheated to 425 F. Place a cooling rack inside a baking sheet.
- ✓ Use some cooking spray to coat the rack and set aside. Get a small bowl and in it, beat the egg whites, adding salt and pepper to taste.
- ✓ Combine the cheese, garlic powder, and breadcrumbs in a separate bowl and mix well.
- ✓ Dip the zucchini sticks into the egg mixture, the breadcrumb and cheese mixture.
- ✓ Transfer the breaded zucchini onto the cooling rack, arranging them in a single layer. Spray additional cooking spray on the top of the breaded zucchini. Allow baking at 425 F for about 15-20 minutes. Withdraw when the zucchini appears golden brown.
- ✓ To serve, combine with Ranch or Marinara sauce for dipping.

748) Zucchini Rounds

Ingredients:

- 1 lb zucchini sliced into rounds
- 2 tbsp extra-virgin olive oil
- 1 tsp garlic powder
- 1 tsp kosher salt
- ½ tsp ground black pepper

Direction: Cooking Time: 40 minutes | Servings: 4

- ✓ Ensure that your air fryer is preheated to 400 F.
- ✓ With the ends of the zucchini cut off, cut them into rounds, each with a thickness of about ¼ inches.
- ✓ Make a mixture of olive oil and seasonings in a clean small bowl.
- ✓ Toss in the zucchini into the olive oil mixture and mix thoroughly.
- ✓ Transfer the zucchini in the basket of the air fryer, and with the drawer closed, allow cooking for 30 minutes.
- ✓ Endeavor to toss twice or thrice during the cooking to make sure that the zucchini browns evenly.

749) Zucchini Fritters

Ingredients:

- 4 oz plain flour
- 1 tbsp mixed herbs
- Salt and ground black pepper to taste
- 1 medium egg beaten
- 5 tbsp milk
- 5 oz zucchini, grated
- 3 oz onion, peeled and diced
- 1 oz cheddar cheese grated

Direction: Cooking Time: 30 minutes | Servings: 8

- ✓ Combine your plain flour and the seasoning in a bowl. Whisk the egg and milk separately and pour in the mixture into the bowl. Stir to make a smooth, creamy batter.
- ✓ Grate the courgette and ensure that no excess moisture is retained before adding the onion. Stir in the cheese.
- ✓ You may add more cheese and flour to make the batter up to the required thickness. Shape the batter into small burgers. Arrange the shaped batter in the air fryer and allow cooking for 20 minutes at 390 F.
- ✓ Withdraw and serve alongside a good dollop of mayonnaise.

750) Zucchini Gratin

Ingredients:

- 2 zucchini
- Salt and ground black pepper to taste
- 2 tbsp bread crumbs
- 4 tbsp grated Parmesan cheese
- 1 tbsp chopped fresh parsley
- 1 tbsp vegetable oil

Direction: Cooking Time: 30 minutes | Servings: 4

- ✓ Ensure that your air fryer is preheated to 360 F.
- ✓ After cutting the zucchini in half lengthways, slice each piece in half again through the middle.
- ✓ Transfer the resulting eight pieces of zucchini into the air fryer basket.
- ✓ Combine the freshly ground black pepper, salt, breadcrumbs, cheese, parsley, and oil in a separate bowl; mix thoroughly.
- ✓ Divide the zucchini into two batches. Transfer the first batch into the air fryer basket and top it with the breadcrumb and cheese mixture.
- ✓ Allow frying for 15 minutes or until the gratin is golden brown. Do the same for the other batch.

751) Broccoli with Cheese Sauce

Ingredients:

- 6 cups broccoli florets (about 12 oz)
- Cooking spray
- 6 lower-sodium saltine crackers
- 4 tsp Aji Amarillo paste
- 1½ oz queso fresco (fresh Mexican cheese), crumbled (about 5 tbsp)
- 10 tbsp low-fat evaporated milk

Direction: Cooking Time: 25 minutes | Servings: 4

- ✓ After coating your broccoli florets generously with cooking spray, divide into batches.
- ✓ Transfer the first batch into the air fryer basket, and allow cooking at 375 F until they are tender-crisp (for about 6-8 minutes).
- ✓ Do the same for the other batch. While the broccoli cooks, combine the saltines, Aji Amarillo paste, queso fresco, and the evaporated milk in a blender and process for about 45 seconds.
- ✓ Withdraw once you have a smooth blend into a microwave bowl.
- ✓ Microwave the blend on 'high' for about 30 seconds.
- ✓ Combine the broccoli with the cheese sauce and serve.

752) Roasted Broccoli and Cauliflower

Ingredients:

- 3 cups broccoli florets
- ¼ tsp sea salt
- ½ tsp garlic powder
- 2 tbsp olive oil
- 3 cups cauliflower florets
- ¼ tsp paprika
- 1/8 tsp ground black pepper

Direction: Cooking Time: 30 minutes | Servings: 6

- ✓ Ensure that your air fryer is preheated to 400 F. Toss the broccoli florets into a large bowl suitable for microwaving. Set your microwave to 'high' and cook the florets for 3 minutes.
- ✓ Remove any accumulated liquid. In the bowl containing the broccoli, combine the sea salt, garlic powder, olive oil, cauliflower, paprika, and black pepper.
- ✓ Transfer the mixture into the air fryer basket.
- ✓ With the timer set at 12 minutes, allow the mixture to cook.
- ✓ After 6 minutes, toss in the vegetables, to ensure even browning.

753) Roasted Cauliflower

Ingredients:

- 3 cloves garlic
- ½ tsp smoked paprika
- ½ tsp salt
- 1 tbsp peanut oil
- 4 cups cauliflower florets

Direction: Cooking Time: 30 minutes | Servings: 2

- ✓ Ensure that your air fryer is preheated to 400 F. Slice your garlic in half before smashing with your knife's blade.
- ✓ Combine the paprika, salt, and oil in a bowl. Finally, add the cauliflower while turning to coat.
- ✓ Transfer the coated cauliflower into the air fryer and allow cooking until you have the desired crispiness.
- ✓ This may take up to 15 minutes, however, endeavor to shake at 5-minute intervals. Serve.

754) Buffalo Cauliflower

Ingredients:

For the Cauliflower:
- 4 cups cauliflower florets
- 1 cup panko breadcrumbs mixed with
- 1 tsp sea salt

For the Buffalo Coating:
- ¼ cup melted vegan butter (¼ cup after melting)
- ¼ cup vegan Buffalo sauce (Check the ingredients for butter. I used Frank's Red Hot)
- For Dipping: Vegan mayo Cashew Ranch, or your favorite creamy salad dressing

Direction: Cooking Time: 25 minutes | Servings: 4

- ✓ Start by melting your vegan butter in the microwave – pour it in a mug and place it in the microwave. Whisk the melted butter in the buffalo sauce. Grab each floret by the stem and dip in the buffalo-butter mixture, ensuring that the floret is well coated in the sauce. Do not worry if the part of the stem you are holding isn't saucy.
- ✓ Hold the floret over the mug until it doesn't drip anymore. Avoiding excessive dripping is necessary to ensure that your panko doesn't get clumpy or sticky.
- ✓ Toss the dipped floret in the salt-panko mixture, while coating generously. Transfer the coated florets into the air fryer basket – a single layer is not compulsory here. Air fry at 350 F, without preheating, for about 14-17 minutes. Shake a few times while cooking and monitor the progress at the same time.
- ✓ Once you can see the florets getting almost browned, the cauliflower is ready to be served.
- ✓ Serve alongside your preferred dipping sauce.

755) Buffalo Cauliflower Bites (ver. 2)

Ingredients:

- 1 large egg white
- 2 tbsp hot sauce (such as Franks Red Hot)
- 3 tbsp no-salt-added ketchup
- ½ head cauliflower, trimmed and cut into
- 1-inch florets (about 4 cups florets)
- ¾ cup panko (Japanese-style breadcrumbs) Cooking spray
- ¼ tsp black pepper
- 1 tsp red wine vinegar
- ¼ cup reduced-fat sour cream
- ¼ oz crumbled blue cheese (about 1 tbsp)
- 1 small garlic clove, grated

Direction: Cooking Time: 55 minutes | Servings: 4

- ✓ Get a clean small bowl and in it, whisk together the egg white, hot sauce, and ketchup until you have a smooth mixture. Toss the panko into a large bowl.
- ✓ Combine the cauliflower florets and ketchup mixture in a separate large bowl and allow the florets coat generously. You may have to work in batches here.
- ✓ Toss the cauliflower into the panko to coat, before coating it again generously with a cooking spray.
- ✓ Move the first batch of the cauliflower into the air fryer basket. Allow cooking at 320 F for about 20 minutes, or until you have crispy and golden brown florets.
- ✓ Do the same for the other batches of the cauliflower. Meanwhile, get a small bowl and in it, combine the pepper, vinegar, sour cream, blue cheese and garlic.
- ✓ Stir well till you have a uniform mixture. Serve the cooked cauliflower alongside the blue cheese sauce.

756) Orange Sesame Cauliflower

Ingredients:

- 2/3 cup water
- 1/3 cup all-purpose flour
- 1/3 cup cornstarch
- ½ tsp salt
- ½ tsp ground black pepper
- 1 medium head cauliflower, cut into florets
- 4 tbsp vegetable oil
- 1 orange
- 2 tbsp soy sauce
- 2 tbsp rice vinegar
- 2 tbsp ketchup
- 2 tbsp brown sugar
- 1 tbsp toasted sesame oil
- 2 cloves garlic, minced
- 1 tsp cornstarch
- Sliced green onion Toasted sesame seeds

Direction: Cooking Time: 1 hour 15 minutes | Servings: 4

- ✓ Get a large, clean bowl and in it, whisk water, flour, cornstarch, salt, and pepper until you have a smooth mixture. Toss in the cauliflower florets and stir until well coated.
- ✓ Remove the cauliflower and place them onto a parchment paper-lined baking sheet.
- ✓ Allow chilling for 30 minutes. Transfer the cauliflower into your air fryer. After drizzling with some vegetable oil, allow to cook for 22 minutes or until you have a tender browned cauliflower.
- ✓ While cooking the cauliflower, measure one teaspoon of zest orange and set aside.
- ✓ Juice the orange to measure up to ¼ of the cup. Get a clean saucepan and in it, make a mixture of the soy sauce, rice vinegar, orange juice, ketchup, brown sugar, sesame oil, and garlic. Place the saucepan containing the mixture on medium heat and allow to simmer.
- ✓ Stir cornstarch with one teaspoon water until dissolved. Whisk into the sauce and allow cooking until you have glossy (takes about 2 minutes). Withdraw the saucepan from the heat and pour in the orange zest.
- ✓ Finally, toss in the cauliflower with the warm sauce. Add green onion and sesame seeds for garnishing. Serve immediately.

757) Honey Glazed Cauliflower Bites

Ingredients:

- 1 small cauliflower
- 1/3 cup gluten free oats
- 1/3 desiccated coconut
- 1/3 cup plain flour
- Salt and ground black pepper to taste
- 1 large egg beaten
- 1 tsp mixed herbs
- 2 tbsp honey
- 1 tsp mixed spice
- 1 tsp garlic puree
- ½ tsp mustard powder
- 2 tbsp soy sauce

Direction: Cooking Time: 30 minutes | Servings: 4

- ✓ Ensure that your air fryer is preheated to 360 F. Make small florets out of your cauliflower by chopping as required. This facilitates easy and fast cooking.
- ✓ Get a clean bowl, and in it, combine the oats, coconut, flour, and add salt and pepper to taste. Set the mixture aside. Get another clean bowl and in it, beat your egg and set aside. Add mixed herbs alongside pepper and salt into the cauliflower to season it.
- ✓ Now roll the cauliflower in the eggs first, then in the oats mixture. Transfer the rolled cauliflower into the air fryer and allow cooking for 15 minutes at 360 F.
- ✓ While it is cooking in a large mixing bowl mix together the rest of your ingredients with a tablespoon.
- ✓ Withdraw the cooked cauliflower and toss it entirely into the mixing bowl alongside the sticky substance. With the aid of thongs (to avoid the cauliflower burning your hands), stir the cauliflower thoroughly to ensure even coating.
- ✓ Return the coated cauliflower into the air fryer dish or a baking mat.
- ✓ Allow cooking for an additional 5 minutes at 360 F.
- ✓ Serve on a bed of lettuce.

758) Spicy Cauliflower Stir-Fry

Ingredients:

- 1 head cauliflower cut into florets
- 3/4 cup onion white, thinly sliced
- 5 cloves garlic finely sliced
- Salt and ground black pepper to taste
- 1 tbsp Sriracha or other favorite hot sauce
- 1½ tbsp tamari or gluten free tamari
- ½ tsp coconut sugar
- 1 tbsp rice vinegar Soy sauce to taste
- 2 scallions for garnish

Direction: Cooking Time: 35 minutes | Servings: 4

- ✓ Place the cauliflower in the air fryer. Use an insert if your air fryer has holes in the base.
- ✓ With the heat set to 350 F and time 10 minutes, allow cooking.
- ✓ Once the timer goes off, open the air fryer and grab the pot by the handle.
- ✓ Withdraw and shake before sliding it back into the compartment.
- ✓ Toss in the sliced onion, stir and cook for ten more minutes. Toss in the garlic too, and stir.
- ✓ Allow cooking for an additional 5 minutes. Get a clean small bowl and in it, combine the pepper, sriracha, salt, coconut sugar, rice vinegar, and soy sauce into a mixture, Pour the mixture on the cauliflower and mix.
- ✓ Allow cooking for five more minutes.
- ✓ All the juice will be retained inside if you use an insert. Sprinkle scallions over the top of the cauliflower as a form of garnish.
- ✓ Serve.

759) Cauliflower Cheese Tater Tots

Ingredients:

- 2 lbs fresh cauliflower
- 1 tbsp oats
- 4 oz bread crumbs
- 1 tbsp desiccated coconut
- 1 large egg
- 1 tsp garlic puree
- Salt and ground black pepper to taste
- 4 oz onion, peeled and thinly diced
- 1 tsp chives
- 1 tsp parsley
- 1 tsp oregano
- 5 oz cheddar cheese

Direction: Cooking Time: 50 minutes | Servings: 12

- ✓ Transfer your chopped cauliflower (now florets) into the soup maker.
- ✓ Add some water and allow steaming for 20 minutes. Meanwhile, prepare the breadcrumbs coating by combining the oats, breadcrumb, and coconut in a separate bowl. Beat your egg in another bowl. Once the cauliflower is cooked, withdraw and drain the water. Return into the soup maker, and add the garlic puree, salt, and pepper.
- ✓ Now blend until you have a mixture with the appearance of breadcrumbs. Transfer the blended mixture into a clean tea towel and squeeze it for few minutes.
- ✓ Stop when you are confident that all the water is drained.
- ✓ Transfer the cauliflower into a mixing bowl alongside the onion and the rest of the herbs, plus the cheese.
- ✓ Mix thoroughly. Shape the mixture into tater tots, and then roll the tots in the breadcrumbs.
- ✓ Move the rolled tater tots into the air fryer and allow cooking at 360 F for 6 minutes.
- ✓ Increase the heat to 390 F and allow cooking for an additional 10 minutes or until the cauliflower is hot in the middle and crispy on the outside.

760) Cauliflower Rice Stuffed Peppers Budget Recipe

Ingredients:

- 1 yellow pepper
- 1 green pepper
- 1 red pepper
- 1 small onion peeled and diced
- 1 tsp garlic puree
- 1 tbsp olive oil
- 1 small courgette very thinly diced
- ¼ yellow pepper very thinly diced
- 1 large carrot very thinly diced
- 1 tsp fennel seeds
- 1 tsp mixed spice
- 1 tsp coriander
- 1 tsp Chinese five spice
- Salt and ground black pepper to taste
- 1 small cauliflower shredded
- 3 tbsp soft cheese

Direction: Cooking Time: 30 minutes | Servings: 3

- ✓ Pinch off the uppermost part of the peppers and pull out the stalk at the center.
- ✓ Arrange pepper bottoms in the Air fryer and apply heat at 390 F for 5 minutes after which the peppers would appear firm and crispy.
- ✓ In a separate pan, sauté the onion with garlic in olive oil at medium heat.
- ✓ Add vegetables and allow to fry for about 4 minutes before seasoning the mixture.
- ✓ After seasoning, put cauliflower in the same pan and mix with the previous contents to make cauliflower rice. In the space from which the middle stalk and top of the peppers were removed, pour in cream cheese and cover with the cauliflower rice.
- ✓ Replace the cover, return the peppers to the air fryer and allow to simmer for about 10 minutes at a heat of 390 F.
- ✓ The Cauliflower Rice Stuffed Peppers can now be served and enjoyed.

761) Sprouts Breaded Mushrooms

Ingredients:

- Breadcrumbs
- 3 oz grams finely grated Parmigiano Reggiano cheese
- 1 egg
- 0.5 oz button mushrooms
- Flour
- Salt and ground black pepper to taste

Direction: Cooking Time: 15 minutes | Servings: 1

- ✓ Get a clean bowl and in it, make a mixture of the breadcrumbs, salt, pepper and the Parmigiano cheese. Set the mixture aside.
- ✓ Get another bowl and beat an egg. Set aside also.
- ✓ Using kitchen papers, pat-dry the mushrooms.
- ✓ Roll the mushrooms in the flour, then dip in the egg, and finally in the breadcrumbs/cheese mixture, making sure that they are well coated.
- ✓ Transfer the coated mushroom into the air fryer and allow cooking for 7 minutes at 360 F. Shake once while cooking. Serve the cooked mushroom while warm, alongside your preferred dipping sauce.

762) Mushroom Croquettes or Meat Croquettes

Ingredients:

- 4 oz mushrooms
- ¼ onion
- 1 oz butter
- 1½ heaped tbsp flour
- ½ liter milk
- Ground nutmeg
- Salt to taste
- 2 oz breadcrumbs
- 2 tbsp vegetable oil

Direction: Cooking Time: 25 minutes | Servings: 8

- ✓ Chop your mushrooms and onions into thin pieces. Get a saucepan and melt the butter in it, toss in the sliced onions and mushrooms and fry. Add the flour and stir well. Warm up the milk and stir it in bit by bit. Continue stirring while the mixture thickens.
- ✓ Add nutmeg and salt to taste. Leave the mixture in the refrigerator for 2 hours to cool. Prepare the breadcrumb coating by combining the oil and the breadcrumbs. Continue stirring until you have a loose and crumbly mixture. Roll 1 tablespoon of filling in the breadcrumbs until they are coated thoroughly.
- ✓ Now place it in the air fryer basket.
- ✓ Do the same for other breadcrumbs, until you have no more filing.
- ✓ Ensure that your air fryer is preheated to 390 F. Place the breadcrumbs into the basket and slide it into the air fryer.
- ✓ Set the timer for 8 minutes and fry the croquettes until they are brown and crispy.
- ✓ Note: You can make meat croquettes by replacing the mushrooms with 4 oz of finely-chopped beef or veal.

763) Stuffed Mushrooms with Sour Cream

Ingredients:

- 24 mushrooms, caps and stems diced
- ½ onion, diced
- 1 small carrot, diced
- ½ orange bell pepper, diced
- 2 slices bacon, diced
- 1 cup shredded Cheddar cheese
- ½ cup sour cream
- 1½ tbsp shredded Cheddar cheese, or to taste

Direction: Cooking Time: 55 minutes | Servings: 24

- ✓ Combine the mushroom stems, onion, carrot, orange bell pepper, and bacon in a skillet.
- ✓ Cook and stir the mixture over medium heat until softened – this takes about 5 minutes. Pour in a cup of Cheddar cheese and sour cream.
- ✓ Continue cooking until the cheese has melted and the stuffing is mixed thoroughly – this takes about 2 minutes.
- ✓ Ensure that your air fryer is preheated to 350 F. Set the mushroom caps on the baking tray carefully. Add the stuffing to each mushroom following the heap style.
- ✓ Add sprinkles of about 1.5 tablespoons Cheddar cheese on top.
- ✓ Transfer the tray of mushrooms into the air fryer basket and allow cooking for about 8 minutes, or until the cheese melts.

764) Shiitake Mushroom Chips

Ingredients:

- 8 oz Shiitake Mushroom
- Salt to taste

Direction: Cooking Time: 20 minutes | Servings: 1-2

- ✓ Start by using cold water to rinse the Shiitake mushroom.
- ✓ Don't make the mistake of leaving it soaked in the water as the mushroom tends to absorb water Bring up the Air fryer to heat of 360 F Depending on your preference, you can either cut off the whole stem from the Shiitake mushroom or only remove the lower part of the stem.
- ✓ Cut the mushroom into slices. There are no hard and fast rules for the size of each slice.
- ✓ But note that if sliced too thin, it starts sticking to the bottom of the Air Fryer pan and burns easily Place the slices of mushroom in the pan and allow to fry for between 9 and 12 minutes or until your desired dryness for the mushroom has been achieved. Mid-way into the frying, you should either stir with a small ladle/spatula or gently shake the pan itself.
- ✓ After frying, sprinkle some salt on the now shrunken mushroom.

765) Stuffed Garlic Mushrooms

Ingredients:

- 1 tsp garlic puree
- 1 oz onion, peeled and diced
- Salt and groundblack pepper to taste
- 1 tbsp olive oil
- 1 tbsp breadcrumbs
- 1 tsp parsley
- 6 small mushrooms

Direction: Cooking Time: 40 minutes | Servings: 4

- ✓ Thoroughly mix the garlic, onion, salt, pepper, olive oil, breadcrumbs, and parsley Rinse the mushrooms properly and pull out the middle stalks, then pour in the breadcrumb mixture to replace the central stalks in the center of the mushrooms.
- ✓ Allow the mushrooms to boil for 10 minutes at a heat of 360 F, and you're done.
- ✓ You can now enjoy your air fryer stuffed Garlic Mushrooms.

766) Stuffed Portobello Mushrooms

Ingredients:

- 3 portobello mushrooms
- 1 tbsp olive oil
- A dash of black pepper
- 1 medium red onion, diced
- 1 tsp minced garlic
- 1 green bell pepper, diced
- 1 tomato, diced Grated cheddar or mozzarella cheese
- 2 slices ham, chopped into small pieces
- Half tsp truffle salt

Direction: Cooking Time: 45 minutes | Servings: 3

- ✓ Heat the Air Fryer or an oven up to a heat of 320 F or 380 F respectively. Get the mushrooms ready by washing them thoroughly and drying.
- ✓ Apply a thick film of olive oil to coat the mushrooms and rub it on your hands as well. Get a big bowl, and mix the other ingredients: black pepper, onions, garlic, bell pepper, tomato, cheese, ham, and truffle salt inside it Split open the mushroom caps and add portions of the mixture from the bowl into it.
- ✓ Depending on your preference, you could layer some more cheese atop the mushroom. Place the mushrooms either in the Air fryer for 8 minutes at its initial heat of 320 F.
- ✓ If you're using an oven, allow the mushroom to get baked for between 12 and 15 minutes, but lower the heat by 10 degrees to 360 F.
- ✓ After the baking or frying is done, the meal is ready to be served with hard boiled eggs and salad.

767) Button Mushroom Melt

Ingredients:

- About 10 button mushrooms
- Salt and ground black pepper to taste Italian dried mixed herbs
- Olive oil Cheddar cheese, shredded Mozzarella cheese, grated
- Dried dill (optional as garnish)

Direction: Cooking Time: 40 minutes | Servings: 4

- ✓ Start by washing the mushrooms and cutting out their stems.
- ✓ You might add a small sprinkle of salt here, black pepper, Italian dried mixed herbs but this is optional. Mushrooms are already tasty on their own, and adding more seasoning may make it turn out too spicy.
- ✓ Also, a little olive oil will aid in not allowing the mushrooms to dry out in the air fryer. Heat the air fryer to a heat of 360 F for between 3 and 5 minutes.
- ✓ As the air fryer gets heated up, place the mushroom in the wire basket within the air fryer, ensure the hollow section is upwards.
- ✓ Sprinkle both cheddar and mozzarella cheese on top of each mushroom cap. Allow the mushrooms to fry for between 7 and 8 minutes at 360 F.
- ✓ The meal is ready to be served. If you so wish, you may add some green herbs like basil, dill, or parleys.

768) Brussels Sprouts

Ingredients:

- ½ tsp ground black pepper
- ½ tsp salt
- 1 tsp avocado oil
- 10 oz Brussels sprouts, trimmed and halved lengthwise
- 1 tsp balsamic vinegar
- 2 tsp crumbled cooked bacon, optional

Direction: Cooking Time: 20 minutes | Servings: 2

- ✓ Ensure that your air fryer is preheated to 350 F. Mix pepper, salt, and oil thoroughly in a clean bowl.
- ✓ Add Brussels sprouts and turn to coat. Allow air frying for 5 minutes.
- ✓ Stop and shake the sprouts, then cook for an extra 5 minutes. Withdraw the sprouts and place in a serving dish.
- ✓ Sprinkle with some balsamic vinegar and turn to coat. Sprinkle with bacon. Serve.

769) Garlic-Rosemary Brussels Sprouts

Ingredients:

- ¼ tsp pepper
- ½ tsp salt
- 3 tbsp olive oil
- 2 garlic cloves, minced
- 1 lb Brussels sprouts, trimmed and halved
- ½ cup panko (Japanese) bread crumbs
- 1-½ tsp fresh rosemary, minced

Direction: Cooking Time: 35 minutes | Servings: 4

- ✓ Ensure that your air fryer is preheated to 350 F. Get a clean microwave-safe bowl, and in it, combine the first four ingredients.
- ✓ Microwave the contents of the bowl for 30 seconds on 'high.' Coat the Brussels sprouts with two tablespoons of the oil mixture, before transferring into the air fryer basket.
- ✓ Set the timer for 4-5 minutes. Stop and stir the sprouts.
- ✓ Resume air-frying while stirring every 4-5 minutes. Only stop when the sprouts are almost soft and are lightened browned (approximately after 8 minutes).
- ✓ Toss the bread crumbs with rosemary and the leftover oil mixture, then sprinkle over sprouts.
- ✓ Cook until you have browned and tender sprouts (for about 3-5 minutes). Withdraw and serve immediately.

770) Brussels Sprouts with Bacon

Ingredients:

- 1 lb Brussels sprouts
- 4 slices back bacon
- Salt and ground black pepper to taste

Direction: Cooking Time: 20 minutes | Servings: 2

- ✓ With the outside skin and the core of your Brussels sprouts removed, transfer them into the air fryer and allow cooking for 10 minutes at 360 F.
- ✓ Meanwhile, dice your bacon and get rid of all the apparent fat.
- ✓ Place them in the bacon once the sprouts have cooked for 10 minutes.
- ✓ With the bacon inside, set the timer for five minutes and 400 F.
- ✓ Serve alongside pepper and salt.

771) Onion Rings

Ingredients:

- 2 tsp baking powder
- ¾ cup all-purpose flour
- ½ cup cornstarch
- 1 tsp salt
- 1 large onion, cut into rings
- 1 egg 1 cup milk
- 1 cup bread crumbs
- Cooking spray
- 2 pinches garlic powder, optional
- 2 pinches paprika, optional

Direction: Cooking Time: 25 minutes | Servings: 4

- Get a small bowl and mix the baking powder, flour, cornstarch, and salt inside it. Roll the sliced onion in the flour mixture until it is covered within it. Break the egg into the flour mixture, add milk, and whisk all together. Pick the coated onion slices and dip them in the batter until they get coated again.
- Drain them by arranging the rings on a wire rack until the batter stops drooping Put the bread crumbs in a dish and add the onion slices to the crumbs successively, place the crumbs on the ring so the onion rings will be well covered with the crumbs.
- While pulling the onion rings out of the bread crumbs, tap them to make the batter and breadcrumb mixture stick properly.
- Heat your air fryer, and get it up to 390 F.
- Keep in mind that instructions from the manufacturer should be followed to prevent damage to the equipment. Arrange the onion rings in the frying basket and add a slight puff of cooking spray.
- Turn the onion rings over to the other side and lower the frying basket into the air fryer. Allow it to fry for between one and one and half minutes, then turn the onion rings over again.
- Allow frying for another one to one and a half minutes. You can then take out the rings and drain them using paper towels.
- Alternatively, you can choose to sprinkle with paprika or garlic powder.

772) Onion Rings With Comeback Sauce

Ingredients:

- ½ tsp kosher salt, divided
- ½ cup (about 2 1/8 oz.) all-purpose flour
- 1 tsp smoked paprika
- 1 large egg 1 tbsp water
- 1 cup whole-wheat panko (Japanese-style breadcrumbs)
- 1 (10-oz.) sweet onion, cut into 1/2-in.-thick rounds and separated into rings
- Cooking spray
- 2 tbsp canola mayonnaise
- 1 tsp Dijon mustard
- ¼ tsp garlic powder
- ¼ tsp paprika
- ¼ cup plain
- 1% low-fat Greek yogurt 1 tbsp ketchup

Direction: Cooking Time: 60 minutes | Servings: 4

- In a shallow dish, thoroughly mix a quarter teaspoon of salt with flour and smoked paprika. Break the egg in another dish and beat it with water.
- In yet another dish, add a quarter teaspoon of salt to panko and stir them together.
- Dip the rings of onion slices in the flour mixture, totally submerging them and shaking off extraneous flour.
- Then drench the onion rings in the egg mixture as well, again, be sure to shake off any extra egg mixture.
- Finally, dip the onion rings in the panko mixture, apply some pressure on it and generously apply cooking spray to both sides of the rings.
- Arrange the onion rings by stacking them on each other and placing them inside the air fryer basket in batches. Then allow them to cook for 5 minutes at 375 F. Turn them over and allow to cook for another five minutes. By this time they would have a golden brown color as well as a crispy texture on both sides.
- While frying other batches, ensure to keep the already fried onion rings covered so as not to let them grow cold. While the onion rings are being fried, make a sauce by mixing mayonnaise, mustard, garlic powder, paprika, yogurt, and ketchup together.
- Each serving may contain two tablespoons of the well-mixed sauce and between 5 and eight onion rings.

773) Roasted Parsnips

Ingredients:

- 6 medium parsnips
- Salt and ground black pepper to taste

Direction: Cooking Time: 20 minutes | Servings: 4

- Skin the Parsnips and cut them up in similarly sized diagonally shaped slices. Arrange the sliced Parsnips inside the Instant Pot Steamer Basket and add a cup of warm water. Then place the basket in the Instant Pot and cover it by shutting the lid.
- The pot should now be put atop the steamer shelf (trivet). The valve setting should be changed to "sealing" and the pressure set at "manual" while the pot is left to steam for 3 minutes.
- As soon as you here the pot beep, bleed off the pressure within it.
- The parsnips should be drained to get rid of as much moisture as possible and placed on a chopping board.
- The drained parsnips should be sprinkled with salt and pepper
- After sprinkling, arrange the parsnips in the air fryer and allow to fry at a heat of 390 F for 8 minutes.

774) Curry Parsnip Fries

Ingredients:
- Large parsnips
- Olive oil Curry powder to taste
- Sea salt to taste

Direction: Cooking Time: 1 hour | Servings: 1

- ✓ Heat the oven to 350 F Skin the parsnips and slice them till they have the similitude of
- ✓ French fries Spread a film of olive oil on a cookie sheet
- ✓ Arrange the parsnips on the cookie sheet and add another film of olive oil on them too.
- ✓ Season the parsnips with curry and some salt.
- ✓ Allow it to bake for between 30 and 50 minutes or until it becomes soft and takes on a light brown color.

775) Celery Root Fries

Ingredients:
- 3 cups water
- 1 tbsp lime juice
- ½ celeriac (celery root), peeled and cut into
- 1/2-inch sticks

Mayo Sauce:
- 1 tsp powdered horseradish
- 1/3 cup vegan mayonnaise
- 1 tbsp brown mustard
- 1 tbsp olive oil
- 1 pinch salt
- Ground black pepper to taste

Direction: Cooking Time: 50 minutes | Servings: 4

- ✓ In a bowl, add water and lime juice to celery roots. Stir the mixture together and leave it for a third of an hour Heat the air fryer to a heat of 390 F Prepare vegan mayo sauce by adding together horseradish powder, vegan mayonnaise, and mustard in a bowl.
- ✓ Cover the mixture and keep it in the refrigerator. Remove water from the celery root sticks and allow to dry before putting in a separate bowl.
- ✓ Add some oil to the fries and sprinkle salt and pepper over it.
- ✓ Turn the fries over to allow a uniform coating to form. Place the drained and dried celery root sticks in the air fryer basket and cook for about 10 minutes after which you can check to see how cooked it is.
- ✓ Shake the basket and cook for eight more minutes till the fries take on a crisp texture and brown color.
- ✓ Now bring out the vegan mayo sauce from the refrigerator and serve alongside the fries.

776) Everything Bagel Kale Chips

Ingredients:
- 6 cups packed torn Lacinato kale leaves, stems and ribs removed
- 1 tbsp olive oil
- 1 tsp lower-sodium soy sauce
- ½ tsp dried minced garlic
- ¼ tsp poppy seeds
- 1 tsp white or black sesame seeds

Direction: Cooking Time: 35 minutes | Servings: 2

- ✓ Rinse the Kale leaves thoroughly, then drain and dry them, totally removing all moisture.
- ✓ Pull the dried leaves apart and tear them into pieces that are between 1 and 0.5 inches long.
- ✓ Toss together kale, olive oil, and soy sauce in a medium bowl, rubbing the leaves gently to be sure they are well coated with mixture.
- ✓ Arrange a third of the Kale leaves in the air fryer basket, and allow to fry at a heat of 375 F for about three minutes. Shake the basket, then fry for another 3 minutes.
- ✓ Place the now fried kale chips on a baking sheet, then season with garlic, poppy seeds, and sesame seeds before it loses the heat of cooking.
- ✓ Repeat with remaining kale leaves.

777) Vegan Stuffed Bell Peppers

Ingredients:
- 2 tsp dried mixed herbs
- 2 cloves garlic, minced
- 1 carrot, diced
- 1 small onion, diced
- ½ cup peas 1 potato, diced
- 1 vegan bread roll, diced
- 6 green bell peppers - tops, seeds, and membranes removed (tops reserved)
- 1/3 cup shredded vegan cheese

Direction: Cooking Time: 50 minutes | Servings: 6

- ✓ In a clean bowl, combine the mixed herbs, garlic, carrot, onion, peas, potato, and bread. After dicing the tops of the green bell pepper, toss them into the bowl.
- ✓ Mix thoroughly. Ensure that your air fryer is preheated to 350 F. Stuff the peppers equally with the filling.

Nutrition:

- ✓ Transfer the stuffed peppers into the air fryer basket. Allow cooking until tender and hot throughout – this takes about 20 minutes.
- ✓ Stir in the shredded vegan cheese and cook until melted – this takes an additional 5 minutes.

778) Roasted Peppers (Bell Peppers)

Ingredients:
- 1 lb mixed bell peppers

Direction: Cooking Time: 15 minutes | Servings: 3

- ✓ Remove the pepper tops by slicing them off. Using a firm grip, pull out the stalk and get rid of all the seeds at once.
- ✓ Now dice the peppers into large and medium pieces.
- ✓ Transfer the pepper pieces in the air fryer and allow cooking for 8 minutes at 360 F.
- ✓ Withdraw after 8 minutes and serve while still warm.

779) Green Salad with Roasted Pepper

Ingredients:
- 1 red bell pepper
- 3 tbsp yoghurt
- 2 tbsp olive oil
- 1 tbsp lemon juice
- Salt to taste
- Freshly ground black pepper to taste
- 2 oz rocket leaves
- 1 romaine lettuce, in broad strips

Direction: Cooking Time: 30 minutes | Servings: 4

- ✓ Ensure that your air fryer is preheated to 390 F.
- ✓ Place the basket containing the bell pepper into the air fryer and allow cooking for 10 minutes.
- ✓ This will roast the bell pepper until you have their skin mildly charred. Withdraw the roasted bell pepper into a bowl and cover it using a plastic wrap or a lid. Allow the covered pepper to rest for 10-15 minutes.
- ✓ After resting, cut the bell pepper into four sections, while removing the skin and the seeds.
- ✓ In a clean bowl, mix a dressing of 2 tablespoons of the moisture from the bell pepper, yogurt, olive oil, and the lemon juice.
- ✓ Add salt and pepper to taste. Add the rocket leaves and the lettuce into the dressing. Finally, garnish your salad with the bell pepper strips.

780) Grilled Tomatoes

Ingredients:

- 3 medium beefcake tomatoes
- Salt and ground black pepper to taste
- 1 tsp oregano

Direction: Cooking Time: 17 minutes | Servings: 3

- ✓ With the tomatoes chopped into two halves, transfer them into the air fryer grill pan. Add sprinkles of salt, oregano, and pepper.
- ✓ Allow cooking for 8 minutes at 360 F. Reduce the heat to 320 F and allow to cook for an extra 5 minutes.
- ✓ This is to let the tomatoes to cook in the middle.
- ✓ Serve.
- ✓ The essence of chopping the tomatoes in half is to get equal sizes and ensure that each tomato has a bottom.

781) Stuffed Tomatoes and Broccoli

Ingredients:

- ¼ cup cheddar cheese, grated
- ¼ cup broccoli, chopped
- 1 organic tomato (preferably big size)
- 4-5 florets broccoli Butter (unsalted)
- Pinch of natural country herbs

Direction: Cooking Time: 25 minutes | Servings: 2

- ✓ Ensure that your air fryer is preheated to 360 F.
- ✓ Get a clean small bowl and in it, mix the grated Cheddar cheese and the chopped broccoli. Remove the pulps and seeds from the tomato.
- ✓ Stuff the empty tomato with the cheddar and broccoli mixture.
- ✓ Transfer the stuffed tomato into the air fryer basket, add the florets of the broccoli, and finally some butter on top.
- ✓ Allow the tomato to air bake for 12 or 15 minutes.
- ✓ Sprinkle some herbs on the melted cheese. Serve.

782) Air Fryer Pickles

Ingredients:

- 32 dill pickle slices
- ½ cup all-purpose flour
- ½ tsp salt
- 3 large eggs, lightly beaten
- ½ tsp garlic powder
- 2 tbsp dill pickle juice
- ½ tsp cayenne pepper
- 2 tbsp snipped fresh dill
- 2 cups panko (Japanese) bread crumbs
- Cooking spray Ranch salad dressing, optional

Direction: Cooking Time: 45 minutes | Servings: 2

- ✓ Ensure that your air fryer is preheated to 425 F.
- ✓ Allow the pickles to stand on a paper towel until the liquid is almost absorbed – this takes about 15 minutes.
- ✓ Get a shallow bowl, and in it, make a mixture of flour and salt.
- ✓ Get another shallow bowl and combine whisked eggs, garlic powder, pickle juice, and cayenne. In a third shallow bowl, mix the dill and panko.
- ✓ Dip the pickles in the flour mixture, ensuring the even coating of both sides and shake to get rid of excess.
- ✓ Dip again in the egg mixture, and finally in the crumb mixture, and pat to ensure that the coating stays. Spray the air fryer basket and the pickles with the cooking spray. You may work in batches if your air fryer is small.
- ✓ Arrange the pickles in a single layer inside the air fryer basket. Allow cooking for 7-10 minutes or until you have crispy and golden brown pickles.
- ✓ Turn the pickles and spray with extra cooking spray. Resume cooking until you have golden brown and crispy pickles – it takes about 7-10 minutes. Serve immediately, with ranch dressing (optional).

783) Spicy Dill Pickle Fries

Ingredients:

- 1½ (16 oz) jars spicy dill pickle spears
- 1 cup all-purpose flour
- ½ tsp paprika
- 1 egg, beaten
- : ¼ cup milk
- 1 cup panko bread crumbs
- Cooking spray

Direction: Cooking Time: 35 minutes | Servings: 10

- ✓ Pat the drained pickles dry. Mix the flour and paprika in a bowl. Get another bowl and in it, mix the beaten egg and milk. Place your panko in a third bowl. Ensure that your air fryer is preheated to 400 F.
- ✓ Dip each pickle in the flour mixture, followed by the egg mixture, and finally in the breadcrumbs. Ensure that the pickles are well coated.
- ✓ Transfer the coated pickles on a plate and do the same for the remaining pickles.
- ✓ Spritz some cooking spray on the coated prickles before placing it in the air fryer basket. You may cook in batches to ensure that the fryer is not overcrowded.
- ✓ Allow cooking for 14 minutes; after 7 minutes, turn the pickles to allow the other side cook.

784) Ratatouille

Ingredients:

- 7 oz courgette and/or aubergine
- 2 tomatoes
- 1 onion, peeled
- 1 yellow bell pepper
- 2 tsp dried Provençal herbs
- 1 clove garlic, crushed
- ½ tsp salt
- Freshly ground black pepper
- 1 tbsp olive oil
- Small, round baking dish, 6-inch diameter

Direction: Cooking Time: 25 minutes | Servings: 4

- ✓ Ensure that your air fryer is preheated to 390 F.
- ✓ Make ½-inch pieces of each of the courgette, aubergine, tomatoes, onion, and bell pepper by cutting.
- ✓ Combine the Provencal herbs, vegetables, garlic, and ½ teaspoon salt and pepper to taste.
- ✓ Stir in a tablespoon of the olive oil. Return the bowl into the air fryer basket and the basket back into the air fryer.
- ✓ Allow the ratatouille to cook for 15 minutes. Stir once when cooking.
- ✓ When cooked, serve the ratatouille alongside fried meat, including a cutlet or entrecote.

785) Ratatouille Italian-Style

Ingredients:
- ½ large yellow bell pepper, cut into cubes
- ½ large red bell pepper, cut into cubes
- ½ onion, cut into cubes
- 1 medium tomato, cut into cubes
- 1 zucchini, cut into cubes
- ½ small eggplant, cut into cubes
- 1 fresh cayenne pepper, diced
- 2 sprigs fresh oregano, stemmed and chopped
- 1 clove garlic, crushed
- 5 sprigs fresh basil, stemmed and chopped
- Salt and ground black pepper to taste
- 1 tsp vinegar
- 1 tbsp white wine
- 1 tbsp olive oil

Direction: Cooking Time: 50 minutes | Servings: 4

- ✓ Ensure that your air fryer is preheated to 400 F.
- ✓ Get a clean bowl and in it, toss in the bell peppers, onion, tomato, zucchini, and the eggplant.
- ✓ Include the cayenne pepper, oregano, garlic, basil, salt, and pepper also.
- ✓ Mix thoroughly to combine properly. Drizzle in vinegar, wine, and oil. Mix the entire mixture to coat all the vegetables.
- ✓ Transfer the vegetable mixture into a baking dish and transfer it into the air fryer basket. Allow cooking for 8 minutes. Stir, and cook for an additional 8 minutes.
- ✓ Stir again and resume cooking until the vegetables are soft. Ensure to stir every 5 minutes, 10 to 15 minutes more.
- ✓ With the dish still inside the air fryer, turn it off for 5 minutes. Remove the dish and allow to rest for 5 minutes. Serve.

786) Air-Fried Asparagus

Ingredients:
- ½ bunch of asparagus, with bottom
- 2 inches trimmed off Avocado or olive oil in an oil mister or sprayer
- Himalayan salt to taste
- Ground black pepper to taste

Direction: Cooking Time: 20 minutes | Servings: 2-4

- ✓ After placing your trimmed asparagus spears in the air-fryer basket, spritz it lightly with cooking oil.
- ✓ Add sprinkles of salt and a tiny bit of black pepper.
- ✓ With the basket inside the air-fryer, allow baking for 10 minutes at 400 F. Serve once baked.

787) Asparagus Fries

Ingredients:
- 1 large egg, beaten
- 1 tsp honey
- ½ cup Parmesan cheese, grated
- 1 cup panko bread crumbs
- 12 asparagus spears, trimmed
- 1 pinch cayenne pepper, optional
- ¼ cup Greek yogurt
- ¼ cup stone-ground mustard

Direction: Cooking Time: 25 minutes | Servings: 6

- ✓ Ensure that your air fryer is preheated to 400 F. Get a long, narrow dish, and in it combing egg and honey.
- ✓ Beat together and set aside. In a separate plate, combine the Parmesan cheese and panko.
- ✓ After coating each asparagus stalk in the egg mixture, roll it also in the panko mix and allow thorough coating.
- ✓ Arrange six spears in the air fryer and allow cooking to the desired brownness – this takes 4 to 6 minutes.
- ✓ Do the same for the other spears. Get a small bowl, and in it, mix the cayenne pepper, yogurt, and mustard.
- ✓ Serve the asparagus spears with the dipping sauce.

788) Roasted Okra

Ingredients:
- ½ lb okra, ends trimmed and pods sliced
- ¼ tsp salt
- 1 tsp olive oil
- 1/8 tsp ground black pepper

Direction: Cooking Time: 25 minutes | Servings: 1

- ✓ Ensure that your air fryer is preheated to 350 F. Get a clean bowl and in it, combine okra, salt, olive oil, and pepper.
- ✓ Stir the mixture gently. Place in a single layer in the air fryer basket.
- ✓ Allow cooking in the air fryer for 5 minutes. Toss and cook for an additional 5 minutes.
- ✓ Toss again and allow cooking for an extra 2 minutes.
- ✓ Withdraw and serve instantly.

789) Tasty Peanut Butter Bars

Ingredients:
- 2 eggs 1 tbsp coconut flour
- 1/2 cup butter, softened
- 1/2 cup peanut butter
- 1/4 cup almond flour
- 1/2 cup swerve

Direction: Preparation Time: 10 minutes Cooking Time: 24 minutes Serve: 9

- ✓ Spray air fryer baking pan with cooking spray and set aside.
- ✓ In a bowl, beat together butter, eggs, and peanut butter until well combined.
- ✓ Add dry ingredients and mix until a smooth batter is formed. Spread batter evenly in prepared pan and place into the air fryer and cook at 325 F for 24 minutes.
- ✓ Slice and serve.

790) Crustless Pie

Ingredients:

- 3 eggs 1/2 cup pumpkin puree
- 1/2 tsp cinnamon
- 1 tsp vanilla
- 1/4 cup erythritol
- 1/2 cup cream
- 1/2 cup unsweetened almond milk

Direction: Preparation Time: 10 minutes Cooking Time: 24 minutes Serve: 4

- ✓ Preheat the air fryer to 325 F. Spray air fryer baking dish with cooking spray and set aside. In a large bowl, add all ingredients and beat until smooth.
- ✓ Pour pie mixture into the prepared dish and place into the air fryer and cook for 24 minutes. Let it cool completely and place into the refrigerator for 1-2 hours. Slice and serve.

791) Cinnamon Ginger Cookies

Ingredients:

- 1 egg 1/2 tsp vanilla
- 1/8 tsp ground cloves
- 1 tsp baking powder
- 3/4 cup erythritol
- 2/4 cup butter
- 1 1/2 cups almond flour
- 1/4 tsp ground nutmeg
- 1/4 tsp ground cinnamon
- 1/2 tsp ground ginger
- Pinch of salt

Direction: Preparation Time: 10 minutes Cooking Time: 12 minutes Serve: 8

- ✓ In a large bowl, mix together all dry ingredients. In a separate bowl, mix together all wet ingredients. Add dry ingredients to the wet ingredients and mix until dough is formed.
- ✓ Cover and place in the fridge for 30 minutes. Preheat the air fryer to 325 F. Make cookies from dough and place into the air fryer and cook for 12 minutes. Serve and enjoy.

792) Chia Chocolate Cookies

Ingredients:

- 2 1/2 tbsp ground chia
- 2 tbsp chocolate protein powder
- 1 cup sunflower seed butter
- 1 cup almond flour

Direction: Preparation Time: 5 minutes Cooking Time: 8 minutes Serve: 20

- ✓ Preheat the air fryer to 325 F. In a large bowl, add all ingredients and mix until combined.
- ✓ Make cookies from bowl mixture and place into the air fryer and cook for 8 minutes. Serve and enjoy.

793) Pumpkin Cookies

Ingredients:

- 1 egg 2 cups almond flour
- 1/2 tsp baking powder
- 1 tsp vanilla
- 1/2 cup butter
- 15 drops liquid stevia
- 1/2 tsp pumpkin pie spice
- 1/2 cup pumpkin puree

Direction: Preparation Time: 10 minutes Cooking Time: 20 minutes Serve: 27

- ✓ Preheat the air fryer to 280 F. In a large bowl, add all ingredients and mix until well combined.
- ✓ Make cookies from mixture and place into the air fryer and cook for 20 minutes. Serve and enjoy.

794) Vanilla Coconut Cheese Cookies

Ingredients:

- 1 egg 1/2 tsp baking powder
- 1 tsp vanilla
- 1/2 cup swerve
- 1/2 cup butter, softened
- 3 tbsp cream cheese, softened
- 1/2 cup coconut flour
- Pinch of salt

Direction: Preparation Time: 10 minutes Cooking Time: 12 minutes Serve: 15

- ✓ In a bowl, beat together butter, sweetener, and cream cheese. Add egg and vanilla and beat until smooth and creamy.
- ✓ Add coconut flour, salt, and baking powder and beat until combined.
- ✓ Cover and place in the fridge for 1 hour. Preheat the air fryer to 325 F. Make cookies from dough and place into the air fryer and cook for 12 minutes.
- ✓ Serve and enjoy.

795) Cheese Butter Cookies

Ingredients:

- 2 eggs 5 tbsp butter, melted
- 1/3 cup sour cream
- 1/3 cup mozzarella cheese, shredded
- 1 1/4 cup almond flour
- 1/2 tsp baking powder
- 1/2 tsp salt

Direction: Preparation Time: 10 minutes Cooking Time: 12 minutes Serve: 8

- ✓ Preheat the air fryer to 370 F.
- ✓ Add all ingredients into a large bowl and mix using a hand mixer.
- ✓ Spoon batter into the mini silicone muffin molds and place into the air fryer and cook for 12 minutes.
- ✓ Serve and enjoy.

796) Pumpkin Custard 2

Ingredients:

- 4 egg yolks 1/2 tsp cinnamon
- 15 drops liquid stevia
- 15 oz pumpkin puree
- 3/4 cup coconut cream
- 1/8 tsp cloves
- 1/8 tsp ginger

Direction: Preparation Time: 10 minutes Cooking Time: 32 minutes Serve: 6

- ✓ Preheat the air fryer to 325 F. In a large bowl, combine together pumpkin puree, cinnamon, swerve, cloves, and ginger. Add egg yolks and beat until combined.
- ✓ Add coconut cream and stir well. Pour mixture into the six ramekins and place into the air fryer. Cook for 32 minutes. Let it cool completely then place in the refrigerator. Serve chilled and enjoy.

797) Cranberry Almond Cake

Ingredients:

- 4 eggs 1 tsp orange zest
- 2 tsp mixed spice
- 2 tsp cinnamon
- 1/4 cup swerve
- 1 cup butter, softened
- 2/3 cup dried cranberries
- 1 1/2 cups almond flour
- 1 tsp vanilla

Direction: Preparation Time: 10 minutes Cooking Time: 16 minutes Serve: 6

- ✓ Preheat the air fryer to 325 F.
- ✓ In a bowl, add sweetener and melted butter and beat until fluffy.
- ✓ Add cinnamon, vanilla, and mixed spice and stir well.
- ✓ Add eggs stir until well combined. Add almond flour, orange zest, and cranberries and stir to combine. Pour batter in a greased air fryer cake pan and place into the air fryer. Cook cake for 16 minutes.
- ✓ Slice and serve.

798) Choco Fudge Cake

Ingredients:
- 6 eggs
- 1 1/2 cup swerve
- 10 oz unsweetened chocolate, melted
- 1/2 cup almond flour
- 10 oz butter, melted
- Pinch of salt

Direction: Preparation Time: 10 minutes Cooking Time: 24 minutes
Serve: 12

- ✓ Preheat the air fryer to 325 F. Spray air fryer cake pan with cooking spray and set aside. In a large bowl, beat eggs until foamy. Add sweetener and stir well.
- ✓ Add melted butter, chocolate, almond flour, and salt and stir to combine. Pour batter into the prepared pan and place into the air fryer and cook for 24 minutes. Slice and serve.

799) Chocolate Coconut Cake

Ingredients:
- 6 eggs 2 tsp baking powder
- 3 oz unsweetened cocoa powder
- 5 oz erythritol
- 3.5 oz coconut flour
- 1 tsp vanilla
- 3 oz butter, melted
- 11 oz heavy cream

Direction: Preparation Time: 10 minutes Cooking Time: 20 minutes
Serve: 9

- ✓ Preheat the air fryer to 325 F. In a bowl, mix together coconut flour, butter, 5 oz heavy cream, eggs, baking powder half cocoa powder, and 3 oz sweetener until well combined. Pour batter into the greased cake pan and place into the air fryer and cook for 20 minutes.
- ✓ Allow to cool completely. In a large bowl, beat remaining heavy cream, cocoa powder, and sweetener until smooth.
- ✓ Spread the cream on top of cake and place in the refrigerator for 30 minutes.
- ✓ Slice and serve.

800) Chocolate Custard

Ingredients:
- 2 eggs 1 tsp vanilla
- 1 cup heavy whipping cream
- 1 cup unsweetened almond milk
- 2 tbsp unsweetened cocoa powder
- 1/4 cup Swerve
- Pinch of salt

Direction: Preparation Time: 10 minutes Cooking Time: 32 minutes
Serve: 4

- ✓ Preheat the air fryer to 305 F. Add all ingredients into the blender and blend until well combined.
- ✓ Pour mixture into the ramekins and place into the air fryer. Cook for 32 minutes. Serve and enjoy.

801) Almond Cinnamon Mug Cake

Ingredients:
- 1 scoop vanilla protein powder
- 1/2 tsp cinnamon
- 1 tsp granulated sweetener
- 1 tbsp almond flour
- 1/2 tsp baking powder
- 1/4 tsp vanilla
- 1/4 cup unsweetened almond milk

Direction: Preparation Time: 5 minutes Cooking Time: 10 minutes
Serve: 1

- ✓ Add protein powder, cinnamon, almond flour, sweetener, and baking powder into the mug and mix well.
- ✓ Add vanilla and almond milk and stir well. Place mug in the air fryer and cook at 390 F for 10 minutes Serve and enjoy.

802) Yummy Brownies

Ingredients:
- 2 tbsp cocoa powder
- 1/4 tsp baking powder
- 1/2 tsp baking soda
- 2 tbsp unsweetened applesauce
- 1 tsp liquid stevia
- 1 tbsp coconut oil, melted
- 3 tbsp almond flour
- 1/2 tsp vanilla
- 1 tbsp unsweetened almond milk
- 1/2 cup almond butter
- 1/4 tsp sea salt

Direction: Preparation Time: 10 minutes Cooking Time: 10 minutes
Serve: 4

- ✓ Preheat the air fryer to 350 F. Grease air fryer baking dish with cooking spray and set aside. In a small bowl, mix together almond flour, baking soda, cocoa powder, baking powder, and salt. Set aside.
- ✓ In a small bowl, add coconut oil and almond butter and microwave until melted.
- ✓ Add sweetener, vanilla, almond milk, and applesauce in the coconut oil mixture and stir well.
- ✓ Add dry ingredients to the wet ingredients and stir to combine. Pour batter into prepared dish and place into the air fryer and cook for 10 minutes. Slice and serve.

30 Day Meal Plan

Day	Breakfast	Lunch	Dinner	Snacks
1	Berry-Oat Breakfast Bars	Sweet Potato, Kale, and White Bean Stew	Salmon with Asparagus	Tuna Salad
2	Whole-Grain Breakfast Cookies	Slow Cooker Two-Bean Sloppy Joes	Shrimp in Garlic Butter	Roasted Portobello Salad
3	Blueberry Breakfast Cake	Lighter Eggplant Parmesan	Cobb Salad	Shredded Chicken Salad
4	Whole-Grain Pancakes	Coconut-Lentil Curry	Seared Tuna Steak	Mango and Jicama Salad
5	Buckwheat Grouts Breakfast Bowl	Stuffed Portobello with Cheese	Beef Chili	Sweet Potato and Roasted Beet Salad
6	Peach Muesli Bake	Lighter Shrimp Scampi	Greek Broccoli Salad	Potato Calico Salad
7	Steel-Cut Oatmeal Bowl with Fruit and Nuts	Maple-Mustard Salmon	Cheesy Cauliflower Gratin	Spinach Shrimp Salad
8	Whole-Grain Dutch Baby Pancake	Chicken Salad with Grapes and Pecans	Strawberry Spinach Salad	Barley Veggie Salad
9	Mushroom, Zucchini, and Onion Frittata	Lemony Salmon Burgers	Cauliflower Mac & Cheese	Tenderloin Grilled Salad

10	Spinach and Cheese Quiche	Caprese Turkey Burgers	Easy Egg Salad	Broccoli Salad
11	Spicy Jalapeno Popper Deviled Eggs	Pasta Salad	Baked Chicken Legs	Cherry Tomato Salad
12	Lovely Porridge	Chicken, Strawberry, And Avocado Salad	Creamed Spinach	Tabbouleh-Arabian Salad
13	Salty Macadamia Chocolate Smoothie	Lemon-Thyme Eggs	Stuffed Mushrooms	Arugula Garden Salad
14	Basil and Tomato Baked Eggs	Spinach Salad with Bacon	Vegetable Soup	Supreme Caesar Salad
15	Cinnamon and Coconut Porridge	Pea and Collards Soup	Misto Quente	Sunflower Seeds and
16	An Omelet of Swiss chard	Spanish Stew	Garlic Bread	Chicken Salad in Cucumber Cups
17	Cheesy Low-Carb Omelet	Creamy Taco Soup	Bruschetta	California Wraps
18	Yogurt And Kale Smoothie	Chicken with Caprese Salsa	Cream Buns with Strawberries	Chicken Avocado Salad
19	Bacon and Chicken Garlic Wrap	Balsamic-Roasted Broccoli	Blueberry Buns	Ground Turkey Salad
20	Grilled Chicken Platter	Hearty Beef and Vegetable Soup	Cauliflower Potato Mash	Scallop Caesar Salad

21	Parsley Chicken Breast	Cauliflower Muffin	French toast in Sticks	Asian Cucumber Salad
22	Mustard Chicken	Cauliflower Rice with Chicken	Muffins Sandwich	Cauliflower Tofu Salad
23	Balsamic Chicken	Ham and Egg Cups	Bacon BBQ	Tuna Salad
24	Greek Chicken Breast	Turkey with Fried Eggs	Stuffed French toast	Roasted Portobello Salad
25	Chipotle Lettuce Chicken	Sweet Potato, Kale, and White Bean Stew	Scallion Sandwich	Shredded Chicken Salad
26	Stylish Chicken-Bacon Wrap	Slow Cooker Two-Bean Sloppy Joes	Lean Lamb and Turkey Meatballs with Yogurt	Mango and Jicama Salad
27	Healthy Cottage Cheese Pancakes	Lighter Eggplant Parmesan	Air Fried Section and Tomato	Sweet Potato and Roasted Beet Salad
28	Avocado Lemon Toast	Coconut-Lentil Curry	Cheesy Salmon Fillets	Potato Calico Salad
29	Healthy Baked Eggs	Stuffed Portobello with Cheese	Salmon with Asparagus	Spinach Shrimp Salad
30	Quick Low-Carb Oatmeal	Lighter Shrimp Scampi	Shrimp in Garlic Butter	Cauliflower Tofu Salad

Conclusion

Thank you for making it to the end. The warning symptoms of diabetes type 1 are the same as type 2; however, in type 1, these signs and symptoms tend to occur slowly over a period of months or years, making it harder to spot and recognize. Some of these symptoms can even occur after the disease has progressed.

Each disorder has risk factors that when found in an individual, favor the development of the disease. Diabetes is no different. Here are some of the risk factors for developing diabetes.

Having a Family History of Diabetes

Usually having a family member, especially first-degree relatives could be an indicator that you are at risk of developing diabetes. Your risk of developing diabetes is about 15% if you have one parent with diabetes while it is 75% if both your parents have diabetes.

Having Prediabetes

Being pre-diabetic means that you have higher than normal blood glucose levels. However, they are not high enough to be diagnosed as type 2 diabetes. Having pre-diabetes is a risk factor for developing type 2 diabetes as well as other conditions such as cardiac conditions. Since there are no symptoms or signs for Prediabetes, it is often a latent condition that is discovered accidentally during routine investigations of blood glucose levels or when investigating other conditions.

Being Obese or Overweight

Your metabolism, fat stores and eating habits when you are overweight or above the healthy weight range contribute to abnormal metabolism pathways that put you at risk for developing diabetes type 2. There have been consistent research results of the obvious link between developing diabetes and being obese.

Having a Sedentary Lifestyle

Having a lifestyle where you are mostly physically inactive predisposes you to a lot of conditions including diabetes type 2. That is because being physically inactive causes you to develop obesity or become overweight. Moreover, you don't burn any excess sugars that you ingest which can lead you to become prediabetic and eventually diabetic.

Having Gestational Diabetes

Developing gestational diabetes which is diabetes that occurred due to pregnancy (and often disappears after pregnancy) is a risk factor for developing diabetes at some point.

Ethnicity

Belonging to certain ethnic groups such as Middle Eastern, South Asian or Indian background. Studies of statistics have revealed that the prevalence of diabetes type 2 in these ethnic groups is high. If you come from any of these ethnicities, this puts you at risk of developing diabetes type 2 yourself.

Having Hypertension

Studies have shown an association between having hypertension and having an increased risk of developing diabetes. If you have hypertension, you should not leave it uncontrolled.

Extremes of Age

Diabetes can occur at any age. However, being too young or too old means your body is not in its best form and therefore, this increases the risk of developing diabetes.

That sounds scary. However, diabetes only occurs with the presence of a combination of these risk factors. Most of the risk factors can be minimized by taking action. For example, developing a more active lifestyle, taking care of your habits and attempting to lower your blood glucose sugar by restricting your sugar intake. If you start to notice you are prediabetic or getting overweight, etc., there is always something you can do to modify the situation. Recent studies show that developing healthy eating habits and following diets that are low in carbs, losing excess weight and leading an active lifestyle can help to protect you from developing diabetes, especially diabetes type 2, by minimizing the risk factors of developing the disorder.

You can also have an oral glucose tolerance test in which you will have a fasting glucose test first and then you will be given a sugary drink and then having your blood glucose tested 2 hours after that to see how your body responds to glucose meals. In healthy individuals, blood glucose should drop again 2 hours post sugary meals due to the action of insulin.

Another indicative test is the HbA1C. This test reflects the average of your blood glucose level over the last 2 to 3 months. It is also a test to see how well you manage your diabetes.

People with diabetes type 1 require compulsory insulin shots to control their diabetes because they have no other option. People with diabetes type 2 can regulate their diabetes with healthy eating and regular physical activity although they may require some glucose-lowering medications that can be in tablet form or in the form of an injection.

All the above goes in the direction that you need to avoid a starchy diet because of its tendency to raise blood glucose levels. Too many carbohydrates can lead to insulin sensitivity and pancreatic fatigue, as well as weight gain with all its associated risk factors for cardiovascular disease and hypertension. The solution is to lower your sugar intake, therefore, decrease your body's need for insulin and increase the burning of fat in your body.

When your body is low on sugars, it will be forced to use a subsequent molecule to burn for energy, in that case, this will be fat. The burning of fat will lead you to lose weight.

I hope you have learned something!

INDEX

A

Air Fried Chicken Schnitzel; 143
Air Fried Guacamole; 183
Air Fried Section and Tomato; 45
Air Fryer Bacon; 159
Air Fryer Chewy Granola Bars; 130
Air Fryer Egg in a Hole; 168
Air Fryer Eggs (Perfect); 110
Air Fryer Lamb Burgers; 160
Air Fryer Meatloaf; 153
Air Fryer Party Meatballs; 154
Air Fryer Pickles; 191
Air fryer Pizza Hut Bread Sticks; 130
Air Fryer Salmon; 163
Air-Fried Asparagus; 192
Air-Fried Chicken Drumettes; 135
Air-Fried Chicken Popcorn; 139
Air-Fried Crumbed Fish; 162
Air-Fried Meatloaf; 159
Air-Fried Pork Dumplings with Dipping Sauce; 156
Airfryer Cheese and Bacon Fries; 128
Airfryer Crispy Roasted Onion Potatoes; 175
Airfryer Turkish Cheese and Leek Koftas; 152
Air-Grilled Honey-Glazed Salmon; 164
Almond Cinnamon Mug Cake; 194
Almond Crunch Granola; 115
Almond Crusted Baked Chili Mahi Mahi; 74
Amazing XXL burger; 120
Apple & Cinnamon Pancake; 30
Apple Omelet; 27
Asian Crispy Chicken Salad; 51
Asian Cucumber Salad; 48
Asparagus Cheese Strata; 115
Asparagus Fries; 192
Asparagus Frittata; 109
Avocado Egg Boat; 182
Avocado Egg Rolls; 110
Avocado Fries; 182
Avocado Lemon Toast; 22
Avocado Mousse; 96
Avocado On Toast; 182
Avocado Slices Recipe; 182
Avocado Turmeric Smoothie; 90

B

Bacon and Chicken Garlic Wrap; 20
Bacon and Egg Sandwiches; 117
Bacon and Eggs; 110
Bacon BBQ; 44
Bacon Cashews; 131
Bacon Egg Muffins; 110
Bacon-Wrapped Chicken Breasts; 139
Baja Fish Taco Recipe; 125
Baked Beans; 105
Baked Chicken Legs; 42
Baked Lamb & Spinach; 66
Baked Mini Spinach Quiches; 118
Baked Potatoes; 174
Baked Salmon with Garlic Parmesan Topping; 69
Baked Veggies Combo; 106
Baked Zucchini Fries; 184
Balsamic Chicken 1; 21
Balsamic Chicken 2; 57
Balsamic Glazed Chicken Breasts; 142
Balsamic Smoked Pork Chops; 157
Balsamic-Roasted Broccoli; 39
Banana Chips; 130
Banana Matcha Breakfast Smoothie; 31
Bang Bang Air Fryer Shrimp; 166
Barbecue Beef Brisket; 59
Barbeque Chicken Wings; 141
Barley Pilaf; 106
Barley Veggie Salad; 50
Basil and Tomato Baked Eggs; 20
Basil And Tomato Baked Eggs; 31
BBQ Chicken Wings; 140
Beans, Walnuts & Veggie Burgers; 107
Beef & Asparagus; 59
Beef Chili; 41
Beef Curry; 63
Beef Salad; 63
Beef Wellington; 155
Beef with Barley & Veggies; 64
Beef with Broccoli; 64
Bell Pepper Pancakes; 26
Berry Mint Smoothie; 89
Berry-Oat Breakfast Bars; 17
Big Fat Veggie Fritters; 180
Black Beans; 105
Blackberry Smoothie; 90
Blackened Shrimp; 69
Blueberries Pudding; 96
Blueberries with Yogurt; 95
Blueberry Breakfast Cake; 17
Blueberry Buns; 44
Blueberry Crisp; 93
Blueberry Lemon Custard Cake; 92
Blueberry Smoothie; 91
Bourbon Bacon Cinnamon Rolls; 158
Braised Lamb with Vegetables; 63
Braised Shrimp; 73
Braised Summer Squash; 82
Brazilian Mini Turkey Pies; 150
Breaded Pork Chops (ver. 2); 156
Breakfast Burrito; 116
Breakfast Casserole Delicious; 114
Breakfast Egg Muffins; 112
Breakfast Egg Rolls; 108
Breakfast Egg Tomato; 113
Breakfast Jalapeno Muffins; 109

Breakfast Mix; 32
Breakfast Muffins; 34
Breakfast Parfait; 29
Breakfast Potatoes; 169
Breakfast Sandwich; 34
Breakfast Smoothie Bowl with Fresh Berries; 23
Breakfast Soufflé; 110
Breakfast Toad-in-the-Hole Tarts; 169
British Fish and Chip Shop Healthy Battered Sausage and Chips; 133
Broccoli Frittata; 113
Broccoli Nuggets; 103
Broccoli Salad 1; 47
Broccoli Salad 2; 50
Broccoli Stilton Soup; 86
Broccoli with Cheese Sauce; 184
Brown Rice & Lentil Salad; 81
Brown Rice Pudding; 97
Bruschetta; 43
Bruschetta Recipe; 132
Brussels Sprouts; 188
Brussels Sprouts with Bacon; 188
Buckwheat Grouts Breakfast Bowl; 18
Buckwheat Porridge; 33
Budget Friendly Air fryer Mini Cheese Scones; 132
Buffalo Cauliflower; 185
Buffalo Cauliflower Bites (ver. 2); 185
Buffalo Chicken Breasts; 143
Buffalo Chicken Strips; 148
Buffalo Style Skinny Chicken Wings; 140
Buffalo-Ranch Chickpeas; 125
Bulgur Porridge; 30
Bunless Burgers; 153
Buttermilk Chicken Thighs; 139
Butternut Squash Roasties; 182
Buttery Dinner Rolls; 171
Buttery Scallops; 114
Button Mushroom Melt; 188

C

Cabbage Soup; 86
Cajun Catfish; 69
Cajun Shrimp & Roasted Vegetables; 69
Cake with Whipped Cream Icing; 99
California Wraps; 49
Caprese Turkey Burgers; 38
Carrot and Pumpkin Recipes; 180
Cauliflower Cheese Tater Tots; 186
Cauliflower Mac & Cheese; 42
Cauliflower Muffin; 40
Cauliflower Potato Mash; 43
Cauliflower Rice Stuffed Peppers Budget Recipe; 186
Cauliflower Rice with Chicken; 40
Cauliflower Tofu Salad; 48
Cauliflower Veggie Burger Recipe; 122
Celery Root Fries; 190
Cheese and Onion Nuggets; 128

Cheese Burger; 121
Cheese Butter Cookies; 193
Cheese Pie; 112
Cheese Stuff Peppers; 114
Cheese Toastie; 169
Cheesy Cauliflower Gratin; 42
Cheesy Garlic Bread; 118
Cheesy Low-Carb Omelet; 20
Cheesy Salmon Fillets; 46
Cherry Tomato Salad; 47
Chia and Coconut Pudding; 23
Chia Chocolate Cookies; 193
Chicken & Broccoli Bake; 54
Chicken & Peanut Stir-Fry; 56
Chicken & Spinach; 56
Chicken & Sweet Potato Hash; 25
Chicken & Tofu; 56
Chicken Avocado Burgers; 121
Chicken Avocado Salad; 48
Chicken Breast Salad; 49
Chicken Breasts in a Bag; 133
Chicken Burgers; 121
Chicken Chili; 53
Chicken Fried Rice; 149
Chicken Parmesan and Fries; 144
Chicken Popcorn; 137
Chicken Quesadillas; 136
Chicken Salad with Grapes and Pecans; 37
Chicken Soup; 53
Chicken Spiedie Recipe; 120
Chicken Tenders; 145
Chicken Wings in Nandos Marinade; 134
Chicken Wings in Orange Sauce; 134
Chicken with Caprese Salsa; 39
Chicken with Chickpeas; 54
Chicken Zoodle Soup; 88
Chicken, Oats & Chickpeas Meatloaf; 55
Chicken, Strawberry, And Avocado Salad; 38
Chick-fil- A Chicken Sandwich; 137
Chickpea Soup; 88
Chili Chicken Wings; 102
Chili Lime Tilapia Healthy; 162
Chili Tuna Puff; 164
Chinese Kebabs and Rice; 159
Chinese Pineapple Pork; 159
Chinese Take Out Sweet 'N Sour Pork; 158
Chipotle Lettuce Chicken; 22
Choco Banana Bites; 95
Choco Fudge Cake; 194
Chocolate & Raspberry Ice Cream; 101
Chocolate Coconut Cake; 194
Chocolate Custard; 194
Chocolate Quinoa Brownies; 93
Cilantro Lime Grilled Shrimp; 70
Cilantro Lime Quinoa; 81
Cinnamon and Coconut Porridge; 20
Cinnamon Cake; 101
Cinnamon Ginger Cookies; 193

Cinnamon Oat Pancakes; 27
Cinnamon Roll Smoothie; 90
Citrus Salmon; 72
Classic Chicken Wings; 140
Classic Mini Meatloaf; 61
Cobb Salad; 41
Coconut and Turmeric Chicken; 136
Coconut Shrimp and Apricot; 165
Coconut Shrimp and Lime Juice; 165
Coconut Spinach Smoothie; 89
Coconut-Lentil Curry; 36
Coffee & Chocolate Ice Cream; 95
Coffee Mousse; 104
Cool Green Beans; 173
Corn Tortilla Chips; 131
Country Fried Steak; 157
Crab Curry; 72
Crab Frittata; 70
Cranberry Almond Cake; 193
Cream Buns with Strawberries; 44
Cream Cheese Pancakes; 31
Cream of Tomato Soup; 86
Creamed Spinach; 42
Creamy Taco Soup; 39
Crispy Airfryer Coconut Prawns; 167
Crispy Breaded Pork Chops; 156
Crispy Crabstick Crackers; 167
Crispy Crunchy Sweet Potato Fries; 179
Crispy Fried Spring Rolls; 149
Crispy Nachos Prawns; 166
Crispy Risotto Balls; 172
Crispy Veggie Quesadillas; 126
Crumbed Chicken Tenderloins; 145
Crunchy Corn Dog Bites; 126
Crunchy Lemon Shrimp; 70
Crustless Pie; 193
Cucumber & Yogurt; 28
Curry Chickpeas; 124
Curry Parsnip Fries; 190
Curry Roasted Cauliflower Florets; 82

D

Dark Chocolate Cake; 94
Delicious & Easy Meatballs; 138
Delicious Rotisserie Chicken; 134
Drunken Ham with Mustard; 159

E

Easy and Delicious Whole Chicken; 141
Easy Chicken Nuggets; 140
Easy Egg Salad; 42
Easy Potato Gratin; 175
Easy Pull Apart Bread; 170
Egg "dough" In A Pan; 28
Egg and Cheese Pockets; 118
Egg Muffins; 32

Egg Muffins with Bell Pepper; 117
Egg Porridge; 29
Eggplant Omelet; 34
Eggs Baked In Peppers; 29
Eggs Florentine; 28
Eggs On The Go; 32
Egg-veggie Scramble; 33
Everything Bagel Chicken Strips; 148
Everything Bagel Kale Chips; 190

F

Fake-On Stew; 87
Falafel; 173
Falafel Burger; 122
Fast Food Hot Dogs; 119
Feta Cheese Dough Balls; 127
Feta Triangles; 128
Figs with Yogurt; 95
Fish and Chips; 160; 161
Fish and Fries; 161
Fish Fingers; 161
Five Cheese Pull Apart Bread; 121
Five Guys Cajun Fries; 178
Five Ingredient Super Simple Fisherman's Fishcakes; 162
Flaky Buttermilk Biscuits; 170
Flavorful Fried Chicken; 140
Flourless Broccoli Cheese Quiche; 115
Flourless Chocolate Cake; 98
Flourless Cordon Bleu; 148
Flourless Crunchy Cheese Straws; 127
Flourless Mashed Potato Cakes; 178
Flourless Mini Zucchini Fritter Bites; 183
Flourless Truly Crispy Calamari Rings; 168
French Lentils; 83
French Onion Soup; 87
French Toast Soldiers; 169
French Toast Sticks; 111
French Toast Sticks (Ver.2); 111
French Toast Sticks With Berries; 112
Fried Calzones; 123
Fried Catfish 3 Ingredient; 162
Fried Hot Prawns with Cocktail Sauce; 167
Fried Meatballs in Tomato Sauce; 154
Fried Mozzarella Sticks; 128
Fried Pizza Sticks; 120
Fried Ravioli; 119
Friendly Airfryer Whole Chicken; 147
Frozen Vanilla Yogurt; 96
Frugal Cheesy Homemade Garlic Bread; 132
Fruit Kebab; 101
Fruit Salad; 95

G

Gambas 'Pil Pil' with Sweet Potato; 166
Garden Wraps; 52
Garlic and Parsley Baby Potatoes; 174

Garlic Bread; 43
Garlic Bread Recipe; 133
Garlic Butter Pork Chops; 157
Garlic Chicken Wings; 102
Garlic Parmesan Breaded Fried Chicken Wings; 138
Garlic Sautée d Spinach; 82
Garlic Shrimp & Spinach; 76
Garlic Sweet Potato Fries; 178
Garlic-braised Short Rib; 62
Garlicky Cabbage; 84
Garlic-Rosemary Brussels Sprouts; 188
Garlic-Sesame Pumpkin Seeds; 52
General Tso's Chicken; 146
Ginger Cake; 100
Gingered Cauliflower; 84
Grain-Free Berry Cobbler; 83
Grains Combo; 105
Granola With Fruits; 32
Greek Broccoli Salad; 41
Greek Chicken Breast; 21
Greek Chicken Lettuce Wraps; 57
Green Beans with Tomatoes; 85
Green Salad with Roasted Pepper; 190
Green Tomato BLT; 169
Greenie Smoothie; 89
Grilled Cajun Salmon; 164
Grilled Cheese; 121
Grilled Fish Fillet with Pesto Sauce; 162
Grilled Herbed Salmon with Raspberry Sauce & Cucumber Dill Dip; 76
Grilled Peaches; 95
Grilled Salmon with Ginger Sauce; 79
Grilled Tomatoes; 191
Grilled Tuna Steaks; 70
Ground Pork with Spinach; 68
Ground Turkey Salad; 48
Guacamole Turkey Burgers; 30
Guilt-Free Ranch Zucchini Chips; 183

H

Halibut with Spicy Apricot Sauce; 75
Ham And Goat Cheese Omelet; 30
Hard Boiled Eggs; 108
Hash Brown Recipe; 178
Hassleback Potatoes; 177
Healthy Baked Eggs; 22
Healthy Carrot Muffins; 28
Healthy Cottage Cheese Pancakes; 22
Healthy Flapjacks Recipe; 130
Healthy Mix Vegetables; 113
Hearty Beef and Vegetable Soup; 39
Herb and Cheese-Stuffed Burgers; 153
Herb Mushrooms; 108
Herb Seasoned Turkey Breast; 134
Herbed Asparagus; 83
Herbed Salmon; 73
Herbed Turkey Breast; 55

Herring & Veggies Soup; 76
Home Bakery Cornish Pasty Recipe; 170
Homemade Fries; 177
Homemade Mozzarella Sticks (ver. 2); 128
Homemade Sausage Rolls; 126
Honey Glazed Cauliflower Bites; 186
Honey Mustard Chicken; 56
Honey Roasted Carrots; 180
Hot Cross Buns; 171
Hot Dogs; 126
Huevos Rancheros; 115

I

Irish Pork Roast; 62
Irish Stew; 87
Italian Beef; 60
Italian Seasoned Chicken Tenders; 141

J

Jalapeño Potato Hash; 117
Jamaican Chicken Meatballs; 149

K

Kale Omelet; 111
Kale, Grape and Bulgur Salad; 51
Kebab Stew; 87
Keto Creamy Bacon Dish; 28
Keto Low Carb Crepe; 27
Ketogenic Cheese Cake; 99
Ketogenic Lava Cake; 98
Ketogenic Orange Cake; 100
Key Lime Pie Smoothie; 90
KFC Easy Chicken Strips in the Air Fryer; 147
KFC Popcorn Chicken in the Air Fryer; 147
Kidney Bean Stew; 86
King Prawns in Ham with Red Pepper Dip; 167

L

Lamb & Chickpeas; 63
Lamb Curry; 65
Lamb Stew recipe 1; 64
Lamb Stew Recipe 2; 87
Lamb with Broccoli & Carrots; 60
Lean Lamb and Turkey Meatballs with Yogurt; 45
Leftover Turkey and Cheese Calzone; 152
Leftover Turkey Muffins; 151
Leftovers Bubble and Squeak; 118
Lemon Cake; 100
Lemon Chicken with Kale; 57
Lemon Cookies; 97
Lemon Custard; 94
Lemon Dill Scallops; 108
Lemon Garlic Green Beans; 81
Lemon Garlic Turkey; 56

Lemon Pepper Chicken Breasts; 144
Lemon Pepper Chicken Wings; 141
Lemon Pepper Salmon; 74
Lemon Pepper Shrimp; 166
Lemon Sole; 74
Lemon-Thyme Eggs; 38
Lemony Brussels Sprout; 84
Lemony Salmon; 71
Lemony Salmon Burgers; 38
Lentils Chili; 106
Lighten up Empanadas; 125
Lighter Eggplant Parmesan; 36
Lighter Shrimp Scampi; 37
Lovely Porridge; 19
Low Carb Roasted Nuts; 131
Low-carb Omelet; 30
Low-Fat Mozzarella Cheese Sticks and marinara sauce; 127

M

Macaroni and Cheese Mini Quiche Recipe; 174
Macaroni and Cheese Toasties in the Air fryer; 173
Make Loaded Potatoes; 175
Mango and Jicama Salad; 51
Maple Custard; 93
Maple-Mustard Salmon; 37
Mashed Butternut Squash; 81
Mashed Cauliflower; 31
Matcha Green Smoothie; 91
Meatball Stew; 87
Meatballs Curry; 54
Meatballs In Tomato Gravy; 61
Meatballs with Feta; 160
Meatless Ball Soup; 87
Mediterranean Fish Fillets; 71
Mediterranean Lamb Meatballs; 60
Mexican-Style Corn on the Cob; 124
Millet Porridge; 24; 33
Mini Frankfurters in Pastry; 129
Mini Peppers with Goat Cheese; 129
Mini Quiche Wedges; 129
Mixed Berry Dutch Pancake; 117
Mixed Chowder; 72
Mixed Veggie Salad; 107
Mocha Pops; 101
Muffins Sandwich; 44
Mushroom and Black Bean Burrito; 116
Mushroom and Spinach Frittata; 109
Mushroom Barley Risotto; 82
Mushroom Croquettes or Meat Croquettes; 187
Mushroom Leek Frittata; 111
Mushroom, Zucchini, and Onion Frittata; 19
Mussels in Tomato Sauce; 72
Mustard Chicken; 21
Mustard Green Beans; 103
Mustard Honey Beef Balls; 155

N

Nando's Chicken Drumsticks; 142

O

Oats Coffee Smoothie; 89
Oil Free Pumpkin French Fries; 181
Oil Free Sticky Pumpkin Wedges; 181
Omelette Frittata with Cheese and Mushrooms; 109
Omelette with Cheese And Onion; 108
Onion Rings; 189
Onion Rings With Comeback Sauce; 189
Orange Carrot Smoothie; 90
Orange Sesame Cauliflower; 185
Oven-Roasted Veggies; 81

P

Pan Grilled Steak; 64
Panko Breaded, Chicken Parmesan, Marinara Sauce; 144
Parmesan Breakfast Casserole; 112
Parmesan Truffle Oil Fries; 177
Parsley Chicken Breast; 21
Parsley Tabbouleh; 82
Party Shrimp; 52
Pasta Salad; 38
Patatas Bravas; 174
Pea and Collards Soup; 39
Peach Muesli Bake; 18
Peanut Butter Banana Smoothie; 90
Peanut Butter Mousse; 104
Peppercorns; 154
Perfect Breakfast Frittata; 114
Philadelphia Herby Chicken Breasts; 144
Pigs In a Blanket; 133
Pizza Dogs; 119
Pizza with Salami and Mushrooms; 119
Popcorn; 124
Popcorn Shrimp; 75
Pork Chops; 156
Pork Chops in Peach Glaze; 67
Pork Chops with Grape Sauce; 58
Pork Salad; 66
Pork Tenderloin with Bell Pepper; 155
Pork with Bell Peppers; 67
Pork with Cranberry Relish; 58
Potato Calico Salad; 51
Potato Hay; 175
Potato Latkes Bites; 177
Potato-Skin Wedges; 176
Poutine; 179
Pulled Pork; 62
Pumpkin Bread; 170
Pumpkin Cookies; 193
Pumpkin Custard 1; 92
Pumpkin Custard 2; 193
Pumpkin Oatmeal with Raisins; 116

Pumpkin Pie Bars; 94
Pumpkin Seeds; 131
Pumpkin Spice Soup; 86
Pumpkin Tortilla Chips; 182

Q

Quick & Easy Chicken Breast; 138
Quick Blend Mexican Chicken Burgers; 120
Quick Low-Carb Oatmeal; 23
Quinoa Bread; 25
Quinoa in Tomato; 106
Quinoa Porridge Recipe 1; 26
Quinoa Porridge Recipe 2; 31

R

Radish Hash Browns; 109
Raspberry Cake With White Chocolate Sauce; 98
Raspberry Chia Pudding; 97
Raspberry Cream Cheese Coffee Cake; 94
Ratatouille; 191
Ratatouille Italian-Style; 192
Red Clam Sauce & Pasta; 70
Restaurant Style Garlic Potatoes; 176
Reuben Calzones; 123
Rib Eye Steak; 153
Rich Fruit Scones; 171
Roasted Balsamic Mushrooms; 102
Roasted Broccoli; 84
Roasted Broccoli and Cauliflower; 185
Roasted Cauliflower; 185
Roasted Chickpeas; 104
Roasted Corn; 130
Roasted Cumin Carrots; 103
Roasted Mangoes; 95
Roasted Okra; 192
Roasted Paprika Potatoes with Greek Yoghurt; 176
Roasted Parsnips; 189
Roasted Pepper Rolls; 129
Roasted Pepper Salad; 114
Roasted Peppers (Bell Peppers); 190
Roasted Pork & Apples; 58
Roasted Pork Loin With Grainy Mustard Sauce; 61
Roasted Pork Shoulder; 67
Roasted Portobello Salad; 47
Roasted Rack of Lamb with a Macadamia Crust; 160
Roasted Stuffed Peppers; 154
Rock Buns; 171
Rosemary Lamb; 60
Rosemary Potato Wedges; 174
Rosemary Roast Potatoes; 175
Rosemary Sausage Meatballs; 158
Rosemary-garlic Lamb Racks; 62
Rotisserie Chicken; 146

S

Salad Preparation; 101
Salmon & Asparagus; 75
Salmon & Shrimp Stew; 79
Salmon and Fennel Salad; 163
Salmon Baked; 80
Salmon Curry; 77
Salmon in Green Sauce; 73
Salmon Milano; 71
Salmon Patties; 164
Salmon Soup; 77
Salmon with Asparagus; 41
Salmon with Bell Peppers; 77
Salt and Vinegar Chickpeas; 124
Salted Nuts; 131
Salty Macadamia Chocolate Smoothie; 19
Sandwich; 137
Sardine Curry; 74
Sausage Cheese Mix; 111
Sausage Egg Cups; 114
Sautéed Veggies; 103
Savory Keto Pancake; 33
Scallion Sandwich; 45
Scallop Caesar Salad; 48
Scallops Wrapped In Bacon; 168
Scampi Shrimp and Chips; 166
Scrambled Eggs; 108
Seared Tuna Steak; 41
Sesame Pork with Mustard Sauce; 58
Sesame Seeds Fish Fillet; 163
Shiitake Mushroom Chips; 187
Shiitake Soup; 86
Shoestring Carrots; 181
Shredded Beef; 60
Shredded Chicken Salad; 47
Shrimp & Artichoke Skillet; 71
Shrimp & Veggies Curry; 78
Shrimp Coconut Curry; 73
Shrimp in Garlic Butter; 41
Shrimp Lemon Kebab; 75
Shrimp Salad; 78
Shrimp Spring Rolls and Sweet Chili Sauce; 165
Shrimp with Broccoli; 79
Shrimp with Green Beans; 72
Shrimp with Zucchini; 78
Simple Grilled American Cheese Sandwich; 120
Simply Fried Chicken Thighs; 139
Sizzling Turkey Fajitas Platter; 151
Skin on French Fries; 178
Skirt Steak With Asian Peanut Sauce; 61
Slimming World Beer Battered Fish and Chips Recipe; 161
Slimming World Carrot Fritters; 181
Slow Cooker Peaches; 92
Slow Cooker Two-Bean Sloppy Joes; 35
Small Jacket Potatoes with Rosemary; 175
Southern Chicken Drumsticks; 141
Southern-Style Chicken; 146

Spanakopita Bites; 123
Spanish Stew; 39
Spatchcock Chicken; 145
Spiced Leg of Lamb; 66
Spiced Nuts; 131
Spiced Overnight Oats; 27
Spiced Pumpkin; 181
Spicy Air Fryer Chicken Breasts; 142
Spicy Air-Fried Chicken Thighs; 138
Spicy and Crispy Chicken Wing Drumettes; 135
Spicy Asian Chicken Thighs; 135
Spicy Buffalo Chicken Wings; 139
Spicy Cauliflower Stir-Fry; 186
Spicy Dill Pickle Fries; 191
Spicy Drumsticks with Barbecue Marinade; 136
Spicy Green Beans; 173
Spicy Jalapeno Popper Deviled Eggs; 19
Spicy Pepper Soup; 86
Spicy Spinach; 83
Spicy Sweet Potato Wedges; 179
Spinach and Cheese Quiche; 19
Spinach and Tomato Egg Cup; 117
Spinach Cheese Pie; 102
Spinach Egg Breakfast; 112
Spinach Frittata; 109
Spinach Salad with Bacon; 38
Spinach Shrimp Salad; 50
Spinach Sorbet; 96
Sprouts Breaded Mushrooms; 187
Steak in the Air Fryer 1; 152
Steak in the Air Fryer 2; 152
Steak with Mushroom Sauce; 59
Steak with Tomato & Herbs; 59
Steamed Kale with Mediterranean Dressing; 24
Steel-Cut Oatmeal Bowl with Fruit and Nuts; 18
Sticky Mushroom Rice; 172
Stir Fried Zucchini; 85
Strawberry & Spinach Smoothie; 26
Strawberry & Watermelon Pops; 96
Strawberry Cheesecake Smoothie; 90
Strawberry Mousse; 96
Strawberry Puff Pancake; 29
Strawberry Salsa; 52
Strawberry Scones; 172
Strawberry Smoothie; 89
Strawberry Spinach Salad; 42
Stuffed Chicken Breasts (Mexican-Style); 134
Stuffed Chicken Breasts Greek-style; 55
Stuffed French toast; 45
Stuffed Garlic Mushrooms; 187
Stuffed Mushrooms; 43
Stuffed Mushrooms with Sour Cream; 187
Stuffed Portobello Mushrooms; 188
Stuffed Portobello with Cheese; 37
Stuffed Potatoes; 176
Stuffed Tomatoes and Broccoli; 191
Stylish Chicken-Bacon Wrap; 22
Sugar Free Carrot Cake; 92

Sugar Free Chocolate Molten Lava Cake; 93
Sunflower Seeds and Arugula Garden Salad; 49
Super Easy Crispy Bacon; 111
Supreme Caesar Salad; 49
Sweet And Sour Soup; 87
Sweet Garlicky Chicken Wings; 140
Sweet Potato and Roasted Beet Salad; 51
Sweet Potato Chips; 180
Sweet Potato Fries; 179
Sweet Potato Hash; 180
Sweet Potato Tots; 180
Sweet Potato Waffles; 25
Sweet Potato, Kale, and White Bean Stew; 35
Swordfish Steak; 74
Swordfish with Tomato Salsa; 79
Syn Free Slimming World Chicken Tikka; 143

T

Tabbouleh- Arabian Salad; 49
Taco Dogs; 119
Tandoori Salmon with Refreshing Raita; 164
Tarragon Scallops; 76
Tasty & Tender Brussels Sprouts; 103
Tasty Harissa Chicken; 102
Tasty Peanut Butter Bars; 192
Tasty Salsa Chicken; 113
Tender Juicy Smoked BBQ Ribs; 158
Tenderloin Grilled Salad; 50
Tex-Mex Hash Browns; 179
Thai Fish Cakes with Mango Salsa; 163
Thai Mango Chicken; 143
Thai Peanut Chicken Egg Rolls; 147
Thanksgiving Turkey Sandwich Recipe; 152
The Best Ever Air Fryer Fries; 177
Three Ingredient Shortbread Fingers; 172
Tofu & Zucchini Muffins; 33
Tofu and Vegetable Scramble; 23
Tofu Scramble; 26
Tofu with Brussels Sprout; 107
Tomato and Spinach Egg Cup; 118
Tomato and Zucchini Sauté; 24
Tomato Mushroom Frittata; 113
Traditional Welsh Rarebit; 168
Trout Bake; 73
Tuna Carbonara; 71
Tuna Patties; 165
Tuna Salad Recipe 1; 47
Tuna Salad Recipe 2; 52
Tuna Sweet corn Casserole; 74
Turkey and Cheese Calzone; 157
Turkey Breast Glazed with Maple Mustard; 150
Turkey Curry Samosas; 151
Turkey Egg Casserole; 116
Turkey Goujons and Sweet Chilli Dip; 150
Turkey Scotch Eggs; 135
Turkey Spicy Rolled Meat; 149
Turkey Spring Rolls; 150

Turkey Stuffed Bread Recipe; 151
Turkey with Fried Eggs; 40
Turkey with Lentils; 55
Turkey-broccoli Brunch Casserole; 30
Two Ingredient Croutons; 132

V

Vanilla Coconut Cheese Cookies; 193
Vanilla Mixed Berry Smoothie; 31
Vegan Croutons; 132
Vegan Lentil Burgers; 122
Vegan Stuffed Bell Peppers; 190
Vegetable Frittata; 32
Vegetable Noodles Stir-Fry; 24
Vegetable Omelet; 32
Vegetable Quiche; 113
Vegetable Rice Pilaf; 82
Vegetable Soup; 43
Veggie Burgers; 122
Veggie Frittata; 25
Veggie Fritters; 33
Veggie Smoothie; 89

W

Walnut-Fruit Cake; 99

Wasabi Crab Cakes; 168
Whole 30 Air fryer Muffins; 110
Whole-Grain Breakfast Cookies; 17
Whole-Grain Dutch Baby Pancake; 18
Whole-Grain Pancakes; 17
Whole-Wheat Pizzas; 125
Wings in a Peach-Bourbon Sauce; 136

Y

Yogurt And Kale Smoothie; 20
Yogurt Cheesecake; 97
Yogurt Raspberry Cake; 116
Yorkshire Pudding Recipe; 172
Yummy Brownies; 194
Yummy Meatballs in Tomato Gravy; 65

Z

Zoodle Won-Ton Soup; 86
Zucchini Cauliflower Fritters; 104
Zucchini Chips; 183
Zucchini Fries; 103
Zucchini Fritters; 184
Zucchini Gratin; 184
Zucchini Mini Pizzas; 52
Zucchini Rounds; 184

Printed in Great Britain
by Amazon